Exogenous Factors in Colonic Carcinogenesis

FALK SYMPOSIUM 128

Exogenous Factors in Colonic Carcinogenesis

Edited by

W. Scheppach
Department of Medicine

and

M. Scheurlen
Medizinische Poliklinik

Klinikum der Universität Würzburg
Würzburg
Germany

Proceedings of Falk Symposium 128 held in Würzburg, Germany,
May 2–3, 2002

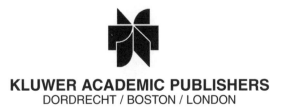

KLUWER ACADEMIC PUBLISHERS
DORDRECHT / BOSTON / LONDON

Library of Congress Cataloging-in-Publication Data is available.

ISBN 0–7923–8780–5

Published by Kluwer Academic Publishers, BV
P.O. Box 17, 3300 AA Dordrecht, The Netherlands.

Sold and distributed in North, Central and South America
by Kluwer Academic Publishers,
101 Philip Drive, Norwell, MA 02061, USA.

In all other countries, sold and distributed
by Kluwer Academic Publishers, Distribution Center,
P.O. Box 322, 3300 AH Dordrecht, The Netherlands.

Printed on acid-free paper

Contents

CONTENTS

CONTENTS

Section VIII: SUMMARY

List of principal contributors

O Al-Taie
Medizinische Poliklinik
Universität Würzburg
Klinikstr. 6-8
D-97070 Würzburg
Germany

LH Augenlicht
Department of Oncology
Albert Einstein Cancer Center
Montefiore Medical Center
111 East 210th St
Bronx, NY 10467
USA

H Bartsch
Deutsches Krebsforschungszentrum
Im Neuenheimer Feld 280
D-69120 Heidelberg
Germany

HK Biesalski
Institut für Biologische Chemie und
  Ernährungswissenschaft
Universität Hohenheim
Frühwirthstr. 12
D-70599 Stuttgart
Germany

H Boeing
Abteilung Epidemiologie
Deutsches Institut für
  Ernährungsforschung
Arthur-Scheunert-Allee 114-116
D-14558 Bergholz-Rehbrücke
Germany

M-C Boutron-Ruault
INSERM U557
ISTNA
5, rue Vertbois
F-75003 Paris
France

RS Bresalier
University of Michigan
Gastrointestinal Cancer Research
  Laboratory
Department of Medicine
Henry Ford Health Sciences Center
2799 West Grand Boulevard
Detroit, MI 48202
USA

R Brigelius-Flohé
Abteilung Vitamine und Atherosklerose
Deutsches Institut für
  Ernährungsforschung
Arthur-Scheunert-Allee 114-116
D-14558 Bergholz-Rehbrücke
Germany

WR Bruce
Department of Nutritional Sciences
University of Toronto
150 College Street
Toronto, ONT M5S 3E2
Canada

R Caspari
Medizinische Klinik
Klinikum der Universität
Sigmund-Freud-Str. 25
D-53105 Bonn
Germany

A Chao
Epidemiology and Surveillance
  Research
American Cancer Society
1599 Clifton Road N.E.
Atlanta, GA 30329-4251
USA

JH Cummings
Department of Molecular and Cellular
Pathology

Ninewells Hospital and Medical School
Dundee, DD1 9SY
UK

H Daniel
Institut für Ernährungswissenschaft
Hochfeldweg 2
D-85350 Freising-Weihenstephan
Germany

R-D Duan
Biomedical Centre, B11
Lund University
S-221 84 Lund
Sweden

RW Hart
Hart Investments, LP
2200 Andover Sq. No. 804
Little Rock, AR 72227
USA

MJ Hill
Nutrition Research Centre
South Bank University
103 Borough Road
London, SE1 0AA
UK

JR Jass
Department of Pathology
McGill University
Duff Medical Building
3775 University Street
Montreal
Quebec, H3A 2B4
Canada

JH Kleibeuker
Academisch Ziekenhuis Groningen
Afd. Interne Geneeskunde
Afd. Gastroenterologie
PO Box 30.001
NL-9700 RB Groningen
The Netherlands

F Kullmann
Klinik und Poliklinik für Innere Medizin I
Klinikum der Universität Regensburg
D-93042 Regensburg
Germany

ME Martinez
Arizona Cancer Center
PO Box 245024
Tucson, AZ 85724-5024
USA

T Menzel
Medizinische Universitätsklinik
Josef-Schneider-Str. 2
D-97080 Würzburg
Germany

V Milovic
2nd Department of Medicine
Johann Wolfgang Goethe University
Theodor Stern Kai 7
D-60590 Frankfurt
Germany

FM Nagengast
Department of Gastroenterology and
 Hepatology
University Medical Centre Nijmegen
Geert Grooteplein Zuid 8
NL-6525 GA Nijmegen
The Netherlands

RW Owen
Deutsches Krebsforschungszentrum
Toxikologie und Krebsrisikofaktoren
Im Neuenheimer Feld 280
D-69120 Heidelberg
Germany

BL Pool-Zobel
Institut für Ernährungswissenschaften
Friedrich Schiller Universität Jena
Dornburger Str. 25
D-07743 Jena
Germany

BS Reddy
Division of Nutritional Carcinogenesis
American Health Foundation
1 Dana Road
Valhalla, NY 10595
USA

IC Roberts-Thomson
Department of Gastroenterology and
 Hepatology
The Queen Elizabeth Hospital
28 Woodville Road
Woodville South, SA 5011
Australia

JL Rombeau
University of Pennsylvania
Medical Center
Department of Surgery
4 Silverstein
3400 Spruce Street
Philadelphia, PA 19105
USA

P Rozen
Department of Gastroenterology
Tel Aviv Medical Center
6 Weizmann St
Tel Aviv 64239
Israel

W Scheppach
Medizinische Poliklinik
Klinikum der Universität Würzburg
Klinikstr. 8
D-97080 Würzburg
Germany

M Scheurlen
Medizinische Poliklinik
Klinikum der Universität Würzburg
Klinikstr. 8
D-97080 Würzburg
Germany

W Schmiegel
Medizinische Klinik
Ruhr-Universität Bochum
Knappschaftskrankenhaus
In der Schornau 23-25
D-44892 Bochum
Germany

HK Seitz
Medizinische Poliklinik
Krankenhaus Salem

Zeppelinstr. 11-33
D-69121 Heidelberg
Germany

DEG Shuker
Department of Chemistry
The Open University
Walton Hall
Milton Keynes, MK7 6AA
UK

ML Slattery
University of Utah
Health Research Center
375 Chipeta Way, Suite A
Salt Lake City, UT 84108
USA

SR Tannenbaum
Biological Engineering Division
Massachusetts Institute of Technology
77 Massachusetts Avenue,
Room 56-731A
Cambridge, MA 02139-4307
USA

JH Weisburger
American Health Foundation
1 Dana Road
Valhalla, NY 10595
USA

Preface

Carcinoma of the colon and rectum is the second most common cause of cancer-related mortality in Western societies. In Germany, over 50 000 new cases and 30 000 deaths are registered annually; these figures are entirely unacceptable. Therapeutic options in advanced stages of disease are rather limited. Therefore, efforts towards cancer prevention must be a major objective of health care systems in industrialized countries. Evidence-based prevention strategies require a profound understanding of the pathogenesis of colorectal cancer and the underlying genetic and environmental factors. Thus, the Falk Symposium 128 in Würzburg (Germany) was dedicated to the important issue of exogenous factors in colonic carcinogenesis and their interplay with the genetic background of this disease.

In approximately 5% of cases, a clear hereditary basis of colorectal cancer has been identified, leading to the description of familial colon cancer syndromes (familial adenomatous polyposis and hereditary non-polyposis colorectal cancer). Although these entities are comparatively rare, they have widened enormously our understanding of colonic carcinogenesis in general. It has also been recognized that sporadic colorectal cancer, which is encountered in 95% of cases, is the consequence of a dynamic process leading from hyperproliferative epithelium through different classes of adenomas to invasive carcinoma. Simultaneously, mutations (APC, K-ras, DCC, p53) are found with increasing frequency during progression through the adenoma-to-carcinoma sequence. Therefore, it has been argued that the pathogenesis of sporadic cancer of the colon and rectum is dominated by genetic events.

On the other hand, epidemiological data clearly indicate that sporadic colorectal cancer has to be considered as a lifestyle tumour, heavily influenced by exogenous factors. A 50% decline of cancer incidence in the case of lifestyle changes such as regular physical activity, maintenance of normal weight, dietary modification (high fruit, high vegetable, low red meat), cessation of smoking, and moderation in alcohol consumption has been predicted on the basis of currently available epidemiological evidence. The question then is how these two aspects (genetics and epidemiology) can be combined to explain comprehensively the phenomenon of colonic carcinogenesis.

PREFACE

The Würzburg Symposium was planned to identify the interfaces between the genetic background and the environment in carcinogenesis. It is noteworthy that the structure and function of a colonic cell may be affected not only by mutations but also by epigenetic events such as hypermethylation of promotor regions eventually leading to gene silencing. Additionally, DNA and histone acetylation have profound effects (upregulation as well as downregulation) on the expression of various genes. *In vitro* studies indicate that defined components of the human diet may act on colonic epithelial cells via these epigenetic events. The modulation of DNA adduct formation is another example of a link between luminal factors and the lining epithelium. Genetic polymorphisms make the situation even more complicated by rendering the individual more or less susceptible to the impact of exogenous factors.

These data show that we are faced with a complex interaction between colonic luminal factors and colonocytes. An understanding of the molecular biology of colorectal cancer may help us to devise prevention stategies, either relying on chemopreventive drugs or nutritional intervention. We hope that the symposium has contributed to the awareness that colorectal cancer is a preventable disease.

Our thanks are due to Dr. Herbert Falk for making this conference in Würzburg possible. We appreciate the continuous and friendly support by the Falk Foundation (especially Mrs. S. Maresch) during two years of preparation. The outstanding contributions by 35 speakers from 9 countries have made this international symposium a great success.

Wolfgang Scheppach, M.D.
Michael Scheurlen, M.D.

Section I
Epidemiology and risk assessment

1
Exposure and disease biomarkers for colorectal cancer risk

W. R. BRUCE

INTRODUCTION

Colorectal cancer risk has been related to diet and lifestyle factors in many ecological, case–control and cohort studies. Risk has been found to increase with
consumption of saturated fat, meat, sugar, overly cooked foods and alcohol, and
a sedentary lifestyle, and to decrease with consumption of vegetables, starch and
fibre[1]. These relationships can be explained in several ways through mechanisms
that relate lifestyle factors and cancer risk, as suggested for instance in refs 2 and 3.
Evaluation of the mechanisms, however, poses a problem. Colorectal cancer
develops over a long period of time and during that time colonic cells are
exposed to circulating and luminal environments that probably depend on diet in
complex, physiological ways.

One approach to bridging the long gap between diet and cancer is to focus on
the development of the disease and on possible surrogate endpoints of cancers,
disease biomarkers. The evaluation of a mechanism relating diet and cancer is
then reduced to two processes: first, the association of the disease biomarker
and cancer; and second, the association between diet and the biomarker.
Considerable progress has been made in the description of the early steps of
tumour development as possible biomarkers. In brief, tumours appear to develop
from enlarging adenomas, though adenomas can remain small and benign or
possibly regress. The development of new adenoma after polypectomy has been
used as a disease biomarker in many studies (e.g. refs 4 and 5). Earlier markers
are also possible. Adenomas appear to develop from enlarging aberrant crypt
foci (ACF)[6]. The foci of aberrant crypts can be identified from the luminal surface by their larger size and their more intense staining with vital stains, such as
methylene blue. The foci begin as single affected crypts and then increase, presumably by crypt fission, to larger and larger foci that eventually become visible
macroscopically as small polyps. The histological appearance of ACF can differ
considerably, from a hyperplastic to a dysplastic structure[7]. The proliferation
rate of cells in ACF can be high[8] and differentiation is frequently incomplete.

This is observed especially on the luminal surface where there are reduced numbers of goblet cells, and columnar cells have fewer microvilli[9], characteristics that may explain the increased vital staining. ACF, like adenomas, can remain benign or regress, and ACF number and size can also be used as clinical disease biomarkers to study the effect of intervention agents[10]. However, the development of these early disease markers does not identify appropriate interventions to reduce the development of human disease.

Another approach to bridging the gap is to focus on the earliest steps in human carcinogenesis, on diet and how it affects exposure to physiological environments; that is, on exposure biomarkers that increase proliferation and mutation in colonic cells. Again, the evaluation of mechanisms relating diet and cancer can be reduced to two processes: first, the association of the exposure biomarker and cancer; and second, the association between diet and the biomarker. Exposure biomarkers are of particular interest if they are closely associated with cancer risk and with dietary factors previously associated with disease. Such biomarkers could support a mechanism relating the diet and cancer. This chapter will consider three groups of exposure biomarkers that appear to fulfil these two conditions, and the corresponding mechanisms that relate diet and cancer risk. It will then consider how the exposure biomarkers might be used to further test the validity of the proposed mechanisms.

INSULIN RESISTANCE

Colon cancer risk has long been associated with abnormalities in glucose and insulin levels and frequently with obesity and a sedentary lifestyle. It was only recently, however, that McKeown-Eyssen[11] and Giovannucci[12] suggested a mechanism that could explain this association. They pointed out that dietary factors, such as increased saturated fat, sugar and high glycaemic carbohydrate and reduced n-3 fatty acids and reduced exercise, are risk factors both for a physiological state referred to as 'insulin resistance' and for colon carcinogenesis. Insulin resistance is a condition in which muscle, liver and fat cells become less sensitive to the metabolic effects of insulin. It is associated with physiologically increased circulating levels of insulin, non-esterified fatty acids and triglycerides, and with the development of type 2 diabetes, obesity, hypertension and atherosclerotic cardiovascular disease[13]. Eyssen and Giovannucci suggested that the dietary and lifestyle factors, by increasing levels of insulin, and perhaps also the circulating energy substrates[11], increase the proliferation of colonic cells and promote colon carcinogenesis.

Experimental animal studies provide support for the proposed mechanism. They show that exogenous insulin increases the proliferation of colonic cells[14] and that repeated injections of insulin promote the growth of ACF[15] and colon cancers[16]. They show that diets increasing insulin resistance, either measured directly or indirectly with postprandial glucose or postprandial insulin, are associated with the promotion of ACF[17,18]. Observational epidemiological studies also provide support for the mechanism. Prospective studies have demonstrated associations between polyps and fasting insulin[19], and colon cancers and C-peptide, a measure of insulin production[20,21]. Associations have also been observed between colon cancers and insulin-like growth factor (IGF)-1 and binding protein (BP)-3[20,22], an association that may be secondary to the effect on insulin[20].

EPITHELIAL BARRIER DEFECTS

Mullin has suggested that failure of the epithelial barrier and increased colonic permeability are early steps in the process of colon carcinogenesis[23]. He showed that tumour promoters produce defects in the tight junctions between epithelial cells grown *in vitro*, and thus increase the membrane permeability, and that the defects are large enough to allow growth factors access to pass from the luminal to the lateral and basal surfaces of the cells[24]. Similar defects can be observed by electron microscopy in epithelial cells of polyps and cancers[25]. Mullin suggested that such defects allowed growth factors, which are typically at a much higher concentration intraluminally than they are in tissues, to reach the basolateral surface of epithelial cells, the site of growth-promoter receptors. Increased epithelial permeability would thus expose the epithelial cells to an increased proliferative stimulus from growth hormones, such as epidermal growth factor (EGF) in the colonic lumen[23].

Increased permeability of the epithelial barrier could also have indirect effects on proliferation through local inflammation. The increased permeability could expose cells in the lamina propria to the 'environment' normally confined to the colonic lumen, for instance, to reduced oxygen tension, to peptides formed in digestion, to viruses and possibly to bacteria[26]. The resulting inflammatory response could induce nitrogen oxide synthase (iNOS) and cyclo-oxygen synthase-2 (COX-2), the accumulation of inflammatory cells and the exposure of the epithelial cells to inflammatory eicosanoids, cytokines and growth factors including IGF[27,28].

Diet could affect the integrity of the colonic epithelium in several ways. Perhaps the most likely is through the effect of dietary calcium and phosphate on concentrations of these ions in the milieu fluid surrounding colonic crypts. A decrease in the concentration of calcium on the basolateral surface of *in-vitro* epithelial cell monolayers is known to increase their permeability by affecting the closure of tight junctions[29]. Similar effects probably occur *in vivo*. Oral boluses of sodium phosphate can produce colonic ulcers and inflammation in humans[30]. The boluses are associated with large increases in serum phosphate, and decreases in the concentration of calcium[31]. Diet may have a similar effect. The Western diet typically provides phosphate in excess of calcium, principally because of the large amounts of phosphate relative to calcium in bread, meat and potatoes, each with a possible 10-fold excess of phosphate[32]. Though the levels of phosphate would never reach those seen following oral gavages, the exposure is repeated thousands of times over a lifetime and could result in focal colonic barrier failure and inflammation.

Colon cancer risk has long been known to be increased in inflammatory bowel disease[33]. Recently a more general association with inflammation has been observed. Patients with colonic polyps and cancers have elevated levels of calprotectin, a protein marker of neutrophils, in their faeces[34,35]. Granulocyte marker protein appears to be elevated prior to the appearance of macroscopic disease[36] and may be present after tumour and polyp resection[37]. The mechanism responsible for the inflammation is not known, though a clinical study demonstrated that colonic inflammation was related to colonic permeability[38].

It seems most likely that repeated exposure to a diet containing an excess of phosphate results in a breakdown of the colonic barrier and an increased permeability. Of course, diet could also decrease the integrity of the colonic epithelium through other mechanisms, such as mechanical injury, selective effects on the growth of toxic bacteria, or effects on the quantity and metabolism of bile acids. However, diets relatively deficient in calcium in relation to phosphate would account for the protective effect of calcium supplements in animal colon carcinogenesis[39] and in clinical studies of polyp recurrence (e.g. ref. 5).

The effects of calcium or other agents could be evaluated with the use of biomarkers for permeability, inflammation and proliferation. Colonic permeability can be assessed with the use of compounds normally excluded by the colonic epithelium[40]. Colonic inflammation can be assessed with faecal calprotectin or, perhaps, a measurement of circulating inflammatory markers such as C-reactive protein. This protein is increased with macroscopic tumours[41]. Colonic proliferation can be assessed by biopsy, though it may be observed to be elevated only under particular circumstances, after consumption of particular foods or only in cells comprising precursor lesions.

The pathways between increased epithelial permeability, increased inflammation and hyperproliferation are probably complex. As noted above, the luminal surface of the ACF is composed of relatively immature cells and appears to be more permeable than other areas of the epithelium. This would expose the epithelial cells at the base of the crypt to growth factors from the lumen, and would lead to inflammation that exposes the epithelial cells to cytokines and growth factors associated with inflammation. Recursive pathways are also possible. Products of inflammation can increase colonic permeability. Strong proliferative stimuli increase mutations and could lead to a failure of cells to fully differentiate before reaching the top of the crypt. Thus both pathways would further reduce the integrity of the epithelial barrier and perpetuate the process, and this could explain the continuing phenotype of the ACF with its hyperproliferation, lack of differentiated cells, and increased permeability. It could also explain the sensitivity of early ACF to agents that break this recursive cycle, such as the demulcent polyethylene glycol[42] and anti-inflammatory agent piroxicam[43].

GENOTOXICITY

Colon cancer is characterized by the accumulation of specific somatic mutations. Thus risk must be closely associated with exposure to factors that increase the frequency of mutations. Somatic mutations can be acquired in the process of normal cell division, increasing age and rate of proliferation. These normal rates can be augmented by endogenous exposures, such as the oxidative stress associated with insulin resistance and inflammation, or exogenous genotoxins such as the heterocyclic amines and polycyclic hydrocarbons. Mutations could also be induced by endogenous products of carbohydrate metabolism and by deficiencies of folate.

In carbohydrate metabolism, six-carbon fructose-1,6-bis phosphate or fructose-1-phosphate is broken down by aldolase into two three-carbon fragments, glyceraldehyde-3-phosphate. There is a by-product in this process, the potentially bifunctional alkylating agent, methylglyoxal[44]. Virtually all cells contain glyoxalases and glutathione that eliminate this potentially toxic compound. However, glutathione levels can decrease with age and diet, with the formation of methylglyoxal adducts most evident in cataracts. The importance of methylglyoxal and related compounds as mutagens in colon carcinogenesis remains to be determined. The ready measurement of methylglyoxal in the blood and its metabolites in the urine should facilitate such studies.

Low levels of dietary folate may be a more important factor in mutagenesis relating to colon cancer. Deficiency of folate, together with B_6, B_{12} and perhaps other methyl donors, has been implicated in colon carcinogenesis[45]. Deficiencies can be assessed through serum or red blood cell folate or increased plasma homocysteine[46].

INTERPLAY OF THE THREE HYPOTHESIZED EXPOSURE RISKS

The three mechanisms described have many interactions. First, food components have possible effects through more than one mechanism. N-3 and n-6 fatty acids can have effects on both insulin resistance/hyperinsulinaemia[18] and on inflammation[47]. Hyperglycaemia/sucrose can have effects on both insulin resistance/hyperinsulinaemia and genotoxicity through the formation of methylglyoxal[44]. Second, mechanisms can interact with each other. Both insulin resistance/hyperinsulinaemia and epithelial barrier defects/inflammation can lead to oxidative stress with genotoxic effects from reactive oxygen species[48,49], as well as increased proliferation. Insulin levels can increase the permeability of epithelial barriers. Inflammatory processes may be involved in the development of type 2 diabetes from an insulin-resistant state[50]. Conversely, insulin levels may affect epithelial permeability[51]. In addition, stress through circulating hydrocortisone can affect both the development of insulin resistance[52] and the integrity of epithelial membranes[53].

TESTS OF THE HYPOTHESES

The hypotheses can be tested most readily with experimental animal studies. Mice could be given a diet with a high level of fat, with a large fraction of n-6 fatty acids and with a high glycaemic index carbohydrate. In addition it could be a diet with a high level of phosphate relative to calcium, with low vitamin D, with low folate, methyl donors and B_{12}. Such a diet might be expected to induce insulin resistance and insulinaemia (high saturated fat and n-6 fatty acids, high glycaemic index carbohydrate) and to increase colonic permeability and inflammation (high phosphate, n-6 fatty acids, deficiency of calcium and vitamin D). It would also increase genotoxicity and mutation frequency (low folate, methionine, choline, B_{12} and high glycaemic index carbohydrate and increased exposure to methylglyoxal). Would such animals develop colon cancer? This experiment has been done by Newmark and colleagues[54]. They used dietary components that were at the lower level of those typical on a Western diet in their 'New Western

Diet'. They found that C57Bl/6 mice, that very infrequently develop colon cancer on usual laboratory diets, develop colon tumours when fed this diet over a period of 18–24 months. It will be interesting to determine whether this diet does induce insulin resistance, colonic inflammation and increased mutations in epithelial cells in animals.

Testing the hypothesis in humans is more difficult. However, it should be possible to do the test in two steps. First, to determine whether dietary factors can be manipulated so as to reduce insulin resistance, colonic inflammation and genotoxicity. Second, to determine whether diets that reduce these measures reduce the development of disease biomarkers and eventually colon cancer. The former intervention studies might be done with guidance from the animal studies, choosing the most readily modified variables. For instance, fish oil might be added to the diet to reduce the ratio of n-6 to n-3 fatty acids and hyperinsulinaemia. Calcium might be added to the diet to reduce the excess of phosphate and the possibility of barrier loss and colonic inflammation. Folate might be added to the diet to reduce the possibility of a deficiency in methyl donors resulting in a decreased mutation frequency. The combined effect of these additions could be on exposure biomarkers for insulin resistance (e.g. postprandial plasma insulin, free fatty acids, triglycerides), colonic inflammation (e.g. faecal calprotectin, serum C-reactive protein) and mutation risk (e.g. serum and red blood cell folate, plasma homocysteine). These studies would be of short duration and could test a wide range of food components to find a protocol that reliably reduces measures of insulin resistance, colonic inflammation and genotoxicity. The most practical and effective protocol could then be tested in longer-term studies aimed at reducing colon carcinogenesis.

Finally, it should be noted that the Western dietary and lifestyle factors identified as risks for colorectal cancer could be similar to those for other cancers[1], for type 2 diabetes and for atherosclerosis. For instance, Stemmermann et al. have described their findings in the autopsies of Japanese–Hawaiian men who had adopted a Western lifestyle[55]. The degrees of atherosclerosis of the coronary arteries and aorta was 'positively and significantly related not only to the presence of adenomatous polyps, but to their size, multiplicity, and degree of atypia as well'. The exposure markers for atherosclerotic cardiovascular disease include: elevated triglycerides and evidence of insulin resistance[13]; C-reactive protein[56] and myeloperoxidase[57], evidence of endothelial dysfunction[58]; and homocysteine[59], evidence of folate and/or B_{12} deficiency. It is evident that the exposure biomarkers for cardiovascular disease are closely related to those for colorectal cancer. Interventions that reduce the levels of the exposure markers for colon cancer could thus have a profound effect on diseases associated with the Western lifestyle.

Acknowledgement

The author is supported by a grant from the Cancer Research Society.

References

1. World Cancer Research Fund. Food, Nutrition and the Prevention of Cancer: A Global Perspective. Washington: American Institute for Cancer Research. 1997:216–51.

2. Bruce WR, Giacca A, Medline A. Possible mechanisms relating diet and risk of colon cancer. Cancer Epidemiol Biomarkers Prev. 2000;9:1271–9.
3. Bruce WR, Giacca A, Medline A. Possible mechanisms relating diet to colorectal cancer risk. IARC Sci Publ. 2002 (In press).
4. Schatzkin A, Lanza E, Corle D et al. Lack of effect of a low-fat, high-fiber diet on the recurrence of colorectal cancer. N Engl J Med. 2000;342:1149–55.
5. Baron JA, Beach M, Mandel JS et al. Calcium supplements for the prevention of colorectal adenomas. Calcium Polyp Prevention Study Group. N Engl J Med. 1999;340:101–7.
6. Bird RP, McLellan EA, Bruce WR. Aberrant crypts, putative precancerous lesions, in the study of the role of diet in the aetiology of colon cancer. Cancer Surv. 1989;8:189–200.
7. Roncucci L, Medline A, Bruce WR. Classification of aberrant crypt foci and microadenomas in human colon. Cancer Epidemiol Biomarkers Prev. 1991;1:57–60.
8. Pretlow TP, Cheyer C, O'Riordan MA. Aberrant crypt foci and colon tumors in F344 rats have similar increases in proliferative activity. Int J Cancer. 1994;56:599–602.
9. Vaccina F, Scorcioni F, Pedroni M et al. Scanning electron microscopy of aberrant crypt foci in human colorectal mucosa. Anticancer Res. 1998;18:3451–6.
10. Takayama T, Katsuki S, Takahashi Y et al. Aberrant crypt foci of the colon as precursors of adenoma and cancer. N Engl J Med. 1998;339:1277–84.
11. McKeown-Eyssen G. Epidemiology of colorectal cancer revisited: are serum triglycerides and/or plasma glucose associated with risk? Cancer Epidemiol Biomarkers Prev. 1994;3:687–95.
12. Giovannucci E. Insulin and colon cancer. Cancer Causes Control. 1995;6:164–79.
13. DeFronzo RA, Ferrannini E. Insulin resistance: a multifaceted syndrome responsible for NIDDM, obesity, hypertension, dyslipidemia, and atherosclerotic cardiovascular disease. Diabetes Care. 1991;14:173–94.
14. Tran TT, Naigamwalla D, Lam L, Giacca A, Bruce RW. Hyperinsulinemia, but not other factors associated with insulin resistance, affects epithelial proliferation in the rat. Proc Am Assoc Cancer Res. 2001;92 (abstract).
15. Corpet DE, Jacquinet C, Peiffer G, Tache S. Insulin injections promote the growth of aberrant crypt foci in the colon of rats. Nutr Cancer. 1997;27:316–20.
16. Tran TT, Medline A, Bruce WR. Insulin promotion of colon tumors in rats. Cancer Epidemiol Biomarkers Prev. 1996;5:1013–15.
17. Tran TT, Gupta N, Goh T et al. Direct measure of insulin sensitivity with hyperinsulinemic–euglycemic clamp and surrogate measures of insulin sensitivity with oral glucose tolerance test: correlations with aberrant crypt foci (ACF) promotion in rats. 2002 (Submitted).
18. Koohestani N, Chia MC, Pham N-A et al. Aberrant crypt focus promotion and glucose intolerance: correlation in the rat across diets differing in fat, n-3 fatty acids and energy. Carcinogenesis. 1998;19:1679–84.
19. Eyssen GEM, Cohen L, Diamandis E et al. Insulin resistance and risk of colorectal neoplasia. 2000 (Submitted).
20. Kaaks R, Toniolo P, Akhmedkhanov A et al. Serum C-peptide, IGF-I, IGF-binding proteins and risk of colorectal cancer in women. J Natl Cancer Inst. 2000;92:34–42.
21. Ma J, Giovannucci E, Pollak M, Leavitt A, Gaziano M, Stampfer MJ. A prospective study of plasma C-peptide and risk of colorectal cancer in men. Proc Am Assoc Cancer Res. 2002;43:2804 (abstract).
22. Ma J, Pollak MN, Giovannucci E et al. Prospective study of colorectal cancer risk in men and plasma levels of insulin-like growth factor (IGF)-I and IGF-binding protein-3. J Natl Cancer Inst. 1999;91:620–5.
23. Mullin JM. Potential interplay between luminal growth factors and increased tight junction permeability in epithelial carcinogenesis. J Exp Zool. 1997;279:484–9.
24. Mullin JM, Ginanni N, Laughlin KV. Protein kinase C activation increases transepithelial transport of biologically active insulin. Cancer Res. 1998;58:1641–5.
25. Soler AP, Miller RD, Laughlin KV, Carp NZ, Klurfeld DM, Mullin JM. Increased tight junctional permeability is associated with the development of colon cancer. Carcinogenesis. 1999;20:1425–31.
26. Swidsinski A, Khilin M, Kerjaschki D et al. Association between intraepithelial Escherichia coli and colorectal cancer. Gastroenterology. 1998;115:281–6.
27. Bjjork J, Nilsson J, Hultcranz R, Johansson C. Growth-regulatory effects of sensory neuropeptides, epidermal growth factor, insulin and somatostatin on non-transformed intestinal epithelial cell line IEC-6 and colon cancer cell line HT 29. Scand J Gastroenterol. 1993;28:879–84.

28. Zimmermann EM, Li L, Hou YT, Mohapatra NK, Puciloska JB. Insulin-like growth factor I and insulin-like growth factor binding protein 5 in Crohn's disease. Am J Liver Physiol. 2001; 280:G1022–9.
29. Ma TY, Tran D, Hoa N, Nguyen D, Merryfield M, Tarnawski A. Mechanism of extracellular calcium regulation of intestinal epithelial tight junction permeability: role of cytoskeletal involvement. Microsci Res Tech. 2000;51:156–68.
30. Driman DK, Preiksaitis HG. Colorectal inflammation and increased cell proliferation associated with oral sodium phosphate bowel preparation solution. Hum Pathol. 1998;29:972–8.
31. DiPalma JA, Buckley SE, Warner BA, Culpepper RM. Biochemical effects of oral sodium phosphate. Dig Dis Sci. 1996;41:749–53.
32. Pennington JAT. Bowes and Church's Food Values of Portions Commonly Used, 17th edn. Lippincott: Philadelphia, 1998.
33. Sandler RS, Eisen GM. Epidemiology of inflammatory bowel disease. In: Kirsner JB, editor. Inflammatory Bowel Disease, 5th edn. Philadelphia: Saunders, 2000:89–112.
34. Tøn H, Brandnes Ø, Dale S et al. Improved method for calprotectin. Clin Chim Acta. 2000;292:41–54.
35. Kronborg O, Ugstad M, Faglerud P et al. Faecal calprotectin levels in a high risk population for colorectal neoplasia. Gut. 2000;46:795–800.
36. Kristinsson J, Røseth AG, Sundseth K et al. Granulocyte marker protein is increased in stool from rats with azoxymethane-induced colon cancer. Scand J Gastroenterol. 1999;34:1216–23.
37. Kristinsson J, Røseth A, Fagerhol MK et al. Fecal calprotectin concentration in patients with colorectal carcinoma. Dis Colon Rectum. 1998;41:316–21.
38. Berstad A, Arslan G, Folvik G. Relationship between intestinal permeability and calprotectin concentration in gut lavage fluid. Scand J Gastroenterol. 2000;35:64–9.
39. Wargovich MJ, Allnutt D, Palmer C, Anaya P, Stephens LC. Inhibition of the promotional phase of azoxymethane-induced colon carcinogenesis in the F344 rat by calcium lactate: effect of simulating two human nutrient density levels. Cancer Lett. 1990;53:17–25.
40. Meddings JB, Gibbons I. Discrimination of site-specific alterations in gastrointestinal permeability in the rat. Gastroenterology. 1998;114:83–92.
41. Mercer DW, Talamo TS. Multiple markers of malignancy in sera of patients with colorectal carcinoma: preliminary clinical studies. Clin Chem. 1985;31:1824–8.
42. Corpet DE, Parnaud G. Polyethylene glycol, a potent suppressor of azoxymethane-induced colonic aberrant crypt foci in rats. Carcinogenesis. 1999;20:915–18.
43. Kawamori T, Rao CV, Seibert K, Reddy BS. Chemopreventive activity of celecoxib, a specific cyclooxygenase-2 inhibitor, against colon carcinogenesis. Cancer Res. 1998;58:409–12.
44. Thornalley PJ. Pharmacology of methylglyoxal: formation, modification of proteins and nucleic acids, and enzymatic detoxification – a role in pathogenesis and antiproliferative chemotherapy. Gen Pharmacol. 1996;27:565–73.
45. Kim Y-I. Folate and carcinogenesis: evidence, mechanisms and implications. J Nutr Biochem. 1999;10:66–88.
46. Herrmann W. The importance of hyperhomocysteinemia as a risk factor for diseases: an overview. Clin Chem Lab Med. 2001;39:666–74.
47. James MJ, Gibson RA, Cleland LG. Dietary polyunsaturated fatty acids and inflammatory mediator production. Am J Clin Nutr. 2000;71(Suppl. 1):343-8S.
48. Paolisso G, Giugliano D. Oxidative stress and insulin action: is there a relationship? Diabetologia. 1996;39:357–63.
49. Shen Z, Wu W, Hazen SL. Activated leukocytes oxidatively damage DNA, RNA, and the nucleotide pool through halide-dependent formation of hydroxyl radical. Biochemistry. 2000;39:5474–82.
50. Pradhan AD, Manson JE, Rifai N, Buring JE, Ridker PM. C-reactive protein, interleukin 6, and risk of developing type 2 diabetes mellitus. J Am Med Assoc. 2000;286:327–34.
51. McRoberts JA, Riley NE. Role of insulin and insulin-like growth factor receptors in regulation of T84 cell monolayer permeability. Am J Physiol. 1994;267 (Gastrointest Liver Physiol. 30):G883–91.
52. Greisen J, Juhl CB, Grofte T, Vilstrup H, Jensen TS, Schmitz O. Acute pain induces insulin resistance in humans. Anesthesiology. 2001;95:578–84.
53. Meddings JB, Swain MG. Environmental stress-induced gastrointestinal permeability is mediated by endogenous glucocorticoids in the rat. Gastroenterology. 2000;119:1019–28.

54. Newmark HL, Yang K, Lipkin M *et al.* A Western-style diet induces benign and malignant neoplasms in the colon of normal C57Bl/6 mice. Carcinogenesis. 2001;22:1871–5.
55. Stemmermann GH, Heilbrun LK, Nomura A, Yano K, Hayashi T. Adenomatous polyps and atherosclerosis: an autopsy study of Japanese men in Hawaii. Int J Cancer. 1986;38:789–94.
56. Libby P, Ridker PM, Maseri A. Inflammation and atherosclerosis. Circulation. 2002; 105:1135–43.
57. Zhang R, Branan ML, Fu X *et al.* Association between myeloperoxidase levels and risk of coronary artery disease. J Am Med Assoc. 2001;286:2136–42.
58. Poredos P. Endothelial dysfunction in the pathogenesis of atherosclerosis. Clin Appl Thromb Hemost. 2001;7:276–80.
59. Malinow MR, Bosom AG, Krauss RM. Homocysteine, diet, and cardiovascular diseases: a statement for healthcare professionals from the Nutrition Committee, American Heart Association. Circulation. 1999;99:178–82.

2
Exogenous factors in colonic carcinogenesis

B. L. POOL-ZOBEL

Colorectal cancers (CRC) are frequent cancers with well-clarified genetic background and high mortality rates, ranking as number one on the incidence list in Germany. They are probably also the tumour types most strongly linked to dietary factors. Epidemiological evidence suggests that high consumption of processed meats and alcohol increases risk. The attempt to identify the carcinogenic compounds involved has traditionally focussed on food-borne toxicants, such as heterocyclic amines or polycyclic aromatic hydrocarbons that are mutagens in *S. typhimurium* or carcinogens in rats. Additionally, endogenous products are expected to contribute. Iron and alcohol metabolism can cause oxidative stress in the gut and the products of oxidative stress [reactive oxygen species (ROS)] induce lipid peroxidation. Both ROS and products of lipid peroxidation cause cell damage in model systems. Basic studies on how these risk factors may interact with the colon epithelium are largely unavailable, mainly due to lack of appropriate testing methods. Research in our laboratory is focussing on using new approaches to study the impact of food-related compounds in the human colon. Methods have been developed to obtain primary human colon cells from biopsies or tissues obtained during surgery. The yield of cells from surgical tissues was 100×10^6 cells/g colon tissue, and from biopsies up to 0.5×10^6 cells per donor, both enough for *in vitro* studies. Using the Comet assay we have assessed sensitivities of primary cells toward different putative risk factors. A novel Comet assay application utilizing fluorescence *in situ* hybridization of isolated DNA with *TP53*-specific probes (Comet FISH) now also enables us to study the potency of risk factors for damage in cancer-relevant genes. The studies showed that colon cells are sensitive to oxidants, products of lipid peroxidation and direct acting carcinogens. H_2O_2 causes genetic damage and steady state levels of oxidized DNA bases are detectable *ex vivo*. The lipid peroxidation products trans-2-hexenal and 4-hydroxynonenal (HNE) are genotoxic at 400 and 100 μM, respectively. *TP53* is more sensitive to the risk factors than global DNA. In conclusion, the quantity and quality of cells from surgery material and even from biopsies is sufficient for *in vitro* investigations of compound-induced genotoxic effects. Cells of colon are susceptible to putative colon cancer risk factors, and the tumour suppressor gene *TP53* is more sensitive than the total cellular DNA. The approach is a useful method to learn more about the effects of risk factors in one of the major target tissues of human carcinogenesis.

3
Definition of cancer susceptibility

M.-C. BOUTRON-RUAULT

INTRODUCTION

Sporadic colorectal cancer represents about 95% of all cases of colorectal cancer, and is mostly associated with dietary or lifestyle risk factors. However, although there is no Mendelian transmission of the disease (contrary to familial adenomatous polyposis (FAP) or hereditary non-polyposis colorectal cancer (HNPCC)), it has been well documented that having a case of colorectal cancer among first-degree relatives approximately doubles the risk of having a colorectal cancer[1]. An interaction between lifestyle risk factors and metabolic polymorphisms is an interesting approach to explain at least part of this association. Over 90 papers have been published between 2000 and 2002 concerning the relationship between common polymorphisms and colorectal cancer, which underlines the interest of the scientific community in this opening field of research. Among these papers, some pointed out ethical issues which must not be forgotten[2]. The use of our knowledge on at-risk polymorphisms must be well regulated in order to avoid possible problems with insurance companies, for example. Several polymorphisms related to colorectal tumours have been identified. Some of them modulate the deleterious effect of dietary factors, whereas others modulate the beneficial effect of other dietary factors. Some polymorphisms are also susceptible to modulating the effect of chemotherapies[3,4]. Knowledge concerning these will be important when planning chemotherapy strategies for patients, but will not be discussed in this chapter.

POLYMORPHISMS ASSOCIATED WITH RISK OF COLORECTAL TUMOURS

A recent review of the literature[5] summarized and meta-analysed the available data on polymorphisms associated with risk of colorectal cancer. Four types of polymorphisms can be identified: those associated with the metabolism of carcinogens, those related to DNA methylation, microenvironment modifiers, and oncogenes and tumour suppressors. From studies published up to 1999 inclusive, the authors of the meta-analysis identified only three polymorphisms which significantly modulated the risk of colorectal cancer, i.e. adenomatous polyposis coli (APC)-I1307K, Harvey ras-1 variable number repeat polymorphism and methylenetetrahydrofolate reductase $(MTHFR)^{Val/Val}$. For other polymorphisms the available data enabled the authors to exclude a relative risk of 1.7 or over, but could not exclude associations at a lower level.

CARCINOGEN METABOLISM GENES

As discussed by Houlston and Tomlinson[5], colonic crypt cells express several of the important xenobiotic metabolizing enzymes, which may modulate the metabolism of precarcinogens present in food, especially in overcooked meat, and in tobacco smoke, i.e. polycyclic aromatic hydrocarbons and heterocyclic amines.

The first step in the activation of these precarcinogens involves phase I enzymes, especially cytochromes P450A1 (CYP1A1) and P450A2 (CYP1A2), which generally produce oxygenated metabolites (epoxy-, hydroxy-, etc.). Phase II enzymes generally detoxify functionalized metabolites produced by the phase I enzymes. Among these, the N-acetyl transferases, NAT1 and NAT2, catalyse N-acetylation of hydroxylized metabolites of aromatic amines. According to reaction size, this leads either to detoxication (N-acetylation) or to carcinogene activation (O- or N,O-acetylation). Thus NATs participate both in the activation and the detoxication of carcinogenes, especially aromatic heterocyclic amines. NAT2 polymorphism determines the slow, or fast/rapid, acetylator status, according to either homozygosity for low-activity alleles, or the presence of at least one fast-activity allele. The glutathione-S transferases detoxify mutagenic electrophiles such as polycyclic aromatic hydrocarbons in diet and tobacco.

Some studies have associated the rapid acetylator status with an increased risk of colorectal cancer (CRC)[6]. Rapid acetylators could be especially exposed to a high risk of CRC when they consume large quantities of overcooked meat, whereas such a dietary habit conveys no particular risk in slow acetylators. The latter could be more susceptible to smoking or high alcohol intake[7]. Such an interaction between the fast acetylator status and consumption of overcooked meat has also been observed for adenomas[8]. However, when summarized in a meta-analysis, the 15 studies on NAT2 polymorphism and the six studies on NAT1 polymorphism did not demonstrate a homogeneous relationship with risk of colorectal neoplasia. Although the studies based on phenotyping demonstrated a combined odds ratio of 1.70 (95% confidence interval 1.23–2.37), those based on genotyping, which constituted the majority of available studies, associated an odds ratio of 1.03 with the rapid acetylator genotype. The NAT1*10 genotype was associated with a combined odds ratio of 1.22, $p > 0.10$. As discussed by Brockton et al. in another recent review of the literature[9], specifically devoted to N-acetyltransferase polymorphisms and colorectal cancer, the lack of consistency can in part be accounted for by methodological factors. It may also be due to interactions between the NAT genes and either environmental exposure or other polymorphic genes, which have not been properly addressed.

Similar inconsistencies were observed when studying GSTM1 and GSTT1 status. Although several studies associated the GSTM1 deletion with an increased risk of colorectal cancer, the association was not significant in most cases[5,10].

According to a meta-analysis[5], no consistent pattern of association was observed among the 12 studies on colorectal cancer and the only one on adenomas. The pooled odds ratio associated with *GSTM1* deficiency was 1.14 for both distal and proximal cancers ($p > 0.10$). Similarly, the pooled odds ratio for *GSTT1* deficiency was 1.10 ($p > 0.10$).

POLYMORPHISM OF THE METHYLENETETRAHYDROFOLATE REDUCTASE (*MTHFR*)

The polymorphism of the enzyme methylenetetrahydrofolate reductase (*MTHFR*) is a good example of the complexity of the involved mechanisms that modulate dietary risk factors. A common polymorphism in the *MTHFR* gene, where a cytosine at nucleotide 677 is replaced by a thymine (677 C→T), results in a modified enzyme where an alanine is replaced by a valine (Ala677Val polymorphism). There is some geographical variation in prevalence of the mutation[11,12]. A north–south gradient of the mutation has been observed in most continents, the mutation being more common in southern regions than in the north. The mutation seems also to be more common in countries with a high intake of dietary folate, such as Latin countries, than in countries with a low mean intake, possibly because, in countries with insufficient intake of folate, the mutation confers a selective disadvantage, especially in terms of human reproduction. The mutation is associated with enzyme thermolability, a reduced activity of the enzyme (homozygotes have about 30% of normal enzyme activity) and a reduction in the conversion of 5,10-methylenetetrahydrofolate (5,10-MTHF) into 5-methyltetrahydrofolate. Thus, according to polymorphism and to folate intake, two opposite effects can be observed: on the one hand, decreased levels of methyl-THF which may adversely affect DNA methylation; on the other hand, depletion of methylene tetrahydrofolate, which interferes with thymidilate biosynthesis, and leads to deoxynucleotide pool imbalances, with an excess of deoxyuridine versus deoxythymidine. Deoxyuridilate DNA may accumulate, and when this abnormal base is removed this may lead to strand breaks. There is some epidemiological evidence that the mutation of the *MTHFR* has a dual effect according to the intake of dietary folate, which could be explained by the above-cited mechanisms. In case of a sufficient folate intake the mutation, compared with the wild type, is beneficial and associated with a reduced risk of colorectal cancer. In that case there would be no deficiency in methyl-THF, whereas there would be more methylene-THF than in non-mutated subjects. The estimated combined odds ratio for *MTHFR*[Val/Val] compared with the other genotypes (Ala/Val or Ala/Ala), in the meta-analysis[5], was 0.77 (95% confidence interval 0.64–0.93). In case of a low folate intake the mutation appears deleterious as compared with the wild type, and this could be explained by a deficiency in methyl-THF, thus leading to DNA hypomethylation[13]. However, one may question the benefit of an accumulation of methylene-THF, i.e. a large availability of bases for DNA synthesis, in cells with a fast division pattern. Epidemiological evidence from the four studies[13–16] which have examined the association of the mutation with colorectal cancer, and of the two which examined the association with adenomas[17,18], tend to demonstrate a protective effect of the mutation only on cancer, i.e. on late-stage tumorigenesis. However, a recent case–control study investigated the association between the mutation and risk of distal colorectal adenoma[19]. Compared with those in the lowest quartiles of red blood cell (RBC) and plasma folate and a wild-type allele, adenoma risk was increased for TT homozygotes in the lowest folate quartiles and decreased in TT homozygotes in the highest quartiles, suggesting an interaction with folate intake similar to that observed for cancers. There was also a significant interaction between TT genotype and the increased adenoma risk associated with alcohol. Another recent case–control study[20] investigated the relationship between *MTHFR* polymorphism, RBC folate and smoking, and high-risk (size ≥10 mm, villous component or severe dysplasia) colorectal adenomas. In case of low RBC folate, risk of 'high-risk adenomas' increased as a function of the number of T alleles. The effect was opposite in case of high RBC folate. Smoking was a strong predictor for high-risk adenomas in cases of CT/TT genotype and low folate. There is a need for further studies to investigate interactions between *MTHFR* polymorphism and environmental factors such as folate intake, alcohol and tobacco.

ONCOGENE AND TUMOUR-SUPPRESSOR GENES

Harvey ras-1 variable number tandem repeat polymorphism (*HRAS1*-VNTR) has been shown to modulate the expression of nearby genes by interacting with transcriptional regulatory elements. The association could also result from linkage disequilibrium[5,21]. The meta-analysis of the five available studies[5] associated carriers of rare alleles with a combined odds ratio of 2.50 (95% confidence limits 1.54–4.05).

A specific polymorphism in the adenomatous polyposis coli gene, the (*APC*)-I1307K variant, has been associated with an increased risk of colorectal cancer in an Ashkenazi population[22]. The meta-analysis of the four available studies led to a combined odds ratio for mutation carriers of 1.61 (95% confidence limits 1.22–2.11). A study in Ashkenazi and non-Ashkenazi Jews identified the I1307K polymorphism in all ethnic Jewish populations, Ashkenazi and non-Ashkenazi, thus supporting the notion of a founder mutation for I1307K[23]. A recent study of colorectal cancer and adenoma patients in the Ashkenazi Jewish community of Ottawa confirmed the association of the mutation with colorectal cancer, but it was not associated with adenoma, suggesting an effect on the malignant transformation of adenoma into carcinoma[24].

MICROENVIRONMENTAL MODIFIERS

A common polymorphism in the gene of the apolipoprotein-E, *APO-E4*, has been associated with a reduced risk of colorectal cancer[25]. It could interact with the colonic microenvironment via bile acids, the faecal bile acid output being lower in individuals with the *APO-E4* allele than in those with other genotypes. The reduction in risk was mostly associated with proximal colorectal cancers as well as adenomas[25]. A recent Australian study also observed a risk reduction for proximal colorectal cancers in *APO-E4* carriers, but the association was not statistically significant[26].

17

OTHER GENES

Vitamin D and calcium have been proposed as protective factors against colorectal neoplasms. A recent study investigated whether vitamin D receptor (VDR) gene polymorphisms influence risk of colorectal adenoma[27]. Although there was no significant association between the studied polymorphisms (BB and FF) and adenoma risk, risk of large (>1 cm) adenomas decreased with increasing copies of the FokI f allele. Compared to the FF genotype, odds ratios for the Ff and ff genotypes were 0.79 (95% CI 0.44–1.41) and 0.32 (95% CI 0.11–0.91), respectively. FokI genotype was more strongly related to large adenoma risk among subjects with low dietary calcium intake or low dietary vitamin D intake or dark skin colour. Another study observed a significant relationship between adenoma risk and the BB genotype[28]. There was no significant association between the BB genotype and risk of colorectal adenomas, but there was a significant interaction between genotype and intake of calcium or of vitamin D. Those with the lowest tertile of vitamin D intake and the BB genotype had a lower risk of colorectal adenoma (OR 0.24, CI 0.08–0.76) than those with the highest tertile of intake and the bb genotype. Similarly, those with the lowest tertile of calcium intake and the BB genotype had a reduced risk of colorectal adenoma (OR 0.34, CI 0.11–1.06).

CONCLUSION

Although the first polymorphisms potentially associated with colorectal neoplasms were identified in the 1980s, this research area has been mostly developed within the past 5 years and is still quite new. Few conclusions can be drawn from available studies so far. This may be due to several factors: limited power of several studies, interactions between polymorphisms and with environmental factors, especially food. Therefore, future studies should be large, should study several polymorphisms as well as diet to be able to investigate potential interactions, and should study subgroups of colorectal cancer, cancer sites or groups based on histology. A better identification of such polymorphisms, and of their interaction with diet, is needed for optimally planning future prevention studies of colorectal cancer.

References

1. Fuchs CS, Giovannucci EL, Colditz GA, Hunter DJ, Speizer FE, Willett WC. A prospective study of family history and the risk of colorectal cancer. N Engl J Med. 1994;25:1669–74.
2. Burn J, Chapman PD, Bishop DT et al. Susceptibility markers in colorectal cancer. IARC Scientific Publication No. 2001;154:131–47.
3. Iacopetta B, Grieu F, Joseph D, Elsaleh H. A polymorphism in the enhancer region of the thymidylate synthase promoter influences the survival of colorectal cancer patients treated with 5-fluorouracil. Br J Cancer. 2001;85:827–30.
4. Stoehlmacher J, Ghaderi V, Iobal S et al. A polymorphism of the XRCC1 gene predicts for response to platinum based treatment in advanced colorectal cancer. Anticancer Res. 2001; 21:3075–9.
5. Houlston RS, Tomlinson IPM. Polymorphisms and colorectal cancer risk. Gastroenterology. 2001;121:282–301.
6. Minchin RF, Kadlubar FF, Ilett F. Role of acetylation in colorectal cancer. Mutat Res. 1993;290:35–42.

7. Welfare MR, Cooper J, Bassendine MF, Daly AK. Relationship between acetylator status, smoking, and diet and colorectal cancer risk in the north-east of England. Carcinogenesis. 1997; 18:1351–4.
8. Roberts-Thompson IC, Ryan P, Khoo KK, Hart WJ, McMichael AJ, Butler RN. Diet, acetylator phenotype, and risk of colorectal neoplasia. Lancet. 1996;347:1372–4.
9. Brockton N, Little J, Sharp L, Cotton SC. N-acetyltransferase polymorphisms and colorectal cancer: a HuGE review. Am J Epidemiol. 2000;151:846–61.
10. Cotton SC, Sharp L, Little J, Brockton N. Glutathione S-transferase polymorphisms and colorectal cancer: a HuGE review. Am J Epidemiol. 2000;151:7–32.
11. Rosenberg N, Murata M, Ikeda Y et al. The frequent 5,10-methylenetetrahydrofolate reductase C677T polymorphism is associated with a common haplotype in whites, Japanese, and Africans. Am J Hum Genet. 2002;70:758–62.
12. Peng F, Labelle LA, Rainey BJ, Tsongalis GJ. Single nucleotide polymorphisms in the methylenetetrahydrofolate reductase gene are common in US Caucasian and Hispanic American populations. Int J Mol Med. 2001;8:509–11.
13. Chen J, Giovannucci E, Kelsey K et al. A methylenetetrahydrofolate reductase polymorphism and the risk of colorectal cancer. Cancer Res. 1996;56:4862–4.
14. Ma J, Stampfer MJ, Giovannucci E et al. Methylenetetrahydrofolate reductase polymorphism, dietary interactions, and risk of colorectal cancer. Cancer Res. 1997;57:1098–102.
15. Slattery ML, Potter JD, Samowitz W, Schaffer D, Leppert M. Methylenetetrahydrofolate reductase, diet, and risk of colon cancer. Cancer Epidemiol Biomarkers Prev. 1999;8:513–18.
16. Park KS, Mok JW, Kim JC. The 677 C > T mutation in 5,10-methylenetetrahydrofolate reductase and colorectal cancer risk. Genet Test. 1999;3:233–6.
17. Chen J, Giovannucci E, Hankinson SE et al. A prospective study of methylenetetrahydrofolate reductase and methionine synthase gene polymorphisms, and risk of colorectal adenoma. Carcinogenesis. 1998;19:2129–32.
18. Marugame T, Tsuji E, Inoue H et al. Methylenetetrahydrofolate reductase polymorphism and risk of colorectal adenomas. Cancer Lett. 2000;151:181–6.
19. Levine AJ, Siegmund KD, Ervin CM et al. The methylenetetrahydrofolate reductase 677 C→T polymorphism and distal colorectal adenoma risk. Cancer Epidemiol Biomarkers Prev. 2000;9:657–63.
20. Ulvik A, Evensen ET, Lien EA et al. Smoking, folate and methylenetetrahydrofolate reductase status as interactive determinants of adenomatous and hyperplastic polyps of colorectum. Am J Med Genet. 2001;101:246–54.
21. Krontiris TG, Devlin B, Karp DD, Robert NJ, Risch N. An association between the risk of cancer and mutations in the HRAS1 minisatellite locus. N Engl J Med. 1993;329:517–23.
22. Laken SJ, Petersen GM, Gruber SB et al. Familial colorectal cancer in Ashkenazim due to a hypermutable tract in APC. Nat Genet. 1997;17:79–83.
23. Shtoyerman-Chen R, Friedman E, Figer A et al. The I1307K APC polymorphism: prevalence in non-Ashkenazi Jews and evidence for a founder effect. Genet Test. 2001;5:141–6.
24. Stern HS, Viertelhausen S, Hunter AG et al. APC I1307K increases risk of transition from polyp to colorectal carcinoma in Ashkenazi Jews. Gastroenterology. 2001;120:392–400.
25. Kervinen K, Sodervik H, Makela J et al. Is the development of adenoma and carcinoma in proximal colon related to apolipoprotein E phenotype? Gastroenterology. 1996;110:1785–90.
26. Butler WJ, Ryan P, Roberts-Thomson IC. Metabolic genotypes and risk for colorectal cancer. J Gastroenterol Hepatol. 2001;16:631–5.
27. Ingles SA, Wang J, Coetzee GA, Lee ER, Frankl HD, Haile RW. Vitamin D receptor polymorphisms and risk of colorectal adenomas (United States). Cancer Causes Control. 2001; 12:607–14.
28. Kim HS, Newcomb PA, Ulrich CM et al. Vitamin D receptor polymorphism and the risk of colorectal adenomas: evidence of interaction with dietary vitamin D and calcium. Cancer Epidemiol Biomarkers Prev. 2001;10:869–74.

4
Epidemiology of colorectal cancer

M. J. HILL

INTRODUCTION

In 1900 the risk of dying of cancer was small. Cancer is, in general, a disease of old age and in 1900 the life expectancy in most countries was less than 50 years; so people simply did not live long enough to be at risk of cancer. With the conquest of infectious disease life expectancy has now increased to more than 70 years for both sexes in most Western countries. We are now, therefore, in the privileged position of needing to worry about cancer risk.

The diseases that caused mortality in 1900 (e.g. typhoid, diphtheria, whooping cough, tuberculosis, smallpox, poliomyelitis, cholera, etc.) are still very serious, but modern preventive medicine enables nearly all of us to go through life without ever having to experience any of them. They have been conquered by prevention. The aim of those of us studying cancer ought to be to put cancer risk into the same category of preventable disease.

In studying the causation, and hence the prevention of cancer, epidemiology is the best instrument available[1], but it is a very imprecise tool. In the case of colorectal cancer we make our task harder by ignoring well-documented differences within that diagnostic group. For example:

1. It has been known for decades that the epidemiology of cancer of the proximal colon differs from that of the distal colon (e.g. ref. 2), and that of both differs from that of rectal cancer. Nevertheless a great many studies of diet and cancer of the large bowel fail to differentiate between the three subsites.
2. It is known that colorectal cancers can arise by a number of histopathological pathways, the most common of which in Western countries is the dysplasia–carcinoma sequence[3], but which also includes the so-called 'flat adenomas' and the 'fringed adenomas'[4].
3. It is known that colorectal cancers can arise via a number of genetic pathways and these will be discussed in detail by Augenlicht (Chap. 9). Cancers arise as a result of multiple gene–environment interactions. Very few epidemiological studies segregate these pathways, even though it should be

20

obvious that, for example, the dietary factors promoting the effects of a particular genetic mutation (e.g. APC) may bear no relation to those promoting the effects of, for example, microsomal instability.

For all of these reasons the epidemiology of colorectal cancer is understandably confused. This will remain the case so long as epidemiologists fail to take account of the work of histologists and geneticists.

This review represents an attempt to summarize what is *known* about the epidemiology of colorectal cancer, rather than what is suspected on the basis of preliminary results. Because of the confounding factors discussed above, results from single studies are extremely unreliable; only when the results are consistent can we have any faith in epidemiological findings.

DESCRIPTIVE EPIDEMIOLOGY

Geographical distribution

The general geographical distribution of the disease has changed progressively during the past 50 years. When I reviewed this topic in 1975[5] the differences were clear. The incidence was high in North America, Australasia and Western Europe and relatively low in Africa, Asia and the Andean countries of South and Central America (Table 1). Within Europe the incidence was higher in the west and north than in the south and east. Within the British Isles the incidence was also higher in the north and west than in the south and east (Table 2). In recent years these differences, though still broadly apparent, have become less clear (Table 1).

Studies of migrants moving from Europe to the United States, from Japan to the United States or from Poland to Australia show that the risk of colorectal cancer is that associated with the final home, and not with the place of birth (reviewed in ref. 5). As will be discussed later, genetic factors are important risk factors for colorectal cancer in individuals. However, the migrant studies demonstrate that the risk of the disease *in a population* is determined by environmental, not genetic, factors. Although occupational factors have occasionally been implicated, diet appears to be the most important risk factor in the environment.

Colon cancer risk within a population increases with socioeconomic status, and is also higher in urban than in rural areas[5]. However, in Western European countries these differences are not large. The risk used to be higher in women than in men[5], with the ratio F/M being higher in the proximal than in the distal colon, but these differences have largely disappeared in recent years.

Associated diseases

The list of associated diseases is long (Table 3), but few of these associations are strong. Table 3 also lists some of the diseases that have proven not to carry an increased risk, despite earlier claims to the contrary.

There are associated cancer sites (reviewed in ref. 5) where a person who has had a primary carcinoma has above the normal risk of developing a subsequent primary colorectal cancer and vice versa.

Table 1 Incidence of colon and rectal cancer in various countries in 1960[19] and 1990[20]

Population	1960		1990	
	Colon	Rectum	Colon	Rectum
Africa				
Nigeria	2.8	2.7	–	–
Gambia	–	–	0.7	0.7
Mozambique	5.3	3.8	–	–
Mali	–	–	2.9	2.5
Asia				
Japan	5.0	4.8	17.1	12.8
India	6.6	4.8	3.2	3.2
Hong Kong	14.5	9.2	21.7	13.8
South and Central America				
Colombia	5.7	4.8	4.4	3.6
Brazil	–	–	17.0	11.2
Chile	5.8	7.0	–	–
Ecuador	–	–	4.9	3.8
Venezuela	7.3	10.2	–	–
North America				
USA – white	26.6	29.6	31.1	15.4
USA – black	25.6	31.9	28.5	10.1
Canada	23.4	29.8	27.8	16.6
Oceania				
New Zealand	30.6	41.3	30.9	20.4
Australia	23.5	27.2	27.4	16.0
Europe				
Switzerland	20.9	19.8	25.7	10.9
Denmark	17.1	20.8	20.3	17.3
France	20.2	18.5	27.2	20.0
Czechoslovakia	12.9	9.4	20.4	22.9

Table 2 Incidence of colon cancer within the British Isles

Country	1960	1990
Scotland	28.2	21.8
Ireland	25.2	21.8
England/Wales	15.8	17.1

Predisposing diseases

Two disease states predispose to colon cancer, namely inflammatory bowel disease (IBD – ulcerative colitis[6] and Crohn's disease[7]) and colon adenomas. For IBD the risk of increasingly severe dysplasia and ultimately carcinoma is maximal if the whole colon is involved, and if the disease has persisted for more than 10 years.

For colon adenomas the most dramatic risks are in the genetically determined diseases familial polyposis coli (FP, where the risk is virtually 100% in those

Table 3 Diseases associated with colon cancer risk in populations and in individuals

Disease	Populations	Individuals
Coronary heart disease	Yes	No
Diabetes	Yes	No
Breast cancer	Yes	Yes
Endometrial cancer	Yes	Yes
Cholecystectomy		Proximal cases
Gastric surgery		Proximal cases
Appendicitis	No	No
Haemorrhoids	No	No
Diverticular disease	No	No

Table 4 Malignant potential of adenomas in relation to their size and histology

	Percentage containing focal areas of malignancy
Size	
Less than 3 mm diameter	0.1
3–10 mm diameter	1.3
10–20 mm diameter	9.5
More than 20 mm diameter	46.0
Histology	
Tubular	4.8
Tubulovillous	22.5
Villous	40.7

carrying the mutant APC gene) and human non-polyposis colorectal cancer (HNPCC). However, between them they account for only about 5% of all colorectal cancers. Discrete, non-familial, adenomas are much more important, since they will be present in about 50% of persons by age 70. The vast majority of colon cancers arise initially in benign adenomas, but the vast majority of adenomas do not progress to cancer. The risk of progression to malignancy (Table 4) increases with adenoma size, villousness, subsite and severity of epithelial dysplasia[3].

These data, together with information on the epidemiology of colon adenomas, led[8] to the postulated mechanism of the dysplasia–carcinoma sequence (Figure 1). The postulate, which has stood the test of time and is still valid, recognized that the environmental factors causing adenoma formation (termed E1) differ from those causing progression through adenoma growth and increasing epithelial dysplasia to carcinoma (termed E2). This is reasonable in the light of the findings of geneticists. In the APC pathway the only gene involved in adenoma formation is the APC gene (plus, perhaps, K-ras); in contrast an array of genes is involved in adenoma progression, and it would be surprising if the same environmental factors amplified the expression of both sets of genes.

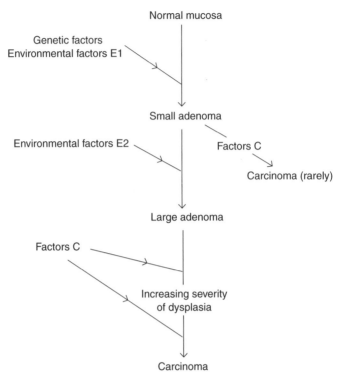

Figure 1 Proposed mechanism of the adenoma (dysplasia)–carcinoma sequence in the colon (based on ref. 8)

On this postulated mechanism the pathway will be via adenoma growth if that is the rate-limiting step. However, if the activity of E2 exceeds that of E1 then the rate of adenoma progression will be faster than that of adenoma formation and (as is seen in many African cohorts) small adenomas will be less common than carcinomas. If the rate of increase in severity of epithelial dysplasia is very rapid (i.e. there is excess factor C) then adenomas will progress directly to carcinomas without an adenoma growth phase (as in cancers arising in flat adenomas).

In HNPCC, where the vast majority of cancers follow the MI pathway, progression from adenoma to carcinoma is very rapid. Since HNPCC arises via the MI pathway there is no reason to suspect that the environmental factors promoting the development or the expression of the genetic changes will be the same as those for the APC pathway. Since most discrete cancers arise via the APC pathway, HNPCC is a poor model for studies of the aetiology and prevention of colon cancer.

Diet and energy balance

The most important risk factors identified to date (i.e. the ones likely to be of use in cancer prevention) are those associated with energy balance and with diet

Table 5   Diet and colorectal cancer

Risk factor	Populations	Case–control	Cohort studies
Cereal fibre (protective)	+++	+++	+
Vegetables (protective)	+++	+++	+
Fish (protective)	++	++	?
Fat (causal)	++	No	No
Red meat (causal)	++	No	No
Calcium (protective)	++	++	+

+++, Evidence is consistently strong; ++, evidence is moderately strong; +, evidence is awaited.

Table 6   Risk factors for adenoma formation and for adenoma progression to cancer (data from refs 8, 12, 13, 14)

Risk factor	Adenoma	Carcinoma
Subsite distribution	Uniform	Mainly distal
Risk in Tromso/Oslo/Liverpool	Similar	2.5-fold range
Tobacco	Correlated	No relation
Alcohol	No relation	Correlated
Cereal fibre	No relation	Inverse
Vegetable intake	No relation	Inverse
Physical activity	No relation	Inverse
Body mass index	Increased risk	Increased risk

composition. The role of energy balance in colon carcinogenesis was reviewed elsewhere[9]. Obesity is a risk factor for colon cancer, and physical activity is inversely related to risk. The protection is greater for males than for females, and is greater for proximal than for distal colon cancer[10].

The dietary factors associated with colon cancer risk were reviewed by Hill[1,11] and are summarized in Table 5. Those most strongly associated with colon cancer risk – vegetables, whole grain cereals and fish – are all inversely related. Much concern was expressed in the millennium year about a group of prospective studies showing no relation between intake of these plant foods and adenoma recurrence rates. These reports were interesting, but were irrelevant to the question of cancer risk[12]. It was recognized more than 20 years ago that the factors causing adenoma formation differ from those causing progression to cancer. Further work, particularly by the group of Jean Faivre[13,14], has confirmed this. The plant foods can now be added to the growing list (Table 6) of examples of risk factors for colon cancer that are not risk factors for adenoma formation.

Although a great deal of heat has been generated by claims that meat is implicated in colorectal carcinogenesis, only the hardened vegetarian would be convinced by the arguments. The evidence has been reviewed by Hill[15].

Other risk factors

There are two other important risk factors for colon cancer. Many studies have now shown beyond doubt that regular aspirin usage protects against colon cancer[16,17].

This has led to an exploration of the role of non-steroidal anti-inflammatory agents (NSAID), and of cyclo-oxygenase 2 (COX-2) inhibitors in the prevention of colon cancer, and this is undoubtedly going to be a major area of interest for colon cancer prevention for the next decade.

The second group of risk factors includes folate[18] and those compounds involved in DNA methylation. Methylation and histone deacetylation are involved in the silencing of tumour-suppressor genes (TSG). This is a genetic pathway the importance of which has still to be quantitated.

CONCLUSIONS

In view of the scope for confounding in our studies of colorectal carcinogenesis it is perhaps surprising that epidemiology can tell us anything at all! It will be able to give us clear guidance only when patients are segregated by tumour sub-site, by genetic pathway, and by histological pathway. In the future the aim must be to identify common risk factors that apply to all (or, at least, most) of these subgroups.

At present all we can say with confidence is that a reduced risk of colorectal cancer is associated with an active lifestyle with plenty of recreational exercise; a diet rich in vegetables, whole grain cereals and fish; and perhaps with the use of prophylactic aspirin. The advantage of all those actions is that they are also associated with decreased risk of cancer at a number of other sites, and a reduced risk of heart disease.

References

1. Hill MJ. Diet and cancer: a review of the scientific evidence. Eur J Cancer Prev. 1995; 4(Suppl. 2):3–42.
2. Faivre J, Boutron MC, Hillon P et al. Epidemiology of colorectal cancer. In: Joossens JV, Hill MJ, Geboers J, editors. Diet and Human Carcinogenesis. Amsterdam: Excerpta Medica, 1985:123–36.
3. Morson BC, Bussey HJR, Day DW, Hill MJ. Adenomas of the large bowel. Cancer Surv. 1983;2:451–78.
4. Jass JR (2002) Molecular pathways of colon cancer development (Chapter 5 of this volume).
5. Hill MJ. The etiology of colon cancer. Crit Rev Toxicol. 1975;4:31–82.
6. MacDougall IPM. Clinical identification of those cases of ulcerative colitis most likely to develop cancer of the bowel. Dis Colon Rectum. 1964;7:447–50.
7. Weedon D, Shorter RG, Ilstrup DM et al. Crohn's disease and cancer. N Engl J Med. 1974;289:1099–1103.
8. Hill MJ, Morson BC, Bussey HJR. Etiology of the adenoma–carcinoma sequence. Lancet. 1978;1:245–7.
9. Hill MJ. Diet, physical activity and cancer risk. Public Hlth Nutr. 1999;2:397–401.
10. Thune I, Lund E. Physical activity and risk of colorectal cancer in men and women. Br J Cancer. 1996;73:1134–40.
11. Hill MJ. ECP dietary advice on cancer prevention. Eur J Cancer Prev. 2001;10:183–90.
12. Hill MJ, Davies GJ, Giacosa A. Should we change our dietary advice on cancer prevention? Eur J Cancer Prev. 2001;10:1–6.
13. Boutron MC, Faivre J, Dop MC et al. Tobacco, alcohol and colorectal cancer. A multi-step process. Am J Epidemiol. 1995;141:1038–46.
14. Boutron-Ruault MC, Senesse P Meance S, Belghiti C, Faivre J. Energy intake, body mass index, physical activity and the colorectal adenoma–carcinoma sequence. Nutr Cancer. 2001;39:50–7.
15. Hill MJ. Meat, cancer and dietary advice to the public. Eur J Clin Nutr. 2002;56:s36–41.

16. Benamouzig R. Do aspirin or non-steroidal anti-inflammatory drugs decrease the risk of colo-rectal cancer? Gastroenterol Clin Biol. 1998;212:S22–7.
17. Benamouzig R, Yoon H, Little J *et al*. APACC, a French prospective study of aspirin efficacy in reducing colorectal adenoma recurrence: design and baseline findings. Eur J Cancer Prev. 2001;10:327–35.
18. Little J, Sharp L. Colorectal neoplasia and genetic polymorphisms associated with folate metabolism. Eur J Cancer Prev. 2002;11:105–10.
19. Doll R. The geographical distribution of cancer. Br J Cancer. 1969;23:1–8.
20. Parkin DM, Muir CS, Whelan SL, Gao YT, Ferlay J, Powell J (1992) Cancer in 5 Continents, Vol. VI. IARC, Lyon.

Section II
Genetics and molecular mechanisms

5
Molecular pathways in colorectal cancer development

J. R. JASS, V. L. J. WHITEHALL, J. YOUNG and
B. A. LEGGETT

INTRODUCTION

The view that most colorectal cancers are initiated by *APC* mutation has been widely promulgated and permeates standard texts as well as the biomedical and clinical literature[1-3]. The concept is based upon the paradigm provided by the adenoma–carcinoma sequence and exemplified by the autosomal dominant condition, familial adenomatous polyposis (FAP)[4]. In FAP, Knudsen's two-hit hypothesis is realized through the demonstration of germline mutation of *APC* followed by somatic mutation or loss of the wild-type copy of this tumour-suppressor gene[5-7]. In sporadic bowel cancer it has been assumed that somatic inactivation of both copies of *APC* would initiate adenomatous change[8]. This premise is based upon the apparent similarity of the adenoma–carcinoma sequence in FAP and common forms of bowel cancer. There is now evidence that this view is incorrect. This is by no means a trivial issue. Cancer prevention is most likely to be successful when applied to the earliest steps in the neoplastic pathway. An understanding of the events occurring at the earliest stages of neoplastic transformation will facilitate the development of appropriately targeted preventive therapy.

FAP – AN APPROPRIATE MODEL FOR SPORADIC COLORECTAL CANCER?

In FAP only a small proportion of the many thousands of adenomas will transform into cancers, and the transition may take decades. Additionally, a unique mode of adenomatous growth involving the apparent combining of microadenomas into a polyclonal lesion has been documented in FAP[9]. In hereditary non-polyposis colorectal cancer (HNPCC) the ratio of adenoma to carcinoma is close to unity and rapid neoplastic evolution is described[10,11]. An intermediate situation is observed in common forms of colorectal cancer. These observations indicate that apparently similar-appearing adenomas may be biologically distinct and have different rates of malignant conversion. Since adenomas occurring in FAP and initiated by bi-allelic inactivation of *APC* are associated with relatively low rates of malignant conversion, the same indolent behaviour would be expected for sporadic adenomas, assuming these are initiated through the same mechanism. By these arguments alone, extrapolation of the FAP model to sporadic colorectal cancer should not be accepted uncritically.

TIMING OF *APC* ALTERATIONS IN SPORADIC ADENOMA AND CARCINOMA

In FAP, either somatic mutation of *APC* or loss of heterozygosity at chromosome 5q is virtually universally present, even within very early lesions[6,7]. It has been assumed that the same would apply to sporadic adenomas. In fact, relatively low frequencies of *APC* mutation are reported in early sporadic neoplasms. In dysplastic aberrant crypt foci (see below), flat tubular adenomas and polypoid tubular adenomas, the frequency of *APC* mutation is reported as 0%, 7% and 36%, respectively[12-14]. A higher frequency (77%) is reported in villous adenomas[15]. A subsequent study demonstrated a trend for *APC* alteration with respect to grade of dysplasia and villous architecture and a significant association with size of adenomas[16]. In three of seven sporadic adenomas with loss of heterozygosity (LOH) at 5q and focal high-grade dysplasia, the LOH was restricted to the high-grade portion of the lesion[17]. These data implicate *APC* inactivation in progression and growth rather than initiation of colorectal adenoma. The findings fit with the suggested role of *APC* mutation in the development of chromosomal instability[18].

In sporadic colorectal cancer *APC* mutation is again not universal, occurring in approximately 60% of cases[19-24]. A higher frequency of *APC* mutation is observed in rectal versus colonic cancers, a finding that is independent of the status of DNA microsatellite stability (MSI)[25]. A relatively low frequency of *APC* mutation is described in flat colorectal cancers (35%)[13], sporadic high-level MSI (MSI-H) cancers (39%)[20-24], and HNPCC cancers (44%)[19-21]. The shortfall of *APC* mutation in HNPCC is, in part, made up by oncogenic β-catenin mutation that is found in around 30% of HNPCC cancers[26,27]. However, β-catenin is rarely detected in sporadic MSI-H cancer[23]. In fact, β-catenin mutation is infrequent in all colorectal cancers other than those complicating HNPCC[27]. These data indicate that *APC* mutation is not obligatory in all cases of colorectal cancer, even as a late event. In view of the usual finding of a normal pattern of β-catenin immunolocalization in sporadic MSI-H colorectal cancer, in which expression is observed along lateral cell membrane[28], it would appear that the WNT (wingless) signalling pathway (in which *APC* and β-catenin participate) might remain intact in this subgroup of colorectal cancers. However, *AXIN2* or downstream WNT targets may be implicated in some cases. The assumption that *APC* mutation initiates the 'vast majority' of colorectal neoplasms is widely believed and promulgated but is not borne out by the facts.

ABERRANT CRYPT FOCI

The term aberrant crypt foci (ACF) was initially applied to the microscopic epithelial lesions observed in experimental animals exposed to carcinogens[29,30]. Similar lesions have been identified in the mucosal surface of human colon after methylene blue staining[31,32]. ACF in humans have been classified as dysplastic and non-dysplastic (hyperplastic)[32,33]. Dysplastic ACF are equivalent to micro-adenomas and probably account for about 5% of all ACF[33]. A subset of non-dysplastic ACF often shows crypt serration and would equate with minute hyperplastic polyps. Some ACF are composed of crypts lined by tall epithelium and showing cystic dilatation. These lack a polypoid counterpart. The mean number of ACF identified in a series of 12 resection specimens from subjects with colorectal cancer has been calculated[31] as $0.37/cm^2$. Given the size of the surface area of the colorectum it is clear that the majority of ACF cannot develop into macroscopic polyps, let alone into malignancies.

It has been suggested that dysplastic aberrant crypt foci (ACF) are initiated by *APC* mutation and may progress to adenoma[33], whereas non-dysplastic ACF are initiated by K-*ras* mutation and some may progress to hyperplastic polyps[33,34]. An alternative view is that non-dysplastic aberrant crypt foci may progress through the advent of adenomatous transformation[35]. The latter is supported in a recent study of dysplastic and non-dysplastic ACF from subjects with and without FAP[12]. With respect to dysplastic ACF from subjects without FAP, 0/15 (0%) showed *APC* mutation, 17/25 (68%) showed K-*ras* mutation and 0/9 (0%) showed β-catenin mutation. An identical mutational spectrum was found in non-dysplastic ACF from subjects without FAP. By contrast, 8/8 (100%) dysplastic ACF from FAP subjects showed *APC* mutation. These data reinforce the concept that *APC* mutation may not be the initiating event in most examples of early sporadic colorectal neoplasia. The earliest mutations in dysplastic ACF implicate K-*ras* and rarely *APC* (except in the condition FAP). However, around 65% of colorectal cancers lack mutation of K-*ras*[21,23,36]. Therefore, it would not be correct to substitute K-*ras* for *APC* mutation as the initiating event in the majority sporadic colorectal cancers.

SERRATED PATHWAY: INTEGRATING DNA METHYLATION AND DNA REPAIR

A necessary proof of the lack of inevitable involvement of *APC* (or K-*ras*) mutation in the initiation of colorectal cancer rests upon the demonstration of an alternative mechanism. Two 'serrated' pathways of sporadic colorectal neoplasia have been proposed. In these pathways 'serrated polyps' are conceived as a morphogenetic continuum encompassing ACF, hyperplastic polyps, admixed polyps and serrated adenomas[37]. Both pathways have been linked to the epigenetic silencing of genes by the methylation of CpG islands within the promoter region. The first and better-characterized serrated pathway culminates in cancers with high-level MSI that occur mainly in the proximal colon. These cancers are distinguished by a number of clinical, demographic, morphological and molecular features[38–41]. A key underlying mechanism is methylation and loss of

33

expression of the DNA mismatch repair gene *hMLH1*[42,43]. The latter is demonstrated in dysplastic subclones within serrated polyps as well as in cancers[44–47]. Extracted DNA from microdissected dysplastic subclones exhibiting loss of hMLH1 protein by immunohistochemistry usually shows MSI-H and mutation of target genes with repetitive coding sequences, for example *TGFβRII*, *IGF2R* and *BAX*[44]. K-*ras* mutation is uncommon[23,28,36] and methylation of a novel gene *HPP1/TPEF* has been suggested as an early event[48,49]. There is little evidence implicating conventional adenomas or the classical mutational spectrum in the evolution of sporadic MSI-H cancer[46]. By contrast, traditional adenomas are considered to serve as precursor lesions in HNPCC[50,51].

The second pathway is more common in the left colon and rectum and is associated with low-level MSI (MSI-L) and silencing of the DNA repair gene O-6-methylguanine DNA methyltransferase (*MGMT*) by promoter methylation[52]. The latter has been demonstrated in around 40% of sporadic colorectal cancers[53]. The function of the suicide enzyme MGMT is to remove pro-mutagenic methyl adducts from guanine[54]. Several methylating compounds predispose to the development of methylguanine adducts, including 4-(methylnitrosamine)-1-(3-pyridyl)-1-butatone (a component of tobacco smoke)[55]. O-6-methylguanine adducts occur more frequently in the normal mucosa of the distal colon and rectum than the proximal colon[56].

K-*ras* mutation occurs relatively frequently in MSI-L cancers[21,28,57], whereas mutation of *TP53* and *APC* occurs at frequencies similar to microsatellite stable colorectal cancer[21]. In the case of K-*ras* and *TP53*, the mutational spectrum associated with *MGMT* inactivation is narrow, mainly G to A and C to T, respectively[58,59]. This pattern is explained by the failure to repair methylguanine : thymine mismatches. The mismatches arise because DNA polymerase β misreads methylguanine as adenine. Therefore, during DNA replication, thymine is mis-paired with methylguanine. In a second round of DNA replication the mismatch may be converted to a stable mutation, for example when adenine is paired with thymine (giving rise to G to A transition)[60]. C to T transition occurs by the same mechanism.

One mechanism for repairing mG : T mismatches would be through excision of the mismatched thymine by a base excision repair enzyme (glycosylase). The resulting single base gap is detected by endonucleases that excise the remaining sugar–phosphate residue as a prelude to DNA repair[61]. However, during the attempted repair of DNA, the same mis-pairing may occur (polymerase β placing T opposite mG). The mismatch leads to a relative delay in further DNA extension and this has been hypothesized to predispose to sister chromatid exchange, double-strand breaks, chromosomal instability and apoptosis. This mechanism of mismatch repair-dependent toxicity to O-6-methylguanine lesions has been described as 'futile cycles of repair'[62–64].

Loss of expression of *MGMT* has been described in traditional adenomas[65] and within dysplastic subclones in serrated polyps (Figure 1)[52]. The latter observation implies that methylation of *MGMT* is not necessarily the initiating event in the evolution of serrated polyps. Additionally, the correlation between *MGMT* methylation and MSI-L status in colorectal cancer is not exact. *MGMT* methylation is associated with the high end of the MSI-L range, frequently implicating two of the five markers in the NCI panel[66]. Such cases may be misdiagnosed as

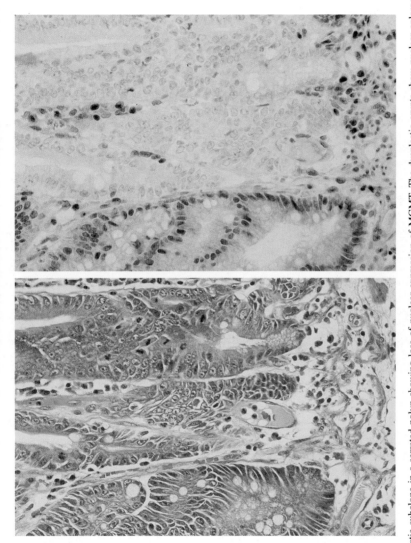

Figure 1 Dysplastic subclone in a serrated polyp showing loss of nuclear expression of MGMT. The dysplastic crypts show nuclear enlargement, prominent nucleoli and numerous mitoses. Nuclei of stromal cells are positive. Left panel H&E; right panel immunostaining for MGMT (MT3.1 NeoMarkers)

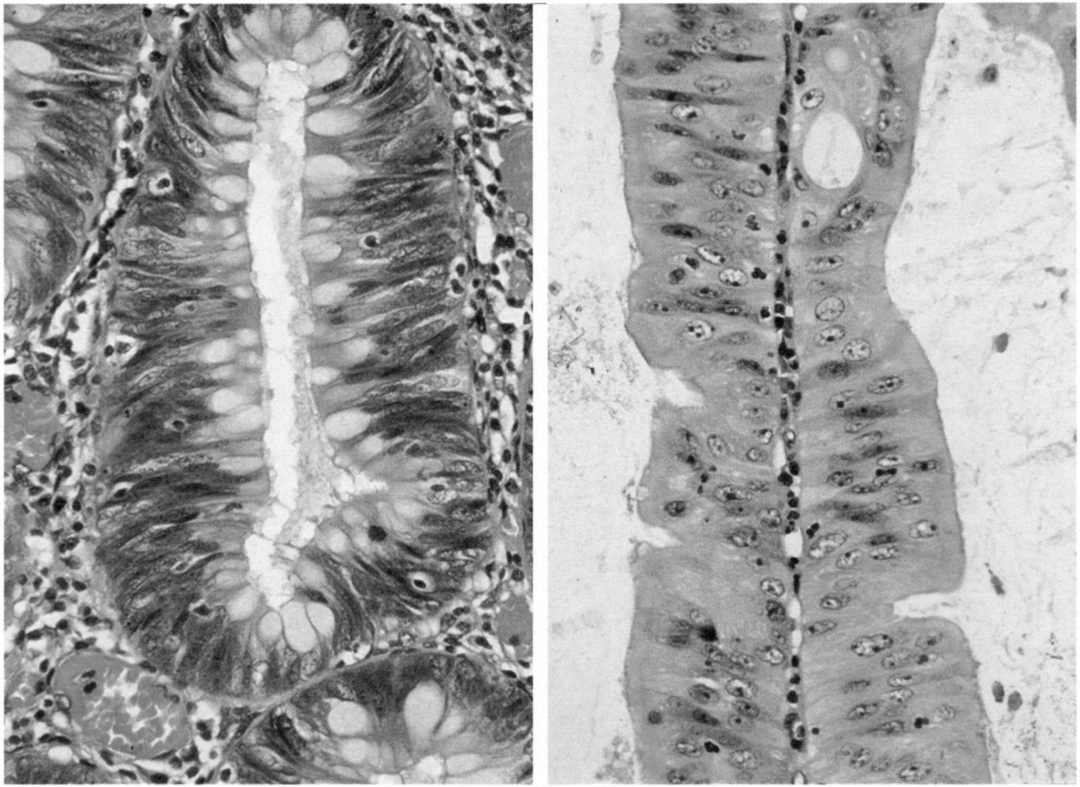

Figure 3 'Blue' or 'top–down' adenomatous dysplasia (left) versus 'pink' or 'bottom–up' hyperplastic dysplasia (right). H&E

36

MSI-H. Importantly, however, DNA instability will not affect mononucleotide markers that are specific for MSI-H.

Other DNA repair genes may be implicated in the initiation of this pathway, explaining the redundancy associated with DNA repair. Additional candidate DNA repair genes include the base excision repair gene methyl purine glycosylase (*MPG*)[67] and polymerase β[68,69]. The role of these genes in the repair of DNA damage related specifically to methylguanine adduct formation is illustrated in Figure 2. A number of explanations, therefore, account for the generation of excessive mG : T mismatches. However, these may yet be repaired by the *hMSH2–hMSH6* heterodimer that recognizes mismatched methylguanine and instigates long-patch repair following the excision of a run of nucleotides around the mismatch site[70,71]. Neither *hMSH2* nor *hMSH6* is a target for promoter methylation or is commonly mutated in tumours outside HNPCC. Since excision occurs preferentially in the daughter strand containing the mismatched thymine, the error may re-occur (futile cycles of repair). Alternatively, the increased long-patch repair that follows generation of numerous mG : T mismatches may simply increase the likelihood of the failed repair of insertional or deletional mismatches, particularly in the error-prone sites represented by the repetitive tracts of DNA found in microsatellite regions. Since the underlying cause is the generation of O-6-methylguanine adducts, polyA tracts (sensitive markers for high-level MSI) would not be specifically targeted by this mechanism. Target sites would be relatively restricted to polyG tracts or (GT)n dinucleotide repeats, for example. The predicted phenotype would be low-level MSI (MSI-L). This would explain the association between *MGMT* methylation and MSI-L status[52].

It is likely that the silencing of DNA repair mechanisms results in an acquired resistance to DNA damage[62–64]. In a DNA-damaging environment such cells will neither stop cycling to repair the damage (through loss of signalling to a cell cycle checkpoint) nor will they undergo apoptosis (through loss of apoptotic signalling)[72]. It is conceivable that the function of some DNA repair genes is to inactivate damaged genes by orchestrating promoter methylation. Released from all such responses to DNA damage, affected cells will acquire a selective growth advantage over their normal counterparts[73]. DNA repair genes may therefore serve as 'gatekeepers'. The silencing of the more familiar 'caretaking' function of DNA repair genes may lead to the accumulation of mutations that add to

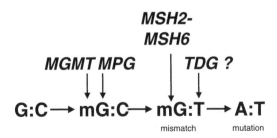

Figure 2   DNA repair genes implicated in repair of methylguanine adducts and mG : T mismatches. Silencing of *MGMT* occurs through methylation whereas loss of function of *hMSH2* or *hMSH6* is largely limited to HNPCC

a cell's growth advantage and accelerate progression to cancer. Therefore, DNA repair genes may serve as both 'gatekeepers' and 'caretakers', a combined role that is now also ascribed to APC^{18}. It is also possible, however, that initiating events are mediated through the epigenetic silencing of alternative genes implicated in the control of differentiation, cell cycle checkpoints or apoptosis, such as $HPP1/TPEF^{48,49}$, $p16^{74}$ or $p14^{75}$. Chance K-*ras* mutation within normal mucosa, by contrast, may result in ACF that have relatively little or no propensity for further evolution. This will apply to the great majority of ACF. However, the ability of K-*ras* mutation to initiate neoplasia may depend on the type of mutation.

TOP–DOWN AND BOTTOM–UP MODELS

Based upon microreconstruction studies in the colorectal mucosa of subjects with FAP, the earliest morphological manifestation of adenomatous neoplasia has been identified as a bud arising from the side of a parent crypt[76]. The bud migrates (in concert with the normal epithelium of the parent crypt) while elongating to form a short tubule composed of an immature and proliferating epithelium. The unicryptal adenoma so formed assumes a superficial position in the mucosa where it 'hangs' from the surface epithelium. Further budding from the base of the neoplastic tubule results in lateral and downward growth and the formation of a microadenoma. This has been described as the 'top–down' model of adenomatous morphogenesis and relates specifically to the silencing of *APC* in FAP[77].

In serrated polyps (hyperplastic polyps and serrated adenomas), the proliferative compartment remains in the lower crypt and cells mature as they migrate into the upper crypt and surface epithelium[78]. A similar 'bottom–up' topography is observed in flat adenomas, villous adenomas, dysplasia in inflammatory bowel disease and intra-epithelial neoplasia in squamous and transitional epithelia. Therefore, 'bottom–up' neoplasia is conventional and 'top–down' neoplasia is exceptional. In 'top–down' neoplasia the epithelium is blue due to the high nuclear : cytoplasmic ratio, condensed state of nuclear chromatin (heterochromatin) and relative lack of cytoplasmic maturation. In 'bottom–up' neoplasia the epithelium may be pink if nuclear chromatin is dispersed (euchromatin) giving a vesicular nucleus, the nuclear : cytoplasmic ratio is low and there is cytoplasmic maturation (Figure 3). 'Bottom–up' neoplasia grows by symmetrical fission rather than budding so that tubules are parallel and perpendicular to the muscularis mucosae.

Dysregulation of the WNT/wingless pathway through mutation of APC or β-catenin is the basis of the asymmetrical budding that characterizes the 'top–down' model of colorectal neoplasia[77,79]. By contrast, 'bottom–up' neoplasia is likely to implicate the dysregulation of cell migration, maturation, adhesion, exfoliation and apoptosis. The specific defect may centre upon a type of apoptosis peculiar to epithelial surfaces and triggered by epithelial exfoliation (anoikis)[80,81]. Different mechanisms may disrupt anoikis, including mutation of K-*ras*[81] and inactivation (by methylation) of the putative anti-adhesion gene $HPP1/TPEF^{48}$.

HYPERPLASTIC POLYPOSIS: A MODEL FOR SPORADIC COLORECTAL CANCER?

If FAP is not an appropriate model for explaining all pathways to sporadic colorectal cancer, is there an alternative familial condition that could serve such a role? Hyperplastic polyposis presents a plausible model for the following reasons: (1) polyps in this condition may show methylation and silencing of relevant DNA repair genes including *hMLH1*[44]; (2) the requisite plasticity in methylator pathways is evident in hyperplastic polyposis in which all types of epithelial polyps may occur (hyperplastic, admixed, serrated adenoma and traditional adenoma)[82] and cancers may be MSI-H, MSI-L or MSS (even within the same subject)[44]; and (3) the condition hyperplastic polyposis may be familial[83,84]. The morphogenetic pathway commences through aberrant crypt foci that may diverge into hyperplastic, mixed and dysplastic lesions as illustrated in Figure 4.

The genetic basis for hyperplastic polyposis is unknown. One mechanism could be a germline mutation or polymorphism conferring an increased tendency to DNA methylation within colorectal epithelial cells. It is conceivable that the responsible genes serve to repair DNA or methylate DNA according to the extent of DNA damage. Polymorphisms in such genes may tilt the balance towards methylation. Association studies employing candidate genes known to play a role in the control of *de-novo* DNA methylation and demethylation would be a reasonable strategy for identifying genes responsible for hyperplastic polyposis and the more frequent attenuated counterparts of this condition. It is conceivable that the majority of colorectal cancers will ultimately be shown to develop on the basis of the hyperplastic polyposis model.

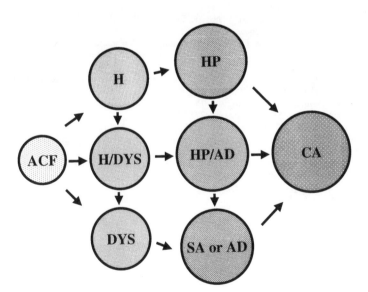

Figure 4 Progression of ACF to cancer through different serrated pathways. ACF may be hyperplastic (H), dysplastic (D) or mixed (H/DYS). These will progress to hyperplastic polyps (HP), admixed polyps (HP/AD) or adenomas that may be serrated (SA) or traditional (AD)

CONCLUSION

A significant proportion of colorectal cancer is initiated not by mutation of *APC*, as is generally supposed, but through the epigenetic silencing of alternative genes implicated in DNA repair mechanisms, epithelial proliferation, maturation, anoikis, and apoptosis. Epithelial hyperplasia and serration are early morphological changes within this alternative pathway. *APC* mutation may result in an early switch to an adenomatous morphology but is not observed in most sporadic MSI-H cancers and is found in only a subset of other types of colorectal cancer. The evolutionary paradigm placing *APC* at the point of initiation of colorectal cancer applies in the specific case of FAP. The failure to discover site-specific genetic pathway models for other solid tumours can now be interpreted as an indirect demonstration of the inadequacy of the single genetic pathway model in colorectal cancer. If new understanding and ultimately cancer prevention is not to be impeded, the single linear pathway spearheaded by *APC* mutation now requires revision with respect to sporadic colorectal cancer.

References

1. Kinzler KW, Vogelstein B. Lessons from hereditary colorectal cancer. Cell. 1996;87:159–70.
2. Fodde R, Smits R, Clevers H. *APC*, signal transduction and genetic instability in colorectal cancer. Nature Rev Cancer. 2001;1:55–67.
3. Tomlinson I, Ilyas M, Johnson V *et al*. A comparison of the genetic pathways involved in the pathogenesis of three types of colorectal cancer. J Pathol. 1998;184:148–52.
4. Bodmer WF, Bailey CJ, Bodmer J *et al*. Localization of the gene for familial adenomatous polyposis on chromosome 5. Nature. 1987;328:614–16.
5. Solomon E, Voss R, Hall V *et al*. Chromosome 5 allele loss in human colorectal carcinomas. Nature. 1987;828:616–19.
6. Rees M, Leigh SEA, Delhanty JDA, Jass JR. Chromosome 5 allele loss in familial and sporadic colorectal adenomas. Br J Cancer. 1989;59:361–5.
7. Ichii S, Horii A, Nakatsuru S, Furyama J, Utsunomiya J, Nakamura Y. Inactivation of both APC alleles in an early stage of colon adenomas in a patient with familial adenomatous polyposis (FAP). Hum Mol Genet. 1992;1:387–90.
8. Vogelstein B, Fearon ER, Hamilton SR *et al*. Genetic alterations during colorectal-tumor development. N Engl J Med. 1988;319:525–32.
9. Novelli MR, Williamson JA, Tomlinson IPM *et al*. Polyclonal origin of colonic adenomas in an XO/XY patient with FAP. Science. 1996;272:1187–90.
10. Järvinen HJ, Aarnio M, Mustonen H *et al*. Controlled 15-year trial on screening for colorectal cancer in families with hereditary nonpolyposis colorectal cancer. Gastroenterology. 2000;118:829–34.
11. Vasen HFA, Nagengast FM, Meera Khan P. Interval cancers in hereditary non-polyposis colorectal cancer (Lynch syndrome). Lancet. 1995;345:1183–4.
12. Takayama T, Ohi M, Hayashi T *et al*. Analysis of K-ras, APC, and beta-catenin in aberrant crypt foci in sporadic adenoma, cancer, and familial adenomatous polyposis. Gastroenterology. 2001;121:599–611.
13. Umetani N, Sasaki S, Masaki T, Watanabe T, Matsuda K, Muto T. Involvement of APC and K-ras mutation in non-polypoid colorectal tumorigenesis. Br J Cancer. 2000;82:9–15.
14. Kim JC, Koo KH, Lee DH *et al*. Mutations at the APC exon 15 in the colorectal neoplastic tissues of serial array. Int J Colorectal Dis. 2001;16:102–7.
15. De Benedetti L, Sciallero S, Gismondi V *et al*. Association of APC gene mutations and histological characteristics of colorectal adenomas. Cancer Res. 1994;54:3553–6.
16. Mulkens J, Poncin J, Arends JW, De Goeij AF. APC mutations in human colorectal adenomas: analysis of the mutation cluster region with temperature gradient gel electrophoresis and clinico-pathological features. J Pathol. 1998;185:360–5.

17. Zauber NP, Sabbath-Solitare M, Marotta SP, Bishop DT. K-ras mutation and loss of heterozygosity of the adenomatous polyposis coli gene in patients with colorectal adenomas with *in situ* carcinoma. Cancer. 1999;86:31–6.
18. Fodde R, Kuipers J, Rosenberg C *et al.* Mutations in the APC tumour suppressor gene cause chromosomal instability. Nat Cell Biol. 2001;3:433–8.
19. Aaltonen LA, Peltomaki PS, Leach FS *et al.* Clues to the pathogenesis of familial colorectal cancer. Science. 1993;260:812–16.
20. Huang J, Papadopoulos N, McKinley AJ *et al.* APC mutations in colorectal tumors with mismatch repair deficiency. Proc Natl Acad Sci USA. 1996;93:9049–54.
21. Konishi M, Kikuchi-Yanoshita R, Tanaka K *et al.* Molecular nature of colon tumors in hereditary nonpolyposis colon cancer, familial polyposis, and sporadic colon cancer. Gastroenterology. 1996;111:307–17.
22. Olschwang S, Hamelin R, Laurent-Puig P *et al.* Alternative genetic pathways in colorectal carcinogenesis. Proc Natl Acad Sci USA. 1997;94:12122–7.
23. Salahshor S, Kressner U, Påhlman L, Glimelius B, Lindmark G, Lindblom A. Colorectal cancer with and without microsatellite instability involves different genes. Genes Chromosomes Cancer. 1999;26:247–52.
24. Shitoh K, Konishi F, Miyaki M *et al.* Pathogenesis of non-familial colorectal carcinomas with high microsatellite instability. J Clin Pathol. 2000;53:841–5.
25. Kapiteijn E, Liefers GJ, Los LC *et al.* Mechanisms of oncogenesis in colon versus rectal cancer. J Pathol. 2001;195:171–8.
26. Miyaki M, Iijima T, Kimura J *et al.* Frequent mutation of β-*catenin* and *APC* genes in primary colorectal tumors from patients with hereditary nonpolyposis colorectal cancer. Cancer Res. 1999;59:4506–9.
27. Mirabelli-Primdahl L, Gryfe R, Kim H *et al.* Beta-catenin mutations are specific for colorectal carcinomas with microsatellite instability but occur in endometrial carcinomas irrespective of mutator pathway. Cancer Res. 1999;59:3346–51.
28. Jass JR, Biden KG, Cummings M *et al.* Characterisation of a subtype of colorectal cancer combining features of the suppressor and mild mutator pathways. J Clin Pathol. 1999;52:455–60.
29. Bird RP. Observation and quantification of aberrant crypts in the murine colon treated with a colon carcinogen: preliminary findings. Cancer Lett. 1987;37:147–51.
30. Bird RP, McLellan EA, Bruce WR. Aberrant crypts, putative precancerous lesions, in the study of the role of diet in the aetiology of colon cancer. Cancer Surv. 1989;8:189–200.
31. Roncucci L, Stamp D, Medline A, Cullen JB, Bruce WR. Identification and quantification of aberrant crypt foci and microadenomas in the human colon. Hum Pathol. 1991;22:287–94.
32. Roncucci L, Medline A, Bruce WR. Classification of aberrant crypt foci and microadenomas in human colon. Cancer Epidemiol Biomarkers Prev. 1991;1:57–60.
33. Jen J, Powell SM, Papadopoulos N *et al.* Molecular determinants of dysplasia in colorectal lesions. Cancer Res. 1994;54:5523–6.
34. Pretlow TP. Aberrant crypt foci and K-ras mutations: earliest recognized players or innocent bystanders in colon carcinogenesis. Gastroenterology. 1995;108:600–3.
35. Nascimbeni R, Villanacci V, Mariani PP *et al.* Aberrant crypt foci in the human colon. Am J Surg Pathol. 1999;23:1256–63.
36. Slattery ML, Curtin K, Anderson K *et al.* Associations between cigarette smoking, lifestyle factors, and microsatellite instability in colon tumors. J Natl Cancer Inst. 2000;92:1831–6.
37. Jass JR. Serrated route to colorectal cancer: back street or super highway? J Pathol. 2001;193:283–5.
38. Ionov Y, Peinado MA, Malkhosyan S, Shibata D, Perucho M. Ubiquitous somatic mutations in simple repeated sequences reveal a new mechanism for colonic carcinogenesis. Nature. 1993;363:558–61.
39. Kim H, Jen J, Vogelstein B, Hamilton SR. Clinical and pathological characteristics of sporadic colorectal carcinomas with DNA replication errors in microsatellite sequences. Am J Pathol. 1994;145:148–56.
40. Jass JR, Do K-A, Simms LA *et al.* Morphology of sporadic colorectal cancer with DNA replication errors. Gut. 1998;42:673–9.
41. Mäkinen MJ, George SMC, Jernvall P, Mäkelä J, Vihko P, Karttunen TJ. Colorectal carcinoma associated with serrated adenoma – prevalence, histological features, and prognosis. J Pathol. 2001;193:286–94.

42. Herman JG, Umar A, Polyak K et al. Incidence and functional consequences of hMLH1 promoter hypermethylation in colorectal carcinoma. Proc Natl Acad Sci USA. 1998;95:6870–5.

43. Cunningham JM, Christensen ER, Tester DJ et al. Hypermethylation of the hMLH1 promoter in colon cancer with microsatellite instability. Cancer Res. 1998;58:3455–60.

44. Jass JR, Iino H, Ruszkiewicz A et al. Neoplastic progression occurs through mutator pathways in hyperplastic polyposis of the colorectum. Gut. 2000;47:43–9.

45. Biemer-Hüttmann A-E, Walsh MD, McGuckin MA, Young J, Leggett BA, Jass JR. Mucin core protein expression in colorectal cancers with high levels of microsatellite instability indicates a novel pathway of morphogenesis. Clin Cancer Res. 2000;6:1909–16.

46. Jass JR, Young J, Leggett BA. Hyperplastic polyps and DNA microsatellite unstable cancers of the colorectum. Histopathology. 2000;37:295–301.

47. Hawkins NJ, Ward RL. Sporadic colorectal cancers with microsatellite instability and their possible origin in hyperplastic polyps and serrated adenomas. J Natl Cancer Inst. 2001;93:1307–13.

48. Young JP, Biden KG, Simms LA et al. HPP1: a transmembrane protein commonly methylated in colorectal polyps and cancers. Proc Natl Acad Sci USA. 2001;98:265–70.

49. Liang G, Robertson KD, Talmadge C, Sumegi J, Jones PA. The gene for a novel transmembrane protein containing epidermal growth factor and follistatin domains is frequently hypermethylated in human tumor cells. Cancer Res. 2000;60:4907–12.

50. Iino H, Simms LA, Young J et al. DNA microsatellite instability and mismatch repair protein loss in adenomas presenting in hereditary non-polyposis colorectal cancer. Gut. 2000;47:37–42.

51. Loukola A, Salovaara R, Kristo P et al. Microsatellite instability in adenomas as a marker for hereditary nonpolyposis colorectal cancer. Am J Pathol. 1999;155:1849–53.

52. Whitehall V, Walsh MD, Young J, Leggett BA, Jass JR. Methylation of O-6-methylguanine DNA methyltransferase characterises a subset of colorectal cancer with low level DNA microsatellite instability. Cancer Res. 2001;61:827–30.

53. Esteller M, Hamilton SR, Burger PC, Baylin SB, Herman JG. Inactivation of the DNA repair gene O^6-methylguanine-DNA methyltransferase by promoter hypermethylation is a common event in primary human neoplasia. Cancer Res. 1999;59:793–7.

54. Pegg AE. Mammalian O^6-alkylguanine-DNA alkyltransferase: regulation and importance in response to alkylating carcinogenic and therapeutic agents. Cancer Res. 1990;50:6119–29.

55. Devereux TR, Belinsky SA, Maronpot RR et al. Comparison of pulmonary O^6-methylguanine DNA adduct levels and Ki-ras activation in lung tumors from resistant and susceptible mouse strains. Mol Carcinogen. 1993;8:177–85.

56. Povey AC, Hall CN, Badawi AF, Cooper DP, O'Connor PJ. Elevated levels of the pro-carcinogenic adduct, O^6-methylguanine, in normal DNA from the cancer prone regions of the large bowel. Gut. 2000;47:362–5.

57. Kambara T, Matsubara N, Nakagawa H et al. High frequency of low-level microsatellite instability in early colorectal cancer. Cancer Res. 2001;61:7743–6.

58. Esteller M, Toyota M, Sanchez-Cespedes M et al. Inactivation of the DNA repair gene O^6-methylguanine-DNA methyltransferase by promoter hypermethylation is associated with G to A mutations in K-ras in colorectal tumorigenesis. Cancer Res. 2000;60:2368–71.

59. Esteller M, Risques RA, Toyota M et al. Promoter hypermethylation of the DNA repair gene O^6-methylguanine-DNA methyltransferase is associated with the presence of G : C to A : T transition mutations in p53 in human colorectal tumorigenesis. Cancer Res. 2001;61:4689–92.

60. Horsfall MJ, Gordon AJ, Burns PA, Zielenska M, van der Vliet GM, Glickman BW. Mutational specificity of alkylating agents and the influence of DNA repair. Environ Mol Mutagen. 1990;15:107–22.

61. Wiebauer K, Jiricny J. Mismatch-specific thymine DNA glycosylase and DNA polymerase beta mediate the correction of G : T mispairs in nuclear extracts from human cells. Proc Natl Acad Sci USA. 1990;87:5842–5.

62. Fink D, Aebi S, Howell SB. The role of DNA mismatch repair in drug resistance. Clin Cancer Res. 1998;4:1–6.

63. Karran P, Bignami M. DNA damage tolerance, mismatch repair and genome instability. BioEssays. 1994;16:833–9.

64. Branch P, Aquilina G, Bignami M, Karran P. Defective mismatch binding and a mutator phenotype in cells tolerant to DNA damage. Nature. 1993;362:652–4.

65. Rashid A, Shen L, Morris JS, Issa JP, Hamilton SR. CpG island methylation in colorectal adenomas. Am J Pathol. 2001;159:1129–35.

66. Boland CR, Thibodeau SN, Hamilton SR et al. A national cancer institute workshop on microsatellite instability for cancer detection and familial predisposition: Development of international criteria for the determination of microsatellite instability in colorectal cancer. Cancer Res. 1998;58:5248–57.

67. Vickers MA, Vyas P, Harris PC, Simmons DL, Higgs DR. Structure of the human 3-methyladenine DNA glycosylase gene and localization close to the 16p telomere. Proc Natl Acad Sci USA. 1993;90:3437–41.

68. Wang L, Patel U, Ghosh L, Banerjee S. DNA polymerase beta mutations in human colorectal cancer. Cancer Res. 1992;52:4824–7.

69. Dobashi Y, Shuin T, Tsuruga H, Uemura H, Torigoe S, Kubota Y. DNA polymerase beta gene mutation in human prostate cancer. Cancer Res. 1994;54:2827–9.

70. Palombo F, Gallinari P, Iaccarino I et al. GTBP, a 160-kilodalton protein essential for mismatch-binding activity in human cells. Science. 1995;268:1912–14.

71. Berardini M, Mazurek A, Fishel R. The effect of O^6-methylguanine DNA adducts on the adenosine nucleotide switch functions of hMSH2–hMSH6 and hMSH2–hMSH3. J Biol Chem. 2000;275:27851–7.

72. Fishel R. Mismatch repair, molecular switches, and signal transduction. Genes Dev. 1998;12:2096–101.

73. Breivik J, Gaudernack G. Genomic instability, DNA methylation, and natural selection in colorectal carcinogenesis. Semin Cancer Biol. 1999;9:245–54.

74. Ahuja N, Mohan AL, Li Q et al. Association between cPG island methylation and microsatellite instability in colorectal cancer. Cancer Res. 1997;57:3370–4.

75. Robertson KD, Jones PA. The human ARF cell cycle regulatory gene promoter is a CpG island which can be silenced by DNA methylation and down-regulated by wild-type p53. Mol Cell Biol. 1998;18:6457–73.

76. Nakamura S, Kino I. Morphogenesis of minute adenomas in familial polyposis coli. J Natl Cancer Inst. 1984;73:41–9.

77. Shih I-M, Wang TL, Traverso G et al. Top–down morphogenesis of colorectal tumors. Proc Natl Acad Sci USA. 2001;98:2640–5.

78. Kang M, Mitomi H, Sada M et al. Ki-67, p53, and Bcl-2 expression of serrated adenomas of the colon. Am J Surg Pathol. 1997;21:417–23.

79. Wasan HS, Park H-S, Liu KC et al. APC in the regulation of intestinal crypt fission. J Pathol. 1998;185:246–55.

80. Shanmugathasan M, Jothy S. Apoptosis, anoikis and their relevance to the pathobiology of colon cancer. Pathol Int. 2000;50:273–9.

81. Frisch SM, Screaton RA. Anoikis mechanisms. Curr Opin Cell Biol. 2001;13:555–62.

82. Leggett BA, Devereaux B, Biden K, Searle J, Young J, Jass J. Hyperplastic polyposis: association with colorectal cancer. Am J Surg Pathol. 2001;25:177–84.

83. Jeevaratnam P, Cottier DS, Browett PJ, Van de Water NS, Pokos V, Jass JR. Familial giant hyperplastic polyposis predisposing to colorectal cancer: A new hereditary bowel cancer syndrome. J Pathol. 1996;179:20–5.

84. Rashid A, Houlihan S, Booker S, Petersen GM, Giardiello FM, Hamilton SR. Phenotypic and molecular characteristics of hyperplastic polyposis. Gastroenterology. 2000;119:323–32.

6
Familial adenomatous polyposis syndrome (FAP): pathogenesis and molecular mechanisms

F. KULLMANN

INTRODUCTION

The impact that modern molecular biology has had on elucidating the genetic basis of neoplasia is best illustrated by the paradigm of sporadic and hereditary colon cancer[1]. The clinical and hereditary characteristics of the familial adenomatous polyposis (FAP) syndrome implied the existence of a single gene that regulates the formation of adenomatous polyps, the precursor for most colorectal cancers. The identification of an interstitial deletion on chromosome 5q in a patient with Gardner's syndrome combined with classical linkage analysis facilitated the positional cloning of the adenomatous polyposis coli (*APC*) gene in 1991[2-5]. FAP is caused by germline mutations in the *APC* gene. Somatic mutations in the *APC* gene are an early event in colorectal tumorigenesis, and can be detected in the majority of colorectal tumours[6]. Recent research has concentrated on the interdependence of *APC* mutations in colorectal tumorigenesis, the biological interactions of the APC protein and its partners and on its connections to the cytoskeleton and microtubulus.

FAMILIAL ADENOMATOUS POLYPOSIS (FAP)

FAP was first described in the literature as a disease with clear dominant inheritance by Lockhart-Mummery in 1925[7]. The hallmark of FAP is the growth of hundreds of adenomatous polyps throughout the colon and rectum by young adulthood. Without intervention, almost all patients develop colorectal cancer (CRC) by age 40[8-10]. FAP is inherited in an autosomal dominant manner, and is responsible for about 0.5% of CRC, affecting 1 in 8000 individuals[11]. Despite the strong selective disadvantage of the disease, the incidence of FAP is maintained by the frequency of new mutations, which contribute about a quarter of all cases[11]. The genetic basis for FAP lies in the germline (inherited or new) mutation of the *APC* gene (OMIM 175100). *APC* germline mutations achieve close to 100% penetrance, although there is marked variation in phenotypic expression of the disease[12–15].

Attenuated FAP (AFAP) is characterized by the presence of less than 100 adenomatous polyps but still carries a significantly increased risk of the development of colorectal cancer[16]. Apart from colorectal tumours, extracolonic lesions are frequently observed in FAP patients. These include desmoid tumours, duodenal and gastric polyps, osteomas, epidermoid cysts, congenital hypertrophy of retinal pigment epithelium (CHRPE), retinal lesions, hepatoblastoma, and brain tumours[17]. CHRPE can be detected by ophthalmoscopy at any age, and thus can be used to identify at-risk family members long before the appearance of polyps[18].

THE *APC* GENE

The identification of a patient with colorectal polyposis in association with mental retardation and other abnormalities, as well as a deletion of the chromosomal band 5q21, was the first clue to localizing the position of the *APC* gene[19]. Linkage analysis of FAP families consequently led to the mapping of *APC* to 5q21[20]. In 1991 the *APC* gene was identified, cloned and characterized[2,4,5].

APC consists of 8535 bp spanning 21 exons (16 translated exons) and encodes a 2861 amino acid (aa) protein that is expressed in specific (frequently postreplicative) epithelial and mesenchymal cells of several fetal and adult human tissues[21]. The APC protein is a large multidomain protein with a molecular mass of 300 kDa (Figure 1)[22,23]. The most abundant *APC* transcript lacks the smallest exon, 10A, and encodes a 2843 aa protein which is the most frequently discussed transcript/protein[24]. Exon 15 comprises more than 75% of the coding sequence of *APC* and is the most frequent target for both germline and somatic mutations[25].

THE STRUCTURE OF THE APC PROTEIN

Several discernible domains have been mapped to *APC* (Figure 1)[26]. The different domains are the homodimerization domain, the homology domain, the armadillo repeats, the 15- and 20-amino-acid repeats, the SAMP repeats, the basic domain, the C-terminal region, and the nuclear import and export signals.

The homodimerization domain at the N-terminus of the APC protein consists of several heptad repeats which mediate oligomerization by a coiled-coil structure[2,27]. The homology domain is localized just upstream of the armadillo repeats and is strongly conserved from fly to humans. However, to date the function of this domain remains elusive.

Amino acids 453 to 767 show some homology to the central repeat region of the *Drosophila* segment polarity protein armadillo. The armadillo repeats consist of seven copies of a 42-amino-acid motif[28]. It is now generally accepted that this domain is a protein–protein interaction domain. Two proteins have been described which bind to APC's armadillo repeats; namely, the B56 regulatory subunit of protein phosphatase 2A (PP2A) and Asef (APC-stimulated guanine nucleotide

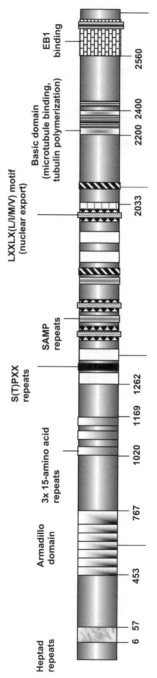

Figure 1 APC protein domains

exchange factor). PP2A is one of the four major serine/threonine protein phosphatases. The regulatory subunit of PP2A, B56, was found to interact with the armadillo repeats of APC while, intriguingly, the catalytic subunit of this enzyme can also bind to Axin[29,30]. Axin and APC are both components of a tetrameric destruction complex of the Wnt signalling pathway. In addition, the armadillo domain binds to Asef, thereby enhancing the interaction of Asef with Rac (a member of the Rho family of small GTPases) that controls cell adhesion and motility via modulation of the actin cytoskeleton[31].

Two motifs in APC have been shown to interact with β-catenin. First, an imperfect repeat of 15 aa (occurring three times between residues 1020 and 1169) and second, an imperfect repeat of 20 aa (occurring seven times between residues 1262 and 2033)[32,33]. Each of the 20 aa repeats contains an SXXXS consensus site that acts as a substrate for glycogen synthase kinase 3β (GSK3β) phosphorylation[34,35]. The 15 and 20 aa repeats show a high degree of homology and are conserved across species[26]. Interspersed between these repeats are three SAMP (Ser-Ala-Met-Pro) repeats that mediate axin binding[36].

The basic domain is roughly localized between aa 2200 and 2400. This region contains many arginine, lysine, and proline residues[26]. This combination suggests that the basic domain is probably a microtubule binding site, a theory that has been corroborated by observations that the C-terminal of APC binds microtubules and stimulates polymerization of tubulin *in vitro*[37,38]. Truncated APC proteins found in colorectal tumours seldom retain the basic domain.

The C-terminal region of APC may play a role in cell cycle progression or growth control through binding to at least three different proteins, namely EB1, hDLG, and PTP-BL[39-41]. EB1, a member of the EB/RP family, represents a highly conserved group of tubulin-binding proteins present in yeast through humans. EB1 has been found to be closely associated with the centromere, mitotic spindle and distal tips of microtubules at all stages of the cell cycle[42-44]. Studies in yeast suggest that EB1 may be involved in a checkpoint mechanism in the cell cycle[45,46]. EB1 itself does not appear to play a direct role in tumorigenesis. Somatic mutations in the EB1 gene have not been found in colorectal tumours, and transgenic mice with a truncated version of APC lacking the EB1 binding site are not at increased risk of gastrointestinal tumours[47,48]. APC's C-terminal amino acids bind through its S/TxV sequence to the PDZ domain of the human suppressor gene hDLG, and the protein tyrosine phosphatase PTP-BL[40,41]. hDLG is a member of the family of membrane-associated guanylate kinases which localize at sites of cell–cell contact of epithelial cells and in the presynaptic nerve termini of the central nervous system. These proteins are involved in the maintenance of cell polarity, migration, and blocking of cell proliferation. The interaction of PTP-BL with APC in the nucleus or at the tips of cellular extensions may indirectly modulate the steady-state levels of tyrosine phosphorylations of APC-associated proteins, such as β-catenin.

GERMLINE MUTATIONS IN *APC*

In FAP, germline mutations are scattered throughout the 5′-half of the *APC* gene (Figure 2). The majority (95%) of these are nonsense or frameshift mutations

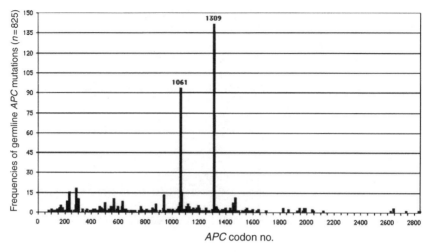

Figure 2 Distribution of germline mutations in the *APC* gene (http://perso.curie.fr/Thierry. Soussi/APC.html)

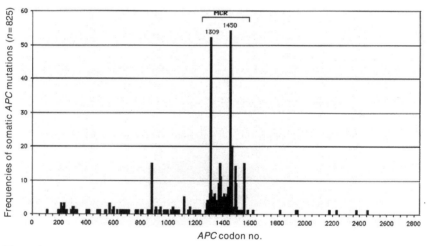

Figure 3 Distribution of somatic mutations in the *APC* gene (http://perso.curie.fr/Thierry.Soussi/ APC.html)

that result in a truncated protein product with abnormal function. In contrast, most somatic mutations are clustered between codons 1286 and 1513, the so-called mutation cluster region[49–51] (Figure 3). In agreement with Knudson's two-hit hypothesis, inactivation of both *APC* alleles can be detected in most intestinal tumours at early stages of tumour development[6,49]. However, in its original formulation, Knudson's hypothesis postulates that the two hits represent independent mutation events, the end result of which is loss of tumour-suppressing function. Detailed mutation analysis of tumour tissue from patients with FAP and *APC*[+/−] mice has shown that *APC* does not entirely follow this model[52–54]. The position and type of the second hit in FAP polyps depends on the localization of the germline mutation. If the germline mutation occurs between codons 1194 and 1392, then there is strong selection for allelic loss of *APC* as the second hit in the development of a colorectal adenoma. If the germline mutation lies outside this region, the second hit in tumorigenesis is most likely to produce a truncating mutation in the MCR[52].

FUNCTIONS OF THE APC PROTEIN

Role of APC in Wnt signalling

The best-known function of the APC protein is the Wnt signalling pathway[55]. Wnt or wingless proteins form a family of highly conserved secreted signalling molecules that regulate cell-to-cell interactions during embryogenesis. In the absence of Wnt signals, free cytoplasmic β-catenin is a target for degradation after phosphorylation through its connection with a multiprotein complex containing axin/conductin, PP2A, glycogen synthase kinase 3β (GSK3β), and APC[36,56,57]. The phosphorylation of β-catenin by GSK3β in this complex leads to the ubiquitination of β-catenin by the β-transducin repeat containing protein (βTRCP) and subsequent degradation by the proteasome pathway[58–60].

Binding Wnt to its receptor, members of the seven-membrane domain receptor family (*frizzled*), a protein called dishevelled (Dsh) is activated[61–63]. To date it is not known how Dsh works. Activated Dsh subsequently inhibits the stabilization of the destruction complex by direct binding to axin, resulting in accumulation of free cytoplasmic and nucleus β-catenin. Inside the nucleus, β-catenin associates with members of the T cell factor (TCF) and lymphoid enhancer factor (LEF) family of transcriptional activators[64]. β-Catenin and TCF/LEF form a complex that activates transcription of target genes such as *MYC, TCF1*, and *cyclinD*[65–67].

In the absence of Wnt signalling, TCF mediates repression of Wnt target genes by binding to transcriptional corepressors. These can be corepressors of the TLE/Groucho family or C-terminal-binding protein CtBP[68,69]. In addition, posttranslational modifications antagonize the activity of the β-catenin/TCF complex.

Role of APC in cell adhesion and migration

The fact that β-catenin binds to APC implies that APC may also play a role in epithelial cell–cell junctions (adherens junctions). The adherens junctions are critical for the establishment and maintenance of epithelial layers. The cytoplasmic domain in cadherins shares the SLSSL sequence found in four of the seven 20 amino acid repeats of APC[70]. β-Catenin binds to the cell adhesion molecule E-cadherin and links E-cadherin to the actin cytoskeleton[71,72]. The former interaction is regulated by tyrosine phosphorylation of β-catenin. In normal mouse intestinal epithelial cells, immunoelectron microscopy showed APC to be localized in the cytoplasm with a significant concentration along the lateral membrane[73], an observation that depends on the presence of an intact microtubule network[74].

Microtubules are dynamic cytoskeletal polymers of α/β tubulin subunits, which are involved in cell migration and polarized cellular morphogenesis. These microtubules serve as a track for microtubule-based motor proteins such as dyneins and kinesins, directional vesicle transport, and organelle positioning of the microtubules themselves. Endogenous APC protein in fixed epithelial cells localizes to clusters at the ends of microtubules, confirming a connection between microtubules and APC *in vivo*[74,75]. These APC clusters localize to areas of cells that are actively migrating[74]. This led to the hypothesis that APC is involved in stabilizing microtubules, thus aiding in the formation of cellular protrusions that are important for cell migration. Recently the stabilizing effect of APC protein on dynamic microtubules *in vitro* and on microtubules in cells transfected to express APC protein was confirmed[76]. Using GFP-tagged APC, it has been shown that the clusters of APC protein at the ends of microtubules observed in fixed cells are likely to result from movement of APC along microtubules towards their growing ends, where APC accumulates near the plasma membrane[75].

A possible explanation for the unique interaction of APC with microtubules might be the presence of multiple binding sites for microtubules and microtubule-binding proteins (Figure 1). In addition to the basic domain in the C-terminal third of APC that binds to microtubules directly, APC contains a binding site for EB1. The binding site for EB1 is missing in the truncated forms of APC found in colorectal tumours, and it has been suggested that EB1 targets APC to microtubule ends[77]. However, the importance of the APC–EB1 interaction is unclear. Truncation of the C-terminus of APC, such as *APC*1638T, will abrogate its interaction with EB1. Fodde *et al.*[78] observed loss of EB1 accumulation at kinetochores in cells that express truncated APC. This implies that the interaction of EB1 with APC is responsible for localizing EB1 at kinetochores. To date it appears that the major portion of cellular EB1 and APC interact with microtubules independently[79]. In contrast, the microtubule tip localization of APC is determined by its binding to EB1 and not its basic domain[77]. In view of these it is possible that the APC–EB1 complex provides a physical link between the growing microtubuli and the kinetochore.

Role of APC in apoptosis and cell-cycle control

In normal human colon APC expression is limited to cells in the luminal part of the crypt[21]. Cells are shed from the luminal surface after undergoing apoptosis (programmed cell death). Single cells from FAP adenomas die by apoptosis, if cell–cell contacts are not maintained. Similarly, removal of survival factors such as serum also induces apoptosis. The ability to survive these two events is a marker of tumour progression[80]. It is possible that APC may also play an indirect role in regulation of apoptosis, as the induction of expression of wild-type APC in the human colon cancer cell line HT-29 (which only expresses truncated forms of APC protein), loss of cell adhesion and strong retardation of cell growth were observed. Analyses demonstrated that cells were not blocked at a particular stage of the cell cycle, but underwent increased apoptosis[81].

In addition, APC may play a role in controlling cell-cycle progression. Recent data show that overexpression of hDLG suppresses cell proliferation by blocking cell-cycle progression from G_0/G_1 to S phase, suggesting that APC–hDLG complex formation plays a significant role in transducing the APC cell cycle blocking signal[82]. Furthermore, the interaction through its C-terminus of APC with the tubulin-binding proteins EB1 and RP1 suggests a role for APC in the cell cycle[39,83]. The yeast EB1 protein is required for a cell cycle checkpoint, while RP1 may play a role in the proliferative control of cells.

Role of APC in chromosomal stability

Chromosomal instability (CIN) is the hallmark of many colorectal cancers, although it is not completely understood at the molecular level. As truncations of the *APC* gene are found in most CRC, this raises the question of whether mutations in *APC* might be responsible for CIN. Recently, two independent groups reported that APC is localized at kinetochores in mitotic cells, the microtubule attachment sites of chromosomes, and that APC mutant cells are defective in spindle formation and chromosome segregation[78,84]. Furthermore, Kaplan *et al.*[84] showed that APC forms a complex with cell cycle checkpoint proteins such as Bub1 and Bub3 at kinetochores, and they proposed a model in which APC monitors the accurate attachment of microtubule ends to kinetochores. These findings led to the intriguing hypothesis that APC (and probably EB1) is essential for microtubules to search for and capture the kinetochores during cell division.

CONCLUSIONS

Mutations in the *APC* gene are the basis of inherited predisposition to CRC in FAP and are also the primary event in initiation of sporadic colorectal tumours. The APC protein is a large multidomain protein with a molecular mass of 300 kDa. The best-known function of the APC protein is the Wnt signalling pathway. Binding Wnt to its receptor, *frizzled*, leads to the inactivation of glycogen synthase kinase 3β (GSK3β) in a cytoplasmic complex with APC, β-catenin, axin and components of the ubiquitin ligation machinery. This leads to a decrease in β-catenin phosphorylation and inhibits its proteasomal degradation. As a consequence, increased β-catenin is available to bind transcription factors, leading to the activation of proliferative genes. In addition, APC has recently emerged as a multifunctional protein that can affect a variety of fundamental cellular processes, in particular cytoskeletal reorganization and chromosomal stability. Improved understanding of both the genetics and biology of APC may, in time, culminate in preventative or therapeutic strategies specifically targeted at reducing the burden of colorectal cancer.

References

1. Kinzler KW, Vogelstein B. Lessons from hereditary colorectal cancer. Cell. 1997;87:159–70.
2. Groden J, Thliveris A, Samowitz W et al. Identification and characterization of the familial adenomatous polyposis coli gene. Cell. 1991;66:589–600.
3. Kinzler KW, Nilbert MC, Vogelstein B et al. Identification of a gene located at chromosome 5q21 that is mutated in colorectal cancers. Science. 1991;251:1366–70.
4. Kinzler KW, Nilbert MC, Su KL et al. Identification of FAP locus genes from chromosome 5q21. Science. 1991;253:661–5.
5. Nishisho I, Nakamura Y, Miyoshi Y et al. Mutations of chromosome 5q21 genes in FAP and colorectal cancer patients. Science. 1991;253:665–9.
6. Powell SM, Zilz N, Beazer-Barclay Y et al. APC mutations occur early during colorectal tumorigenesis. Nature. 1992;359:235–7.

7. Lockhart-Mummery A. Cancer and heredity. Lancet. 1925;1:427–9.
8. Foulkes WD. A tale of four syndromes: familial adenomatous polyposis, Gardner syndrome, attenuated APC and Turcot syndrome. Q J Med. 1995;88:853–63.
9. Kinzler KW, Vogelstein B. Lessons from hereditary colorectal cancer. Cell. 1996;87:159–70.
10. White RL. Tumor suppressing pathways. Cell. 1998;92:591–2.
11. Bisgaard ML, Fenger K, Bulow S, Niebuhr E, Mohr J. Familial adenomatous polyposis (FAP): frequency, penetrance, and mutation rate. Hum Mutat. 1994;3:121–5.
12. Giardiello FM, Krush AJ, Petersen GM et al. Phenotypic variability of familial adenomatous polyposis in 11 unrelated families with identical APC gene mutation. Gastroenterology. 1994;106:1542–7.
13. Nugent KP, Phillips RK, Hodgson SV et al. Phenotypic expression in familial adenomatous polyposis: partial prediction by mutation analysis. Gut. 1994;35:1622–3.
14. Wu JS, Paul P, McGannon EA, Church JM. APC genotype, polyp number, and surgical options in familial adenomatous polyposis. Ann Surg. 1998;227:57–62.
15. Rozen P, Samuel Z, Shomrat R, Legum C. Notable intrafamilial phenotypic variability in a kindred with familial adenomatous polyposis and an APC mutation in exon 9. Gut. 1999;45:829–33.
16. Spirio L, Olschwang S, Groden J et al. Alleles of the APC gene: an attenuated form of familial polyposis. Cell. 1993;75:951–7.
17. van Es JH, Giles RH, Clevers HC. The many faces of the tumor suppressor gene APC. Exp Cell Res. 2001;264:126–34.
18. Diaz-Llopis M, Menezo JL. Congenital hypertrophy of the retinal pigment epithelium in familial adenomatous polyposis. Arch Ophthalmol. 1988;106:412–13.
19. Herrera L, Kakati S, Gibas L, Pietrzak E, Sandberg AA. Gardner syndrome in a man with an interstitial deletion of 5q. Am J Med Genet. 1986;25:473–6.
20. Bodmer WF, Bailey CJ, Bodmer J et al. Localization of the gene for familial adenomatous polyposis on chromosome 5. Nature. 1987;328:614–16.
21. Midgley CA, White S, Howitt R et al. APC expression in normal human tissues. J Pathol. 1997;181:426–33.
22. Groden J, Joslyn G, Samowitz W et al. Response of colon cancer cell lines to the introduction of APC, a colon-specific tumor suppressor gene. Cancer Res. 1995;55:1531–9.
23. Kraus C, Reina-Sanchez J, Sulekova Z, Ballhausen WG. Immunochemical identification of novel high-molecular-weight protein isoforms of the adenomatous polyposis coli (APC) gene. Int J Cancer. 1996;65:383–8.
24. Horii A, Nakatsuru S, Ichii S, Nagase H, Nakamura Y. Multiple forms of the APC gene transcripts and their tissue-specific expression. Hum Mol Genet. 1993;2:283–7.
25. Beroud C, Soussi T. APC gene: database of germline and somatic mutations in human tumors and cell lines. Nucl Acids Res. 1996;24:121–4.
26. Polakis P. The adenomatous polyposis coli (APC) tumor suppressor. Biochim Biophys Acta. 1997;1332:F127–47.
27. Joslyn G, Richardson DS, White R, Alber T. Dimer formation by an N-terminal coiled coil in the APC protein. Proc Natl Acad Sci USA. 1993;90:11109–13.
28. Peifer M, Berg S, Reynolds AB. A repeating amino acid motif shared by proteins with diverse cellular roles. Cell. 1994;76:789–91.
29. Seeling JM, Miller JR, Gil R, Moon RT, White R, Virshup DM. Regulation of beta-catenin signaling by the B56 subunit of protein phosphatase 2A. Science. 1999;283:2089–91.
30. Hsu W, Zeng L, Costantini F. Identification of a domain of Axin that binds to the serine/threonine protein phosphatase 2A and a self-binding domain. J Biol Chem. 1999;274:3439–45.
31. Kawasaki Y, Senda T, Ishidate T et al. Asef, a link between the tumor suppressor APC and G-protein signaling. Science. 2000;289:1194–7.
32. Su LK, Vogelstein B, Kinzler KW. Association of the APC tumor suppressor protein with catenins. Science. 1993;262:1734–7.
33. Rubinfeld B, Souza B, Albert I et al. Association of the APC gene product with beta-catenin. Science. 1993;262:1731–4.
34. Munemitsu S, Albert I, Souza B, Rubinfeld B, Polakis P. Regulation of intracellular beta-catenin levels by the adenomatous polyposis coli (APC) tumor-suppressor protein. Proc Natl Acad Sci USA. 1995;92:3046–50.
35. Rubinfeld B, Albert I, Porfiri E, Fiol C, Munemitsu S, Polakis P. Binding of GSK3beta to the APC–beta-catenin complex and regulation of complex assembly. Science. 1996;272:1023–6.

36. Kishida S, Yamamoto H, Ikeda S *et al*. Axin, a negative regulator of the wnt signaling pathway, directly interacts with adenomatous polyposis coli and regulates the stabilization of beta-catenin. J Biol Chem. 1998;273:10823–6.
37. Munemitsu S, Souza B, Muller O, Albert I, Rubinfeld B, Polakis P. The APC gene product associates with microtubules *in vivo* and promotes their assembly *in vitro*. Cancer Res. 1994;54:3676–81.
38. Smith KJ, Levy DB, Maupin P, Pollard TD, Vogelstein B, Kinzler KW. Wild-type but not mutant APC associates with the microtubule cytoskeleton. Cancer Res. 1994;54:3672–5.
39. Su LK, Burrell M, Hill DE *et al*. APC binds to the novel protein EB1. Cancer Res. 1995;55:2972–7.
40. Matsumine A, Ogai A, Senda T *et al*. Binding of APC to the human homolog of the *Drosophila* discs large tumor suppressor protein. Science. 1996;272:1020–3.
41. Erdmann KS, Kuhlmann J, Lessmann V *et al*. The adenomatous polyposis coli-protein (APC) interacts with the protein tyrosine phosphatase PTP-BL via an alternatively spliced PDZ domain. Oncogene. 2000;19:3894–901.
42. Berrueta L, Kraeft SK, Tirnauer JS *et al*. The adenomatous polyposis coli-binding protein EB1 is associated with cytoplasmic and spindle microtubules. Proc Natl Acad Sci USA. 1998;95:10596–601.
43. Morrison EE, Wardleworth BN, Askham JM, Markham AF, Meredith DM. EB1, a protein which interacts with the APC tumour suppressor, is associated with the microtubule cytoskeleton throughout the cell cycle. Oncogene. 1998;17:3471–7.
44. Juwana JP, Henderikx P, Mischo A *et al*. EB/RP gene family encodes tubulin binding proteins. Int J Cancer. 1999;81:275–84.
45. Beinhauer JD, Hagan IM, Hegemann JH, Fleig U. Mal3, the fission yeast homologue of the human APC-interacting protein EB-1 is required for microtubule integrity and the maintenance of cell form. J Cell Biol. 1997;139:717–28.
46. Muhua L, Adames NR, Murphy MD, Shields CR, Cooper JA. A cytokinesis checkpoint requiring the yeast homologue of an APC-binding protein. Nature. 1998;393:487–91.
47. Jais P, Sabourin JC, Bombled J *et al*. Absence of somatic alterations of the EB1 gene adenomatous polyposis coli-associated protein in human sporadic colorectal cancers. Br J Cancer. 1998;78:1356–60.
48. Smits R, Kielman MF, Breukel C *et al*. Apc1638T: a mouse model delineating critical domains of the adenomatous polyposis coli protein involved in tumorigenesis and development. Genes Dev. 1999;13:1309–21.
49. Miyoshi Y, Nagase H, Ando H *et al*. Somatic mutations of the APC gene in colorectal tumors: mutation cluster region in the APC gene. Hum Mol Genet. 1992;1:229–33.
50. Miyaki M, Konishi M, Kikuchi-Yanoshita R *et al*. Characteristics of somatic mutation of the adenomatous polyposis coli gene in colorectal tumors. Cancer Res. 1994;54:3011–20.
51. Ichii S, Takeda S, Horii A *et al*. Detailed analysis of genetic alterations in colorectal tumors from patients with and without familial adenomatous polyposis (FAP). Oncogene. 1993;8:2399–405.
52. Lamlum H, Ilyas M, Rowan A *et al*. The type of somatic mutation at APC in familial adenomatous polyposis is determined by the site of the germline mutation: a new facet to Knudson's 'two-hit' hypothesis. Nat Med. 1999;5:1071–5.
53. Rowan AJ, Lamlum H, Ilyas M *et al*. APC mutations in sporadic colorectal tumors: A mutational 'hotspot' and interdependence of the 'two hits'. Proc Natl Acad Sci USA. 2000;97:3352–7.
54. Smits R, Hofland N, Edelmann W *et al*. Somatic Apc mutations are selected upon their capacity to inactivate the beta-catenin downregulating activity. Genes Chromosomes Cancer. 2000;29:229–39.
55. Peifer M, Polakis P. Wnt signaling in oncogenesis and embryogenesis – a look outside the nucleus. Science. 2000;287:1606–9.
56. Behrens J, Jerchow BA, Wurtele M *et al*. Functional interaction of an axin homolog, conductin, with beta-catenin, APC, and GSK3beta. Science. 1998;280:596–9.
57. Hart MJ, de Los SR, Albert IN, Rubinfeld B, Polakis P. Downregulation of beta-catenin by human Axin and its association with the APC tumor suppressor, beta-catenin and GSK3 beta. Curr Biol. 1998;8:573–81.
58. Jiang J, Struhl G. Regulation of the Hedgehog and Wingless signalling pathways by the F- box/WD40-repeat protein Slimb. Nature. 1998;391:493–6.
59. Marikawa Y, Elinson RP. Beta-TrCP is a negative regulator of Wnt/beta-catenin signaling pathway and dorsal axis formation in *Xenopus* embryos. Mech Dev. 1998;77:75–80.

60. Aberle H, Bauer A, Stappert J, Kispert A, Kemler R. Beta-Catenin is a target for the ubiquitin-proteasome pathway. EMBO J. 1997;16:3797–804.
61. Axelrod JD, Miller JR, Shulman JM, Moon RT, Perrimon N. Differential recruitment of Dishevelled provides signaling specificity in the planar cell polarity and Wingless signaling pathways. Genes Dev. 1998;12:2610–22.
62. Boutros M, Mlodzik M. Dishevelled: at the crossroads of divergent intracellular signaling pathways. Mech Dev. 1999;83:27–37.
63. Boutros M, Mihaly J, Bouwmeester T, Mlodzik M. Signaling specificity by Frizzled receptors in *Drosophila*. Science. 2000;288:1825–8.
64. Roose J, Clevers H. TCF transcription factors: molecular switches in carcinogenesis. Biochim Biophys Acta. 1999;1424:M23–37.
65. He TC, Sparks AB, Rago C *et al*. Identification of c-MYC as a target of the APC pathway. Science. 1998;281:1509–12.
66. Roose J, Huls G, van Beest M *et al*. Synergy between tumor suppressor APC and the Beta-catenin-Tcf4 target Tcf1. Science. 1999;285:1923–6.
67. Tetsu O, McCormick F. Beta-catenin regulates expression of cyclin D1 in colon carcinoma cells. Nature. 1999;398:422–6.
68. Roose J, Molenaar M, Peterson J *et al*. The *Xenopus* Wnt effector XTcf-3 interacts with Groucho-related transcriptional repressors. Nature. 1998;395:608–12.
69. Brannon M, Brown JD, Bates R, Kimelman D, Moon RT. XCtBP is a XTcf-3 co-repressor with roles throughout *Xenopus* development. Development. 1999;126:3159–70.
70. Jou TS, Stewart DB, Stappert J, Nelson WJ, Marrs JA. Genetic and biochemical dissection of protein linkages in the cadherin–catenin complex. Proc Natl Acad Sci USA. 1995;92:5067–71.
71. Knudsen KA, Soler AP, Johnson KR, Wheelock MJ. Interaction of alpha-actinin with the cadherin/catenin cell–cell adhesion complex via alpha-catenin. J Cell Biol. 1995;130:67–77.
72. Rimm DL, Koslov ER, Kebriaei P, Cianci CD, Morrow JS. Alpha 1(E)-catenin is an actin-binding and -bundling protein mediating the attachment of F-actin to the membrane adhesion complex. Proc Natl Acad Sci USA. 1995;92:8813–17.
73. Miyashiro I, Senda T, Matsumine A *et al*. Subcellular localization of the APC protein: immuno-electron microscopic study of the association of the APC protein with catenin. Oncogene. 1995;11:89–96.
74. Nathke IS, Adams CL, Polakis P, Sellin JH, Nelson WJ. The adenomatous polyposis coli tumor suppressor protein localizes to plasma membrane sites involved in active cell migration. J Cell Biol. 1996;134:165–79.
75. Mimori-Kiyosue Y, Shiina N, Tsukita S. Adenomatous polyposis coli (APC) protein moves along microtubules and concentrates at their growing ends in epithelial cells. J Cell Biol. 2000;148:505–18.
76. Zumbrunn J, Kinoshita K, Hyman AA, Nathke IS. Binding of the adenomatous polyposis coli protein to microtubules increases microtubule stability and is regulated by GSK3 beta phosphorylation. Curr Biol. 2001;11:44–9.
77. Askham JM, Moncur P, Markham AF, Morrison EE. Regulation and function of the interaction between the APC tumour suppressor protein and EB1. Oncogene. 2000;19:1950–8.
78. Fodde R, Kuipers J, Rosenberg C *et al*. Mutations in the APC tumour suppressor gene cause chromosomal instability. Nat Cell Biol. 2001;3:433–8.
79. Dikovskaya D, Zumbrunn J, Penman GA, Nathke IS. The adenomatous polyposis coli protein: in the limelight out at the edge. Trends Cell Biol. 2001;11:378–84.
80. Hague A, Hicks DJ, Bracey TS, Paraskeva C. Cell–cell contact and specific cytokines inhibit apoptosis of colonic epithelial cells: growth factors protect against c-myc-independent apoptosis. Br J Cancer. 1997;75:960–8.
81. Morin PJ, Vogelstein B, Kinzler KW. Apoptosis and APC in colorectal tumorigenesis. Proc Natl Acad Sci USA. 1996;93:7950–4.
82. Ishidate T, Matsumine A, Toyoshima K, Akiyama T. The APC–hDLG complex negatively regulates cell cycle progression from the G0/G1 to S phase. Oncogene. 2000;19:365–72.
83. Renner C, Pfitzenmeier JP, Gerlach K *et al*. RP1, a new member of the adenomatous polyposis coli-binding EB1-like gene family, is differentially expressed in activated T cells. J Immunol. 1997;159:1276–83.
84. Kaplan KB, Burds AA, Swedlow JR, Bekir SS, Sorger PK, Nathke IS. A role for the adenomatous polyposis coli protein in chromosome segregation. Nat Cell Biol. 2001;3:429–32.

7
Hereditary non-polyposis colorectal cancer: pathogenesis and mechanisms

P. ROZEN

INTRODUCTION

Hereditary non-polyposis colorectal cancer (HNPCC) is a clinical syndrome that was recognized in a 1913 publication by the American pathologist, A. S. Warthin[1]. Since then H. T. Lynch of Omaha has best characterized it, and, it is thus often referred to as the Lynch syndrome[2,3]. Based on studies identifying the responsible somatic and germline mutations in serial colorectal cancer (CRC) patients, HNPCC is believed to be responsible for 1–5% of all CRC[4-6]. Clinically it manifests as early-onset (<50 years old), proximal-sited (60–70%) CRC and, compared to sporadic cancer, there is a high risk for rapidly developing synchronous (7% vs. 1%) and metachronous neoplasia (30% at 10 years vs. 5%), but with a better prognosis than similar stage sporadic CRC. The tumours are frequently poorly differentiated, diploid, mucinous cancers, and densely infiltrated by lymphocytes[7,8] (Figure 1). Adenomatous polyps do occur, but are not numerous[9]. There is a high risk for endometrial cancer (40% lifetime risk) and an increased risk for small bowel, ureter, ovary, and brain neoplasia, but probably not breast cancer as had previously been considered[2,3,10-18].

Genetically it is a highly penetrant, autosomal, dominant genetic disease[2,3]. It lacks characteristic phenotypic manifestations, so it is identified clinically by obtaining a family history of early-onset HNPCC-associated neoplasia occurring in three or more relatives, over two or more generations (modified 'Amsterdam' Criteria)[19]. In 1993 and soon after, in a series of multicentred, independent, ground-breaking studies, it was recognized that some cases of CRC demonstrated the presence of insertions or deletions in the DNA of repetitive microsatellite sequences, a state which is now termed microsatellite instability (MSI) and results in a replication error (RER) phenotype, some of whose features had been identified clinically as occurring in HNPCC[20-24]. This state of MSI had previously been recognized as occurring in yeast and bacteria, and was due to a genetic loss in the DNA mismatch repair (MMR) system[20].

Table 1 The chromosomal sites of known mismatch repair (MMR) genes and their heterodimer combinations occurring during mitosis and meiosis[26]

Chromosomal site	MMR gene	MutSα	MutSβ	Other heterodimers	MutLα	MutLβ	Other heterodimers	Meiosis repair
2p21–22	MSH2	×	×					
5q11–12	MSH3		×					
1p31	MSH4			×				×
6p21.3	MSH5			×				×
2p16	MSH6	×						
3p21.3	MLH1				×	×	×	×
14q24.3	MLH3					×		×
2q31–33	PMS1					×		
7p22	PMS2				×			

THE MISMATCH REPAIR PATHWAY

Genes had been identified in yeast and bacteria that control proteins responsible for repairing errors in DNA replication that can occur during the cell cycle DNA synthetic (S) phase. Similar human mutations were identified on chromosomes 1, 2, 3, 5, 6, 7 and 14[21–26] (Table 1). When the function of the second, normal (wild-type), allele is lost in a target organ, then the hypermutable cell accumulates mutations at an accelerated rate, so allowing neoplasia to occur. This could be the result of hypermethylation, mutation or loss of heterozygosity (personal communication, Dr J. Jass, Queensland, Australia).

MMR pathway in HNPCC

In addition to involvement of *PMS1*, *PMS2*, *MLH3* and *MSH6* (see below), to date the *MSH2* and *MLH1* mutations are equally the most commonly occurring germline mutations in clinically identified HNPCC[4,20,24]. However, not all patients having these somatic mutations in their cancer cells carry the germline mutation; conversely, not all patients clinically classified as HNPCC have yet had a MMR mutation identified. Another genetic perturbation responsible for clinical features simulating HNPCC may be the loss of the tumour suppressor transforming growth factor receptor (TGFβ$_1$ *R11*)[27].

What happens at the cellular level?

During synthesis of new DNA strands, errors may occur in DNA replications that are usually corrected by DNA polymerase[28]. If this is still inadequate, then the MMR system continues to repair the mutations, especially those occurring in microsatellite-paired mononucleotide or dinucleotide repeats. The error deforming the DNA double-helix is recognized during the cell cycle and it is then bound to a complex, which is a heterodimer of *MSH2* and *MSH6* (MutSα which repairs one base-pair insertions or deletions) or *MSH2* and *MSH3* (MutSβ which

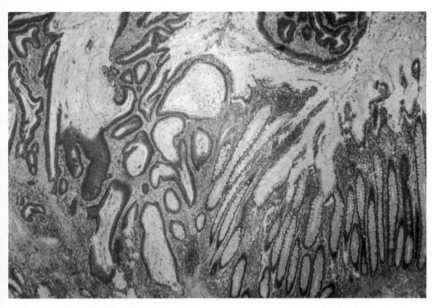

Figure 1 HNPCC colorectal cancer demonstrating the typical mucinous features and dense infiltration with lymphocytes

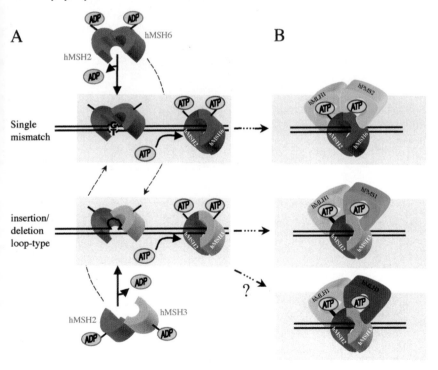

Figure 2 Complexes of the MMR proteins. ADP-bound when resting, binds to ATP when a heterodimer. **A**: Left upper, corrects a single mismatch; below corrects a loop deletion or insertion. **B**: The final heterodimer complexes. Figure provided by Dr R. Fishel and reprinted with permission of *Cancer Research*[31]

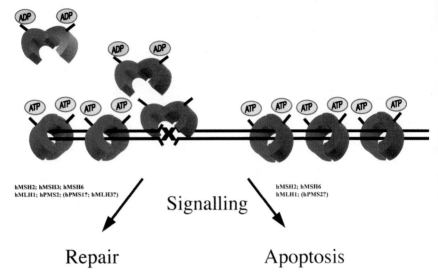

Figure 3 Signalling by activated MMR 'sliding clamps', leading either to repair or apoptosis. Figure provided by Dr R. Fishel and reprinted with permission of *Cancer Research*[31]

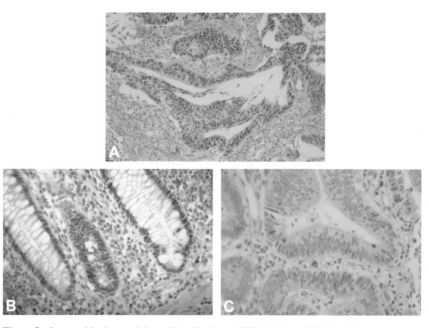

Figure 5 Immunohistology staining with antibody to *MSH2*. **A**: Sporadic CRC, with brown nuclear staining, indicating an intact *MSH2*; **B**: stained normal colonic epithelium from a HNPCC patient, indicating an intact *MSH2* in the tissue; **C**: no staining of the HNPCC cancer, indicating a mutation of *MSH2* in chromosome 2

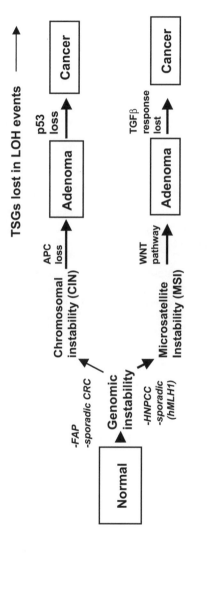

Figure 4 Differing stepwise genetic changes and pathways found in sporadic and HNPCC oncogenesis. Figure provided by Dr R. Boland, San Diego

helps repair longer defects) (Table 1)[26–31]. This is then complexed to the second heterodimer of *MLH1* and *PMS2* (MutLα) or *MLH1* and *PMS1* (MutLβ), or *MLH1* and *MLH3* that helps complete the resynthesis of the newly corrected DNA strand[26]. The *MSH4* and *MSH5* and *MLH1* and *MLH3* complexes are active during meiotic recombination[26] (Table 1). The complexes probably have overlapping and redundant MMR activity. They act as sensors to lead either to DNA repair or to apoptosis. They were believed to act as functional switches to exchange ADP to ATP, but are now considered to act as 'sliding clamps' (Figures 2 and 3). These and the subsequent chain of events are still being established[31].

Thus, a cell carrying a mutated and normal MMR gene is phenotypically normal. When a second, somatic inactivation occurs in the wild-type gene, then the cell is phenotypically hypermutable[20,21,32,33]. This can be recognized histochemically by identifying the absence of staining for presence of the normal gene – *MLH1*, *MSH2*, *PMS2*, or *MSH6*, etc.[2,34–37].

HOW DOES THE MUTATED CELL PROGRESS TO CANCER?

The usual pathway for sporadic CRC involves *K-RAS* and *p53* mutations[38]. These are significantly less frequent in microsatellite instability tumours, whether in those occurring sporadically or those of HNPCC patients. In familial adenomatous polyposis, *APC* mutations appear to occur as the initial 'gatekeeper' event, while it is a later finding in approximately 60% of sporadic CRC and high-grade dysplastic, villous polypoid adenomas (70%)[8,20,38–41] (Figure 4). However, *APC* mutations are found in only 44% of HNPCC CRC, but β-catenin is mutated in 31%[41]. Loss of heterozygosity (LOH) of the *APC* gene is uncommon in HNPCC[41].

Microsatellite instability (MSI) in HNPCC tumours, sporadic neoplasia and ulcerative colitis

MSI has been described as occurring in about 15% of sporadic (especially right-sided) CRC patients, also in some adenomas detected in HNPCC patients, in most HNPCC CRC and their extracolonic neoplasia[2,32,37,42–47]. MSI is also described as occurring in many non-gastrointestinal cancers, as a somatic finding, without evidence of a germline perturbation[44]. These sporadic and HNPCC CRC, with MSI, frequently do not have a normal *MLH1* due to methylation of the gene's promoter region which can lead to a low degree of MSI[20,23,48]. Most sporadic CRC with MSI have an abnormal *MLH1* due to this methylation that apparently increasingly occurs with ageing[37,49]. This has not yet been reported to occur in other genes[20]. While methylation of the DNA repair gene *MGMT* is found in MSI-L cancers, typically occurring in the distal colon and having a high frequency of K-ras mutations[41], MSI is often found in the non-neoplastic colonic mucosa of chronic ulcerative colitis (UC) patients[50]. Similarly, it occurs in the UC-associated dysplasia and cancers.

Other somatic mutations in MSI cells

Mutations in the coding regions of other genes involved in growth control (pro-liferation or apoptosis) have also been identified. It has been postulated that a cascade of such changes occurs as a consequence of inadequate MMR[41]. These involve *MSH3, MSH6, APC*, or β-catenin, TGF-β*RII, E2F4, BAX*, insulin-like growth factor receptor II (IGF*IIR*), and *PTEN*[27,51–55]. These allow for the escape from growth control[31,56]. β-Catenin mutations are described in about 30% of HNPCC cancers but rarely found in sporadic MSI (high) CRC[41].

Biological characteristics of MSI cells

MMR defective cells have increased resistance to DNA alkylation (which requires an intact MMR system) as compared to the wild-type cell[26,57,58]; there-fore they may be relatively resistant to cytotoxic chemotherapy[59]. Even so, the HNPCC CRC patients have longer survival than stage-equivalent sporadic CRC patients[18].

IDENTIFYING, TESTING AND CLASSIFICATION OF MSI

Based on the conclusions of two consensus meetings that took place in Bethesda, Maryland, to recommend guidelines to test for and quantify the occurrence of MSI, five microsatellite markers were chosen to evaluate the degree of MSI[60,61]. These comprised two mononucleotide sequences (BAT 25 and 26) and three din-ucleotide repeats (D2S123, D5S346 and D17S250). It was concluded that if none of the five microsatellite markers is unstable, then the tumour is classified as microsatellite stable (MS-S); if one is unstable then it is MS low (MSI-L); if two or more microsatellites are unstable, then the tumour is classified as MS high (MSI-H). As with most consensus conclusions, various researchers have accepted these markers or chosen others or added markers according to their own experience[37,61–63].

DIAGNOSIS OF HNPCC AND ITS GERMLINE MUTATION

Most CRC demonstrating MSI are sporadic cancers and do not have a germline DNA mutation[5,37,45,47]. Identifying the responsible germline HNPCC mutation is technically difficult because of the large number of exons at risk and the occur-rence of non-coding polymorphisms, alternative splicing, insertions, deletions, nonsense mutations and missense mutations that have all been described as occurring[20,64]. In order to limit this search and workload, many centres use an initial immunohistochemical screening test of the tumour to identify the mutated gene (if present) (Figure 5), and maybe follow this up with a test for MSI in the DNA extracted from carefully microdissected tumour tissue so as to confirm that it is a MSI-H or L tumour[2,34–37]. The combination of immunohistochemistry and BAT-26 polymerase chain reaction (PCR) has been shown to detect most MSI tumours. This then limits the laborious laboratory search for the mutation look-ing for a truncated protein by denaturing gel electrophoresis (DGGE), and/or by heteroduplex or fluorescent multiplex PCR or direct sequencing[31,64-66]. If the mutation is successfully identified (60–70%), then it becomes an important and clinically useful tool for screening the family at risk and identifying those who need lifetime clinical screening and follow-up[2,67].

QUESTIONS THAT NEED TO BE ADDRESSED

The above text represents a summary of our knowledge concerning the clinical and biological features of HNPCC. These are reviewed in references 2, 3, 20, 26 and 41. However, the knowledge is incomplete and our understanding is still in a state of flux.

Can we differentiate clinically between sporadic and HNPCC CRC?

Young et al. recently addressed this question[37]. About 15% of CRC are known to exhibit MSI, but only a minority is due to a HNPCC germline mutation. A clinical, pathological and genetic comparison of these cancers demonstrated that sporadic MSI-H tumours were more likely to occur in women, at an older age (mean 75 years) and have a loss of MLH1[37,67,68]. This is a phenomenon that occurs with age by progressive methylation of the promoter area. The sporadic MSI-H tumours were almost always proximal sited, mucinous, poorly differentiated with serrated features. Similarly, serrated adenomas were likely to be found adjacent to the cancer. Conversely, the HNPCC CRC were more likely to occur at a younger age (mean 47 years), are also found in the distal colon and possibly lack MSH2 or MLH1, to express β-catenin, be infiltrated by lymphocytes and have adjacent tubular adenomas[37].

Sporadic CRC, having MSI-L, do occur in the distal colon and are due to methylation of the DNA repair gene MGMT[37,47]. They also demonstrate the presence of k-ras mutations and apparently pass through the hyperplastic polyp-serrated adenoma pathway.

What is the incidence of HNPCC in the general population?

The figures quoted for HNPCC in population studies vary from 3% in Finland, which has a stable population with a known founder effect, to only 1% in a large sample of the US CRC population, but certainly not representative of the entire multi-ethnic US population[4-6,69]. The estimation usually depends on clinical criteria to identify families suggestive of HNPCC and then confirmation of the diagnosis by mutation analysis. However, just as in familial adenomatous polyposis we now recognize that attenuated or atypical manifestations may occur, we must assume that this is also likely for HNPCC, e.g. with mutations in MSH6 and occurrence of an excess of endometrial carcinoma in the pedigree. Thus, the clinical criteria have changed, and broaden as we further identify mutator genes in HNPCC that lead to atypical phenotypic manifestations, including age of onset and site of neoplasia[70,71]. In contrast, other researchers have taken sequential cases of CRC and tried to identify the presence of MSI and the germline mutation[4,5,69]. This is also limited by our ever-changing criteria for HNPCC diagnosis and increasing understanding of HNPCC cancer biology (see below).

Do we need to change our criteria for evaluating MMR?

Using the standard panel of microsatellite markers, many patients having a *MSH6* mutation have been shown to have a MSI-L phenotype[30,72,73]. This has been attributed to the major function of *MSH6*, which is to correct base–base mismatches that do not result in MSI[72]. The presence of *MSH6* immunostaining in some cases has been attributed to its relatively small effect on protein structure and lack of LOH. In the case of *MLH3* mutations a minority of tumours exhibits MSI-H using the standard panel, but more do so by testing with additional dinucleotide and tetranucleotide repeats[43,53,71].

Thus, it is clear that we cannot definitively assess the CRC burden size due to HNPCC until we have a fuller understanding of the range of its clinical and genetic manifestations.

Can environment modulate the phenotypic manifestations of MSIP

Exposing cell lines deficient in *MLH1* or *MSH6* genes to heterocyclic amines (e.g. PhIP) significantly increased their mutation rate[74]. In contrast, growing *MLH1*- and *MSH3*-deficient cell lines in the presence of the antioxidant ascorbate reduced MSI and number of mutants induced by added H_2O_2 (see ref. 75). Mice that had been genetically manipulated to have germline MSI equivalent to human HNPCC[76] had their tumorigenesis inhibited by oral supplementation of their diets with calcium and vitamin D (Dr M. Lipkin, New York, personal communication).

There is clinical evidence that patients with MSI-positive sporadic CRC were more likely to have had a higher lifetime exposure to tobacco smoking than were MSI-negative CRC patients. Similarly, they were more likely to have had a high intake of carcinogenic heterocyclic amines[77]. A study of HNPCC patients having differing polymorphisms for carcinogen metabolism showed a correlation between the occurrence of these polymorphisms and their tumour location and its age of onset[78].

How can we adapt chemoprevention and therapy to HNPCC biology?

It has been proposed that environmental exposures, e.g. to tobacco smoke, high temperature red meat/fat cooking, could silence tumour-suppressor genes in humans[77]. Conversely, it remains to be seen if changing lifestyle, diet and/or some chemopreventive agent could influence the human mutator phenotype. The lack of COX-2 expression in HNPCC, as compared to sporadic CRC, could limit the chemopreventive usefulness of COX-2 inhibitor drugs in those patients[79].

The CRC found in HNPCC patients is typified histologically by its dense infiltration with lymphocytes[7,37], thus suggesting an immunological reaction to the tumour and a target for preparing a prophylactic cancer vaccine for these patients[80].

Can we indirectly use HNPCC biology to help in clinical diagnosis and assessing prognosis?

MSI has been detected in the serum of a few patients having MSI-positive CRC with immunohistochemical evidence of mutations in *MSH2* or *MLH1*[81]. Faecal DNA testing for BAT 26, as a marker of MSI, has been successful in pilot studies[82,83], and now in an applied manner to patients having MSI-positive right-sided CRC[84]. These tests might be useful for pre-evaluation for HNPCC and performing germline analysis, and for the follow-up of HNPCC patients.

HNPCC patients with CRC have a better prognosis than similar-stage sporadic CRC patients[3,18,85,86]. This has been attributed to the presence of MSI in the cancer cells. Identification of this MSI has been correlated with longer-term survival, and could be a useful tool at the time of surgery, to assess outcome and likelihood of developing a metachronous cancer[87,88].

CONCLUSIONS

The astute clinical observation of Warthin and the definitive clinical delineation of HNPCC by H. T. Lynch, led to the recognition of HNPCC as being an entity separate from sporadic CRC, and that it is an oncogenetic disorder. This in turn led to identification of the hypermutable microsatellite-unstable cell as being the specific pathway for carcinogenesis in HNPCC patients. Not all the clinical and biological facets of HNPCC have been determined in terms of aetiology, genetic diagnosis and clinical management. Even so, with the knowledge we already have, targeted genetic and systematic clinical screening significantly reduces the morbidity and mortality from CRC in carriers[80,89]. Further knowledge will help in identifying biological pathways susceptible to chemopreventive modulation of the HNPCC phenotype. Just as the study of familial adenomatous polyposis led to the development of oncogenetics, so our understanding of HNPCC has taken us another step forward in the battle with cancer.

Acknowledgements

Thanks are due to Drs J. Jass, Queensland, Australia, and R. Boland, San Diego, USA for reviewing this text and providing useful information; also to Drs R. Fishel and R. Boland for allowing publication of their figures.

References

1. Warthin A. Heredity with reference to carcinoma. Arch Intern Med. 1913;12:546–55.
2. Rozen P, Levin B, Young G. Who are at risk for familial colorectal cancer and how can they be managed? In: Rozen P, Young G, Levin B, Spann S, editors. Colorectal Cancer in Clinical Practice: Prevention, Early Detection and Management. London: Dunitz, 2002:55–66.
3. Lynch HT, Smyrk TC. Hereditary colorectal cancer. Semin Oncol. 1999;26:478–84.
4. Aaltonen LA, Salovaara R, Kristo P et al. Incidence of hereditary nonpolyposis colorectal cancer and the feasibility of molecular screening for the disease. N Engl J Med. 1998;338:1481–7.
5. Cunningham JM, Kim C-Y, Christensen ER et al. The frequency of hereditary defective mismatch repair in a prospective series of unselected colorectal carcinomas. Am J Hum Genet. 2001;69:780–90.
6. Katballe N, Christensen M, Wikman FP et al. Frequency of hereditary non-polyposis colorectal cancer in Danish colorectal cancer patients. Gut. 2002;50:43–51.
7. Jass JR, Smyrk TC, Steward SM et al. Pathology of hereditary non-polyposis colorectal cancer. Anticancer Res. 1994;14:1631–4.
8. Kim H, Jen J, Vogelstein B et al. Clinical and pathological characteristics of sporadic colorectal carcinomas with DNA replication errors in microsatellite sequences. Am J Pathol. 1994; 145:148–56.

9. Lanspa ST, Lynch HT, Smyrk TC *et al*. Colorectal adenomas in the Lynch syndromes: results of a colonoscopy screening program. Gastroenterology. 1990;98:1117–22.
10. Rodriguez-Bigas MA, Vasen H, Lynch H *et al*. Characteristics of small bowel carcinoma in hereditary nonpolyposis colorectal carcinoma. Cancer. 1998;83:240–4.
11. Müller A, Edmonston TB, Corao DA *et al*. Exclusion of breast cancer as an integral tumor of hereditary nonpolyposis colorectal cancer. Cancer Res. 2002;62:1014–19.
12. Aarnio M, Mecklin JP, Aaltonen LA *et al*. Life-time risk of different cancers in hereditary nonpolyposis colorectal cancer (HNPCC) syndrome. Int J Cancer. 1995;64:430–3.
13. Watanabe T, Muto T, Sawada T *et al*. Flat adenoma as a precursor of colorectal carcinoma in hereditary nonpolyposis colorectal carcinoma. Cancer. 1996;77:627–34.
14. Vasen HFA, Nagengast FM, Khan PM. Interval cancers in hereditary non-polyposis colorectal cancer (Lynch syndrome). Lancet. 1995;345:1183–4.
15. Menko FH, Te Meerman GJ, Sampson JR. Variable age of onset in hereditary nonpolyposis colorectal cancer: clinical implications. Gastroenterology. 1993;104:946–7.
16. Vasen HFA, Wijnen JT, Menko FH *et al*. Cancer risk in families with hereditary nonpolyposis colorectal cancer diagnosed by mutation analysis. Gastroenterology. 1996;110:1020–7.
17. Rodriguez-Bigas MA, Vasen HFA, Pekka-Mecklin J *et al*. Rectal cancer risk in hereditary nonpolyposis colorectal cancer after abdominal colectomy. Ann Surg. 1997;225:202–7.
18. Watson P, Lin KM, Rodriguez-Bigas M *et al*. Colorectal carcinoma survival among hereditary nonpolyposis colorectal carcinoma family members. Cancer. 1998;83:259–66.
19. Vasen HFA, Watson P, Mecklin J-P, Lynch HT and the ICG-HNPCC. New clinical criteria for hereditary nonpolyposis colorectal cancer (HNPCC, Lynch syndrome) proposed by the international collaborative group on HNPCC. Gastroenterology. 1999;116:1453–6.
20. Boland CR. Hereditary nonpolyposis colorectal cancer (HNPCC). In: Scriver CR, Beaudet AL, Sly WS, Valle D, Childs B, Kinzler KW, Vogelstein B, editors. The Metabolic and Molecular Bases of Inherited Disease, 8th edn. New York: McGraw-Hill, 2001:769–83.
21. Hemminki A, Peltomaki P, Mecklin J-K. Loss of the wild type MLH1 gene is a feature of hereditary nonpolyposis colorectal cancer. Nat Genet. 1994;8:405–10.
22. Lindblom A, Tannergard P, Werelius B *et al*. Genetic mapping of a second locus predisposing to hereditary non-polyposis colon cancer. Nat Genet. 1993;5:279–82.
23. Parsons R, Li G-M, Longley M *et al*. Mismatch repair deficiency in phenotypically normal human cells. Science. 1995;268:738–40.
24. Liu B, Nicolaides NC, Markowitz S *et al*. Mismatch repair gene defects in sporadic colorectal cancers with microsatellite instability. Nat Genet. 1995;9:48–55.
25. Nicolaides N, Littman S, Modrich P *et al*. A naturally occurring hPMS2 mutation can confer a dominant negative mutator phenotype. Mol Cell Biol. 1998;18:1635–41.
26. Bellacosa A. Functional interactions and signaling properties of mammalian DNA mismatch repair proteins. Cell Death Differ. 2001;8:1076–92.
27. Lu SL, Kawabata M, Imamura T *et al*. HNPCC associated with germline mutation in the TGF-β type II receptor gene. Nat Genet. 1998;19:17–18.
28. Sancar A. DNA repair in humans. Annu Rev Genet. 1995;29:69–105.
29. Acharya S, Wilson T, Gradia S *et al*. hMSH2 forms specific mispair-binding complexes with hMSH3 and hMSH6. Proc Natl Acad Sci USA. 1996;93:13629–34.
30. Akiyama Y, Sato H, Yamada T *et al*. Germ-line mutation of the hMSH6/GTBP gene in an atypical hereditary nonpolyposis colorectal cancer kindred. Cancer Res. 1997;57:3920–3.
31. Fishel R. The selection for mismatch repair defects in hereditary nonpolyposis colorectal cancer: revising the mutator hypothesis. Cancer Res. 2001;61:7369–74.
32. Leach FS, Polyak K, Burrell M *et al*. Expression of the human mismatch repair gene hMSH2 in normal and neoplastic tissues. Cancer Res. 1996;56:235–40.
33. Marra G, Chang CL, Laghi LA *et al*. Expression of the human MutS homolog 2 (hMSH2) protein in resting and proliferating cells. Oncogene. 1996;13:2189–96.
34. Thibodeau SN, French AM, Roche PC *et al*. Altered expression of hMSH2 and hMLH1 in tumors with microsatellite instability and genetic alterations in mismatch repair genes. Cancer Res. 1996;56:4836–40.
35. Perrin J, Gouvernet J, Parriaux D *et al*. MSH2 and MLH1 immunodetection and the prognosis of colon cancer. Int J Oncol. 2001;19:891–5.
36. Muller W, Burgart LJ, Krause-Paulus R *et al*. The reliability of immunohistochemistry as a prescreening method for the diagnosis of hereditary nonpolyposis colorectal cancer (HNPCC) – results of an international collaborative study. Famil Cancer. 2001;1:87–92.

37. Young J, Simms LA, Biden KG *et al*. Features of colorectal cancers with high-level microsatellite instability occurring in familial and sporadic settings. Parallel pathways of tumorigenesis. Am J Pathol. 2001;159:2107–16.
38. Fearon ER, Vogelstein B. A genetic model for colorectal tumorigenesis. Cell. 1990;61:759–67.
39. Konishi M, Kikuchi-Yanoshita R, Tanaka K *et al*. Molecular nature of colon tumors in hereditary nonpolyposis colon cancer, familial polyposis, and sporadic colon cancer. Gastroenterology. 1996;111:307–17.
40. Huang J, Papadopoulos N, McKinley *et al*. APC mutations in colorectal tumors with mismatch repair deficiency. Proc Natl Acad Sci USA. 1996;93:9049–54.
41. Jass JR, Young J, Leggett BA. Evolution of colorectal cancer: change of pace and change of direction (Review). J Gastroenterol Hepatol. 2002;17:17–26.
42. Jacoby RF, Marshall DJ, Kailas S *et al*. Genetic instability associated with adenoma to carcinoma progression in hereditary colon cancer. Gastroenterology. 1995;109:73–82.
43. Aaltonen LA, Peltomaki P, Mecklin J-P *et al*. Replication errors in benign and malignant tumors from hereditary nonpolyposis colorectal cancer patients. Cancer Res. 1994;54:1645–8.
44. Yin J, Kong D, Wang S *et al*. Mutation of hMSH3 and hMSH6 mismatch repair genes in genetically unstable human colorectal and gastric carcinomas. Hum Mutat. 1997;10:474–8.
45. Samowitz WS, Slattery ML, Kerber RA. Microsatellite instability in human colonic cancer is not a useful clinical indicator of familial colorectal cancer. Gastroenterology. 1995;109:1765–71.
46. Liu B, Farrington SM, Petersen GM *et al*. Genetic instability occurs in the majority of young patients with colorectal cancer. Nat Med. 1995;1:348–52.
47. Kambara T, Matsubara N, Nakagawa H *et al*. High frequency of low-level microsatellite instability in early colorectal cancer. Cancer Res. 2001;61:7743–6.
48. Thibodeau SN, French AJ, Cunningham JM *et al*. Microsatellite instability in colorectal cancer: Different mutator phenotypes and the principle involvement of hMLH1. Cancer Res. 1998;58:1713–18.
49. Cunningham JM, Christensen ER, Tester DJ *et al*. Hypermethylation of the hMLH1 promoter in colon cancer with microsatellite instability. Cancer Res. 1998:58:3455–60.
50. Brentnall TA, Crispin DA, Bronner MP *et al*. Microsatellite instability is present in non-neoplastic mucosa from patients with longstanding ulcerative colitis. Cancer Res. 1996;56:1237–40.
51. Akiyama Y, Iwanaga R, Saitoh K *et al*. Transforming growth factor β type II receptor gene mutations in adenomas from hereditary nonpolyposis colorectal cancer. Gastroenterology. 1997;112:33–9.
52. Souza R, Appel R, Yin J *et al*. Microsatellite instability in the insulin-like growth factor II receptor gene in gastrointestinal tumours. Nat Genet. 1996;14:255–7.
53. Ikeda M, Orimo H, Moriyama H *et al*. Close correlation between mutation of E2F4 and hMSH3 genes in colorectal cancers with microsatellite instability. Cancer Res. 1998;58:594–8.
54. Yagi OK, Akiyama Y, Nomizu T *et al*. Proapoptotic gene BAX is frequently mutated in hereditary nonpolyposis colorectal cancers but not in adenomas. Gastroenterology. 1998;114:268–74.
55. Shin K-H, Park YJ, Park J-G. *PTEN* gene mutations in colorectal cancers displaying microsatellite instability. Cancer Lett. 2001;174:189–94.
56. Perucho M. Microsatellite instability: the mutator that mutates the other mutator. Nat Med. 1996;2:630–1.
57. Aebi S, Kurdi-Haidar B, Gordon R *et al*. Loss of DNA mismatch repair in acquired resistance to cisplatin. Cancer Res. 1996;56:3087–90.
58. Carethers JM, Chauhan DP, Fink D *et al*. Mismatch repair proficiency and *in vitro* response to 5-fluorouracil. Gastroenterology. 1999;117:123–31.
59. Marcelis CLM, van der Putten HWHM, Tops C *et al*. Chemotherapy resistant ovarian cancer in carriers of an hMSH2 mutation? Famil Cancer. 2001;1:107–9.
60. Rodriguez-Bigas MA, Boland CR, Hamilton SR *et al*. A National Cancer Institute workshop on hereditary nonpolyposis colorectal cancer syndrome: meeting highlights and Bethesda guidelines. J Natl Cancer Inst. 1997;89:1758–62.
61. Boland CR, Thibodeau SN, Hamilton SR *et al*. A National Cancer Institute workshop on microsatellite instability for cancer detection and familial predisposition: development of international criteria for the determination of microsatellite instability in colorectal cancer. Cancer Res. 1998;58:5248–57.
62. Bocker T, Diermann J, Friedl W *et al*. Microsatellite instability analysis: a multicenter study for reliability and quality control. Cancer Res. 1997;57:4739–43.

63. Bapat BV, Madlensky L, Temple LKF *et al.* Family history characteristics, tumor microsatellite instability and germline *MSH2* and *MLH1* mutations in hereditary colorectal cancer. Hum Genet. 1999;104:167–76.
64. Luce MC, Marra G, Chauhan DP *et al. In vitro* transcription/translation assay for the screening of hMLH1 and hMSH2 mutations in familial colon cancer. Gastroenterology. 1995; 109:1368–74.
65. Xia L, Shen W, Ritacca F *et al.* A truncated hMSH2 transcript occurs as a common variant in the population: implications for genetic diagnosis. Cancer Res. 1996;56:2289–92.
66. Charbonnier F, Olschwang S, Wang Q *et al. MSH2* in contrast to *MLH1* and *MSH6* is frequently inactivated by exonic and promoter rearrangements in hereditary nonpolyposis colorectal cancer. Cancer Res. 2002;62:848–53.
67. Nystrom-Lahti MN, Kristo P, Nicolaides NC *et al.* Founding mutations and Alu-mediated recombination in hereditary colon cancer. Nat Med. 1995;1:1203–6.
68. Nakagawa H, Nuovo GJ, Zervos EE *et al.* Age-related hypermethylation of the 5' region of *MLH1* in normal colonic mucosa is associated with microsatellite-unstable colorectal cancer development. Cancer Res. 2001;61:6991–5.
69. Samowitz WS, Curtin K, Lin HH *et al.* The colon cancer burden of genetically defined hereditary nonpolyposis colon cancer. Gastroenterology. 2001;121:830–8.
70. Vasen HFA, Wu Y, Sijmons RH *et al.* Clinical definition of hereditary non-polyposis colorectal cancer: a search for the impossible? Scand J Gastroenterol. 2001;36(Suppl. 234):61–7.
71. Wu Y, Berends MJW, Sijmons RH *et al.* A role for *MLH3* in hereditary nonpolyposis colorectal cancer. Nat Genet. 2001;29:137–8.
72. Berends MJW, Wu Y, Sijmons RH *et al.* Molecular and clinical characteristics of *MSH6* variants: an analysis of 25 index carriers of a germline variant. Am J Hum Genet. 2002;70:26–37.
73. Edelmann W, Yang K, Umar A *et al.* Mutation in the mismatch repair gene Msh6 causes cancer susceptibility. Cell. 1997;92:467–77.
74. Glaab WE, Kort KL, Skopek TR. Specificity of mutations induced by the food-associated heterocyclic amine 2-amino-1-methyl-6-phenylimidazo-[4,5-*b*]-pyridine in colon cancer cell lines defective in mismatch repair. Cancer Res. 2000;60:4921–5.
75. Glaab WE, Hill RB, Skopek TR. Suppression of spontaneous and hydrogen peroxide-induced mutagenesis by the antioxidant ascorbate in mismatch repair-deficient human colon cancer cells. Carcinogenesis. 2001;22:1709–13.
76. Karaguchi M, Edelmann W, Yang K *et al.* Tumor-associated *Apc* mutations in *Mlh1$^{-/-}$Apc$^{16.38N}$* mice reveal a mutational signature of Mlh1 deficiency. Oncogene. 2000;19:5755–63.
77. Wu AH, Shibata D, Yu MC *et al.* Dietary heterocyclic amines and microsatellite instability in colon adenocarcinomas. Carcinogenesis. 2001;22:1681–4.
78. Moisio A-L, Sistonen P, Mecklin J-P *et al.* Genetic polymorphisms in carcinogen metabolism and their association to hereditary nonpolyposis colon cancer. Gastroenterology. 1998;115: 1387–94.
79. Sinicrope FAA, Lemoine M, Xi L *et al.* Reduced expression of cyclooxygenase 2 proteins in hereditary nonpolyposis colorectal cancers relative to sporadic cancers. Gastroenterology. 1999;117:350–8.
80. Sæterdal I, Bjørheim J, Gjertsen MK *et al.* Frameshift-mutation peptides as tumor-specific antigens in inherited and spontaneous colorectal cancer. Proc Natl Acad Sci USA. 2001;98: 13255–60.
81. Kölble K, Ulrich OM, Pidde H *et al.* Microsatellite alterations in serum DNA of patients with colorectal cancer. Lab Invest. 1999;79:1145–50.
82. Ahlquist DA, Skoletsky JE, Boynton KA *et al.* Colorectal cancer screening by detection of altered human DNA in stool: feasibility of a multitarget assay panel. Gastroenterology. 2000;119:1219–27.
83. Dong SM, Traverso G, Johnson C *et al.* Detecting colorectal cancer in stool with the use of multiple genetic targets. J Natl Cancer Inst. 2001;93:858–65.
84. Traverso G, Shuber A, Olsson L *et al.* Detection of proximal colorectal cancers through analysis of fecal DNA. Lancet. 2002;359:403–4.
85. Sankila R, Aaltonen LA, Järvinen HJ *et al.* Better survival rates in patients with *MLH1*-associated hereditary colorectal cancer. Gastroenterology. 1996;110:682–7.
86. Lynch HT, Smyrk T. Colorectal cancer, survival advantage, and hereditary nonpolyposis colorectal cancer (Editorial). Gastroenterology. 1996;110:943–7.

87. Gryfe R, Kim H, Hsieh ETK *et al.* Tumor microsatellite instability and clinical outcome in young patients with colorectal cancer. N Engl J Med. 2000;342:69–77.
88. Masubuchi S, Konishi F, Togashi K *et al.* The significance of microsatellite instability in predicting the development of metachronous multiple colorectal carcinomas in patients with nonfamilial colorectal carcinoma. Cancer. 1999;85:1917–24.
89. Jarvinen HJ, Aarnio M, Mustonen H *et al.* Controlled 15-year trial on screening for colorectal cancer in families with hereditary non-polyposis colorectal cancer. Gastroenterology. 2000;118:829–34.

8
Possible molecular targets for exogenous factors

R. W. OWEN, B. SPIEGELHALDER and H. BARTSCH

The genetics of colorectal cancer is reasonably well defined via the adenoma–carcinoma sequence in people with germline mutations, e.g. familial polyposis coli. This is not the case in the development of sporadic adenoma, resulting as a process of somatic mutations which account for over 90% of the disease incidence. The prevention of colorectal cancer can only be achieved in the general population by protection of DNA in the intestinal epithelium. A lack of protection leads to the formation of DNA-adducts which are potent preneoplastic lesions and ultimately lead to carcinogenesis. Recent clinical intervention trials of mooted favourite anticancer agents, especially fibre, have been disappointing, however. Perhaps it is time for a different approach. Evidence is emerging that the major aetiological modulators of colorectal cancer in the diet are antioxidants which mediate their effects by inhibition of lipid peroxidation and the formation of DNA adducts. Therefore, in general, protection could be effected by adopting a healthy diet, e.g. Mediterranean with its high content of monounsaturated fatty acids and phenolic antioxidants (simple phenols, secoiridoids, lignans and tocopherols). We have developed methods to test this hypothesis. Using as a model the generation of reactive oxygen species (ROS) by the faecal matrix, we have demonstrated potent inhibition of the process by the major classes of phenolic antioxidants within olive oil. As an example, tyrosol mediates its effects *in vitro* by interacting with the hydroxyl radical (HO$^{\bullet}$) to form hydroxytyrosol. Pilot studies in human volunteers, intervened with olive oil, show that relative to dietary intake, urinary excretion of tyrosol decreases while hydroxytyrosol increases, supporting a scavenging effect of the former. In conclusion, phenolic antioxidants in olives and olive oil display potent antioxidant properties, and their interaction with ROS in humans is confirmed. Clinical intervention trials with olive oil and purified phenolic antioxidants therein are therefore recommended, to fully establish their potential in the chemoprevention of colorectal cancer.

Section III
Identification of genetically determined risk groups

9
Hereditary versus environmental factors in colorectal cancer

L. H. AUGENLICHT, W. YANG, A. WILSON, B. HEERDT,
J. MARIADASON and A. VELCICH

INTRODUCTION

The unfortunate existence of population groups that are at high genetic risk for development of colorectal cancer (i.e. familial adenomatous polyposis coli, or FAP, and hereditary non-polyposis colon cancer, or HNPCC) has led to profound insight into the genes responsible for development of the disease, and the pathways through which these genes normally participate in mucosal homeostasis that are aberrant when the genes are mutated[1]. However, despite this understanding of the causal mechanisms of initiation and progression of colon cancer, it can be readily demonstrated that environmental factors are the major determinants of risk for colon cancer for the 95% of the patients who are not in the FAP and HNPCC genetic high-risk groups. The principal evidence for this statement comes from epidemiological studies, especially of migrant populations. For example, Japanese who move to Hawaii exhibit a rapid change in site specificity of cancer, from that of stomach to colon, within one or two generations[2]. Even within the HNPCC high-risk group, environmental factors can play a major role. In the initial studies of high-risk individuals by Warthin in the early 1900s, 'family G' displayed a high incidence of stomach cancer but low incidence of colon cancer[3]. By the 1960s, when this family was reinvestigated by Lynch in his defining studies of HNPCC, colon cancer incidence in the family had become frequent and stomach cancer much reduced[4]. This mirrored the shift of intestinal cancer site in the general population over this time from stomach to colon. Thus, a gene defect in this family that we now know causes a deficiency in DNA mismatch repair determined the high rate of cancer, but environmental factors, most likely diet, determined site specificity. This predominant role of diet in the determination of risk for colon cancer development is also reflected in hundreds of studies in rodent systems that have defined a role for a large number of micro- and macro-nutrients in modulation of cancer development initiated by chemical carcinogens or, more recently, by genetic factors.

Thus, the challenge we face is to understand how nutritional factors modulate the pathways that genetic studies have identified as the *sine qua non* of colon cancer development. This is a difficult task because, despite its high prevalence, development of colon cancer is, in reality, a rare event. Outside of the very high genetic risk groups, the vast majority of patients develop a single tumour over five or six decades of life. During this time there are approximately a trillion cell divisions in the intestinal mucosa. Since tumours most likely develop clonally from a single initiated cell, only one of these cell divisions leads to the full development of a cancer. Thus, the pathways involved determine the probability of abnormal growth, and the numbers suggest that very subtle shifts in this probability can profoundly influence whether or not an individual develops a tumour during the normal seven decades allotted to most humans. Therefore, in patient populations it is very difficult to discern significant shifts in the biochemistry or molecular biology of pathways that regulate homeostasis, especially against the backdrop of genetic and dietary variation in the population. However, the use of rodent genetic models abrogates at least three of these problems: genetic background, and hence variation among 'subjects', can be much better controlled; diets can be rigorously formulated; and the influence of particular pathways can be dissected.

COMPLEXITY OF PATHWAYS

The initiator of almost all human colon cancer is mutational inactivation of the *APC* gene, the same gene that causes FAP when inherited in mutant form[1]. This gene encodes a multifunctional protein which can influence several important pathways[5]. Significant evidence suggests the role that the product of this gene plays in Wnt signalling is a key to intestinal homeostasis and tumour development (e.g. refs 5 and 6). Wnt signalling is a developmentally important pathway for vertebrates. APC participates by binding to, and targeting, β-catenin, for degradation through ubiquitination and proteosome degradation[7–10]. This occurs in a complex with GSK kinase and axin, among other molecules, and functionally maintains relatively low levels of β-catenin in colonic epithelial cells. In the absence of APC, β-catenin levels increase significantly, and in turn form a complex with a transcription factor, TCF, in the nucleus[11–13]. This complex can activate a number of genes. Among those that have been identified as transcriptional targets of β-catenin-TCF are cyclin D1 and c-myc, two genes involved in growth whose activation by this mechanism would tend to move cells into and through the cell cycle and therefore contribute to transformation[14–16].

However, inactivation of TCF-4 in a mouse model is lethal soon after parturition, and the mechanism of this lethality is revealing[17]. There is a degeneration of the mucosa of the small intestine, and animals essentially bleed to death. This degeneration is due to loss of the stem cell population and hence failure to repopulate the mucosa. The stem cell population is lost because the cells differentiate, not because they undergo apoptosis. Therefore, a functional downregulation of this pathway due to inactivation of TCF is related to premature cell differentiation.

To determine whether the down-regulation of the pathway by wild-type APC function also normally targets cell differentiation, we turned to a model system in culture. We and others have shown that the Caco-2 colon carcinoma cell line undergoes normal cell maturation as a function of time in culture (e.g. ref. 18). This includes cell cycle arrest in G_0/G_1 and differentiation along the absorptive cell lineage. Importantly, the cells do not undergo apoptosis. This is similar to the maturation of intestinal epithelial cells *in vivo*. Rates of apoptosis in the intestinal mucosa are very low, ranging from less than 1% in the colon to 2–3% in the small intestine. Thus, the increase in expression of APC that cells exhibit as they migrate towards the lumen from the crypt, which inversely affects β-catenin-TCF signalling, is normally correlated with cessation of cell proliferation and differentiation, rather than apoptosis. This is also reflected in the Caco-2 cell line. As the cells undergo cell cycle arrest and express markers of differentiation, there is a decrease in both β-catenin-TCF complex formation and activity[19]. In these cells, which have a mutant APC gene, this is due to a decrease in TCF-4 expression, as well as a sequestering of β-catenin by increased expression of E-cadherin[19]. As previously mentioned, two targets of this pathway are the cyclin D1 and c-myc genes. Therefore, down-regulation of this signalling pathway is probably directly involved in the cell cycle arrest that is seen. In order to determine if the pathway is also involved in the lineage-specific differentiation, we first asked whether genes that are up-regulated in the absorptive cell are transcriptionally regulated during Caco-2 cell differentiation. Up-regulation of the promoters of four such genes – alkaline phosphatase (ALP), intestinal fatty acid binding protein (iFABP), carcinoembryonic antigen (CEA), and sucrase-isomaltase (SI) – was indeed seen in conjunction with the down-regulation of β-catenin-TCF signalling. We then demonstrated that premature down-regulation of this pathway by three different mechanisms – introduction of wild-type APC, forced over-expression of E-cadherin, or introduction of a dominant-negative for TCF4 – were all effective in increasing ALP and iFABP promoter activity, but not that of CEA and SI[19].

Therefore, β-catenin-TCF signalling can clearly play a role in stimulating some aspects of intestinal cell differentiation. The heterogeneity in response among the genes investigated was not unexpected, since it is clear that a large number of signalling pathways can influence markers of intestinal differentiation. We had already shown that the short-chain fatty acid butyrate, a physiological regulator of colonic cell maturation, can induce aspects of Caco-2 cell differentiation and growth regulation that are not stimulated as a function of contact inhibition[18]. Thus, as might be predicted, the complete programme of intestinal cell maturation is probably complex and highly integrated.

In order to gain insight into this complexity, in the early 1980s we began to devise methods to interrogate the level of expression of each of large numbers of genes. In 1982 we reported on the expression of each of 400 cDNA sequences in mouse colon and other tumours, comparing and contrasting patterns of expression[20], and discovered cell cycle linked over-expression of an endogenous retroviral sequence in a chemically induced mouse colon tumour[21–23]. We then extended this approach to the measurement of each of more than 4000 sequences using RNA isolated from human tissue. These assays utilized a computerized scanning and image-processing system, a forerunner of modern microarray approaches to profiling of gene expression[24]. The data revealed a pattern of gene expression that was characteristic of human colonic tissue at elevated risk for development of colon cancer (e.g. FAP and HNPCC[25]), and that mitochondrial gene expression was coordinately decreased in human colonic tumours and increased when colonic carcinoma cell lines were induced to differentiate[26]. This latter observation led to a series of experiments which demonstrated that mitochondrial function and, in particular, regulation of the mitochondrial membrane potential, was necessary for normal pathways of colonic cell differentiation and apoptosis[27-34].

SHORT-CHAIN FATTY ACIDS AS PHYSIOLOGICAL REGULATORS OF COLONIC CELL MATURATION

We have more recently used microarray analysis of gene expression for investigation of the response of colonic cells to a number of agents potentially important in regulation of intestinal homeostasis and chemoprevention[35]. First, we continued our investigations into the mechanism of action of butyrate, a 4-carbon short-chain fatty acid (SCFA) produced by microbial fermentation of dietary fibre in the large intestine. Such SCFA are the principal energy source for colonic epithelial cells (e.g. ref. 36), and we have shown that utilization of these agents by β-oxidation in the mitochondria is necessary to stimulate pathways of colonic cell maturation both *in vitro* and *in vivo* (e.g. ref. 32, and references therein). Utilizing an 8000 member cDNA array, butyrate was compared to three other agents: trichostatin A, like butyrate an inhibitor of histone deacetylase activity; sulindac, a non-steroidal anti-inflammatory drug (NSAID) with significant chemopreventive activity; and curcumin, a widely consumed component of curry and turmeric that has chemopreventive activity for colon and other cancers.

The first observation was that, although all of the agents induced changes in gene expression, butyrate, unlike the other agents, induced a monotonic increase in the number of sequences that were elevated or repressed in expression as a function of time[35]. We believe that this continuous expansion of altered gene expression is the hallmark of a programmed response of the cells, leading to a cascade of events that ultimately results in a well-defined and integrated outcome. Since, among these agents, this is seen only with butyrate, a clear physiological regulator of colonic epithelial cell maturation, we interpret this as indicating that cells have evolved to undergo preprogrammed well-integrated responses to physiological agents that they normally encounter. This is similar to a conclusion we reached from the observation that efficient utilization of SCFA in the mouse colon was required for maintaining an apoptotic pathway, but that this was not necessary in the small intestine, in which cells are not exposed to the same high concentrations of SCFA[32]. In contrast, such integrated cascades of events are not triggered by pharmacological agents to which the cells have not been exposed, and to which they have no well-defined programme of response. We believe that this is one reason such agents probably have unwanted side-effects. A specific example of this involving multiple levels of regulation of the c-myc gene will be presented below.

More in-depth analysis of the responses to the agents revealed a complex recruitment by butyrate of gene sets as a function of time that was much different from those genes recruited by the other agents[35]. The butyrate response was most similar to that of trichostatin A. This may be due to the fact that both are inhibitors of histone deacetylase activity; indeed, a subset of genes was identified in which changes in expression closely paralleled the kinetics of change in histone acetylation, and which may therefore be coordinately regulated by this mechanism. However, despite this, the overall observation was that of the differences in response to the agents, which was also seen when specific subsets of genes involved in cell signalling or the machinery of the cell cycle were investigated. Therefore, although butyrate, trichostatin A and sulindac all induce what appear at the cellular level to be a similar G_0/G_1 cell cycle arrest and apoptosis, at the molecular level the cells respond very differently[35].

A specific example of this was investigated more closely. We had reported that butyrate, trichostatin A and sulindac all up-regulate β-catenin-TCF activity[37]. However, since c-myc is a direct target of this signalling pathway[14], the well-known down-regulation of c-myc by butyrate was seemingly incompatible with the up-regulation of this pathway. To investigate this further, we employed a novel method that permitted us to image the transcription site of c-myc in the nucleus of colon cells in culture[38]. Probes were used which interrogated either the 5' or the 3' end of the growing mRNA precursors. We were able to conclude that the increase in β-catenin-TCF activity induced by butyrate did indeed elevate initiation of c-myc transcription, but in terms of c-myc mRNA synthesis, this increased initiation was abrogated by a block to transcriptional elongation in exon 1[39]. Sulindac also increased β-catenin-TCF activity and initiation of c-myc transcription but, in contrast, the transcriptional block was not recruited, and full-length c-myc mRNA could be produced[39]. As a consequence, in response to butyrate, c-myc mRNA steady-state levels decreased, as has been reported, but in response to sulindac, c-myc levels increased. We believe that this is another specific example of our hypothesis that cells have evolved to respond in a well-integrated fashion to physiological regulators they normally encounter, but cannot do so in response to new pharmacological agents. In this case, as a consequence, sulindac elevated c-myc despite the cell cycle arrest it induced. We suggest that this inappropriate elevation of c-myc in the context of cell cycle arrest is one of the reasons for the serious side-effects of sulindac. For example, elevated expression of c-myc in growth-inhibited cells can lead to apoptosis, which may contribute to the ulceration and bleeding seen with this drug (e.g. refs 40 and 41).

MECHANISMS OF RESPONSE TO SULINDAC

Although sulindac has serious side-effects, it is also highly effective as a chemo-preventive agent for colon cancer in both humans and rodents[42–45]. Therefore, it is important to understand its mechanisms of action in this regard, so that agents and strategies can be designed to capitalize on this activity while minimizing toxicity. The response of colonic carcinoma cells to sulindac *in vitro* evaluated by microarray analysis was highly complex. In order to help focus on specific gene sets that might be critical in this response, we repeated the array analysis utilizing RNA isolated from rectal biopsies of three patients taken either before drug treatment, or following 1 month of daily treatment with 300 mg sulindac[46].

Again, for each patient the number of genes altered in expression was high; moreover, the altered gene sets differed considerably among the three patients. We compared these *in-vivo* databases to the similar databases on changes in gene expression induced by sulindac *in vitro*. We first focused on those genes that were differentially affected *in vivo* and *in vitro*, and identified a gene set which was down-regulated *in vivo*, but either not expressed, or not altered in expression, *in vitro*[46]. All of these genes are normally expressed in lymphocytes. This was interesting since sulindac is an anti-inflammatory drug. Therefore, it was not surprising that lymphocyte-associated sequences were down-regulated by the drug, since the representation of lymphocytes in the rectal biopsies should decrease following sulindac treatment. The lack of expression or change in these sequences *in vitro* is consistent with the lack of lymphocytes in the epithelial cell cultures. Thus, the gene profiling approach accurately reflects aspects of tissue physiology.

The second set of sequences we focused on was those that are altered similarly both *in vivo* and *in vitro* by sulindac[46]. Only eight sequences, or 0.1% of the total, satisfied this criterion. Among these were the cyclin kinase-dependent inhibitor, $p21^{WAF1/cip1}$. The significance of this observation is that this gene had already been shown by others to be induced in colon cells *in vitro* by NSAID (e.g. refs 47 and 48). Thus, our data extended this to cells in the intestinal mucosa *in situ*. Moreover, this gene, whose product inhibits cyclin-dependent kinase activity and therefore cell cycle progression, is normally expressed in the intestinal mucosa only as cells exit the proliferative compartment[49]. There was therefore good reason to hypothesize that it could play a fundamental role in pathways of colonic cell maturation that might be important in the response to sulindac.

In order to determine if the induction of p21 by sulindac was functionally important in the response to the drug, we designed a mouse experiment. Others had developed a mouse model in which the p21 gene had been targeted for inactivation[50]. Although fibroblasts derived from these $p21-/-$ mice have deficiencies in cell cycle checkpoints, the mice are generally healthy. We reasoned that the loss of p21 function might be interactive with a genetic initiation of intestinal tumour formation. Therefore, we crossed the p21 mice with a model in which the Apc gene is inactivated, the Apc1638 mouse[51,52]. We examined mice which were $Apc+/-$, to initiate tumour formation, and either $p21+/+$, $+/-$ or $-/-$[53]. Inactivation of the p21 gene increased tumour formation initiated by Apc, and this was related to gene dosage. The mechanism seemed to be perturbation of normal patterns of cell maturation in the mucosa, since the mucosa of mice with inactivation of p21 showed increased cell proliferation, decreased apoptosis, and decreased number of cells differentiated along the goblet cell lineage. This was also a function of p21 gene dosage[53].

Since there were significant effects of loss of p21 on the intestinal mucosa, pointing to an early event mediated by p21, we also fed other genetically identical groups a Western-style diet (i.e. high fat and phosphate, low calcium and vitamin D) that had been shown to increase Apc-induced intestinal tumours, but at a later stage of tumour growth[54]. As predicted, the combination of the loss of p21 and the Western diet was completely additive on increasing tumour incidence and frequency, therefore reinforcing the hypothesis that the two modulators of Apc-initiated tumour formation act by different mechanisms, and probably at different stages of tumourigenesis[53].

The critical experiment was then to determine if sulindac could inhibit tumour formation in the absence of p21. Mice that were Apc+/−, and either p21 wild-type, or with a single or both p21 alleles inactivated, were fed a diet containing sulindac for 36 weeks. As had been shown by others, in the p21 wild-type mice, sulindac was effective in reducing intestinal tumour incidence and frequency initiated by Apc. However, loss of even a single p21 allele completely abrogated this response[46]. More recently we have used quantitative real-time polymerase chain reaction to assay p21 expression in the duodenal mucosa of these mice. Sulindac effectively induced p21 in the p21 wild-type animals, but not in the p21+/− mice (W.C. Yang *et al.*, unpublished). Therefore, it appears that loss of a single p21 allele can influence the response of the remaining wild-type allele by an epigenetic mechanism. The important conclusion is that p21 induction by sulindac is necessary for its inhibitory affect on intestinal tumour formation[46].

THE IMPORTANCE OF MUCIN SYNTHESIS

The concept that intestinal cell differentiation is critical in normal homeostasis, and that its disruption is causal in tumour formation, has clear experimental precedence for colon cancer. Aberrant crypt foci (ACF) are considered preneoplastic lesions for colon cancer in humans, in mice treated with colon carcinogens, and in the Apc1638 mouse[55]. One characteristic of ACF is a depletion in goblet cells and hence a reduction in the mucin they produce[55]. Our long-standing interest in the structure and regulation of Muc2, the gene which encodes the principal colonic mucin, provided us the reagents for addressing the question of the importance of loss of this cell type in tumourigenesis[56–58]. Accordingly, we targeted the mouse Muc2 gene for inactivation by substituting a neo-cassette for exons 2–4 of Muc2[59]. Although a mRNA was produced from the locus in the mice that were Muc2−/−, we showed that this was a non-functional hybrid molecule that read through the neo-cassette downstream into the Muc2 gene. Staining of the intestinal crypts and villi with haematoxylin and eosin, alcian blue, or with an antibody specific for the Muc2 apomucin, showed the absence of recognizable goblet cells and the Muc2 mucin. The architecture of the crypts was also perturbed in the Muc2−/− mice. Crypts were narrower and significantly longer than in wild-type mice[59].

Most important, the Muc2−/− mice form adenomas and adenocarcinomas in the small and large intestine, and in the rectum[59]. This takes place in the absence of any other known genetic or chemical initiator. Thus, the loss of recognizable goblet cells, and of the mucin they produce, is sufficient to cause intestinal tumour formation. This appears to be due to a disruption in tissue homeostasis: there is increased mucosal proliferation, decreased apoptosis, and a profound increase in rate of cell migration along the crypt–villus axis[59]. In light of these data, the decrease in goblet cell number in the Apc+/−, p21−/− mice, in which the loss of p21 accelerates and increases tumour formation, becomes particularly interesting[53].

The molecular mechanisms that underlie this tumour formation are not yet clear. First, although there are no recognizable goblet cells, the lineage is not totally ablated, since the mucosa of Muc2$-/-$ mice is similar to wild-type mice in the staining for Itf, another marker of the goblet cell lineage[59]. A critical question, therefore, is the extent to which the lineage is altered, or whether inactivation of Muc2 is limited to effects on only this gene. This will be approached through microarray analysis, with comparison of the Muc2$-/-$ mucosa to that of wild-type mice, as well as to model systems in culture that differentiate either along the goblet or the absorptive cell lineage, for which we have already generated microarray data bases (Velcich et al., unpublished). Second, although c-myc is over-expressed in the Muc2$-/-$ tumours, as it is in the tumours due to inactivation of Apc, there does not appear to be an alteration of β-catenin signalling, pointing to different mechanisms that target c-myc in the Apc and Muc2 models[59].

It does not appear that a decreased number of terminally differentiated goblet cells itself is sufficient to cause tumour formation, since such goblet cell loss is seen, but tumours do not form, in a transgenic mouse strain in which goblet cells are targeted for destruction by linkage of promoter elements of Itf – a specific marker of this lineage – to an attenuated diphtheria toxin gene[60]. Therefore, of even greater fundamental interest is the question of whether the disruption in homeostasis in the Muc2$-/-$ intestinal mucosa, and the resulting tumourigenesis, is due to the loss of mucin, and perhaps its barrier function. An alternative hypothesis is that the loss of mucin causes alterations in signalling pathways of the mucosal cells, either due to a previously unappreciated role of MUC2 protein, or to the disrupted architecture of the crypt that may be sufficient to alter cell–cell and cell–matrix interactions in the mucosa.

SUMMARY AND CONCLUSIONS

The genetics of intestinal tumour formation are increasingly well understood, and this has identified molecular and biochemical pathways that are fundamental in regulating mucosal homeostasis and normal function. However, less is understood regarding the mechanisms through which dietary factors can modulate or circumvent these pathways to generate the profound effects that such environmental influences can have on risk for, and progression of, cancer. The use of novel mouse models, coupled with new genomic approaches that permit analysis of the complexity and interaction of genetic and dietary affects, has already provided insight into these questions, and should continue to increase our understanding of the integration of the multiple factors that normally maintain a functioning intestinal mucosa, and whose disruption leads to tumourigenesis. Finally, our development of the Muc2$-/-$ mouse model provides a means of dissecting the fundamental importance that mucin synthesis plays in intestinal homeostasis, and in potentially regulating the interaction of the mucosa with its environment.

References

1. Kinzler KW, Vogelstein B. Lessons from hereditary colorectal cancer. Cell. 1996;87:159–70.
2. Potter. 4.10 Colon, Rectum. In, ed. (Food, Nutrition and the Prevention of Cancer: A global perspective. 1997 American Institute for Cancer Research, Washington, DC. pp. 216–251.

3. Warthin AS. Heredity with reference to carcinoma. Arch Intern Med. 1913;12:546–55.
4. Lynch HT, Krush AJ. Cancer family G revisited: 1895–1970. Cancer. 1971;27:1505–11.
5. van Es JH, Giles RH, Clevers HC. The many faces of the tumor suppressor gene APC. Exp Cell Res. 2001;264:126–34.
6. Shih I-M, Yu J, He T-C, Vogelstein B, Kinzler KW. The B-catenin binding domain of adenomatous polyposis coli is sufficient for tumor suppression. Cancer Res. 2000;60:1671–6.
7. Rubinfeld B, Souza B, Albert I et al. Association of the APC gene product with b-catenin. Science. 1993;262:1731–4.
8. Rubinfeld B, Albert I, Porfiri E, Fiol C, Munemitsu S, Polakis P. Binding of GSL3b to the APC–b-catenin complex and regulation of complex assembly. Science. 1996;272:1023–6.
9. Ikeda S, Kishida S, Yamamoto H, Murai H, Koyama S. Axin, a negative regulator of the Wnt signalling pathway, forms a complex with GSK-3B and B-catenin and promotes GSK-3B-dependent phosphorylation of B-catenin. EMBO J. 1998;17:1371–84.
10. Sakanaka C, Weiss JB, Williams LT. Bridging of B-catenin and glycogen sythase kinase-3B by axin and inhibition of B-catenin-mediated transcription. Proc Natl Acad Sci USA. 1998;95:3020–3.
11. Morin PJ, Sparks AB, Korinek V et al. Activation of b-catenin-Tcf signaling in colon cancer by mutations in b-catenin or APC. Science. 1997;275:1787–90.
12. Korinek V, Barker N, Morin PJ et al. Constitutive transcriptional activation by a b-catenin-Tcf complex in APC$-/-$ colon carcinoma. Science. 1997;275:1784–7.
13. Rubinfeld B, Albert I, Porfiri E, Munemitsu S, Polakis P. Loss of B-catenin regulation by the APC tumor suppressor protein correlates with loss of structure due to common somatic mutations of the gene. Cancer Res. 1997;57:4624–30.
14. He T-C, Sparks AB, Rago C et al. Identification of c-MYC as a target of the APC pathway. Science. 1998;281:1509–12.
15. Tetsu O, McCormick F. B-catenin regulates expression of cyclin D1 in colon carcinoma cells. Nature. 1999;398:422–6.
16. Shtutman M, Zhurinsky J, Simcha I et al. The cyclin D1 gene is a target of the B-catenin/LEF-1 pathway. Proc Natl Acad Sci USA. 1999;96:5522–7.
17. Korinek V, Barker N, Moerer P et al. Depletion of epithelial stem-cell compartments in the small intestine of mice lacking Tcf-4. Nature Genet. 1998;19:379–83.
18. Mariadason JM, Rickard KL, Barkla DH, Augenlicht LH, Gibson PR. Divergent phenotypic patterns and commitment to apoptosis of Caco-2 cells during spontaneous and butyrate-induced differentiation. J Cell Physiol. 2000;183:347–54.
19. Mariadason JM, Bordonaro M, Aslam F et al. Down-regulation of B-catenin-TCF signaling is linked to colonic epithelial cell differentiation. Cancer Res. 2001;61:3465–71.
20. Augenlicht LH, Kobrin D. Cloning and screening of sequences expressed in a mouse colon tumor. Cancer Res. 1982;42:1088–93.
21. Royston ME, Augenlicht LH. Biotinated probe containing a long-terminal repeat hybridized to a mouse colon tumor and normal tissue. Science. 1983;222:1339–41.
22. Augenlicht LH, Kobrin D, Pavlovec A, Royston ME. Elevated expression of an endogenous retroviral long terminal repeat in a mouse colon tumor. J Biol Chem. 1984;259:1842–7.
23. Augenlicht LH, Halsey H. Expression of a mouse long terminal repeat is cell cycle-linked. Proc Natl Acad Sci USA. 1985;82:1946–9.
24. Augenlicht LH, Wahrman MZ, Halsey H, Anderson L, Taylor J, Lipkin M. Expression of cloned sequences in biopsies of human colonic tissue and in colonic carcinoma cells induced to differentiate in vitro. Cancer Res. 1987;47:6017–21.
25. Augenlicht LH, Taylor J, Anderson L, Lipkin M. Patterns of gene expression that characterize the colonic mucosa in patients at genetic risk for colonic cancer. Proc Natl Acad Sci USA. 1991;88:3286–9.
26. Heerdt BG, Halsey HK, Lipkin M, Augenlicht LH. Expression of mitochondrial cytochrome c oxidase in human colonic cell differentiation, transformation, and risk for colonic cancer. Cancer Res. 1990;50:1596–600.
27. Heerdt BG, Augenlicht LH. Effects of fatty acids on expression of genes encoding subunits of cytochrome c oxidase and cytochrome c oxidase activity in HT29 human colonic adenocarcinoma cells. J Biol Chem. 1991;266:19120–6.
28. Heerdt BG, Houston MA, Augenlicht LH. Potentiation by specific short-chain fatty acids of differentiation and apoptosis in human colonic carcinoma cell lines. Cancer Res. 1994;54:3288–94.

29. Heerdt BG, Houston MA, Rediske JJ, Augenlicht LH. Steady-state levels of mitochondrial messenger RNA species characterize a predominant pathway culminating in apoptosis and shedding of HT29 human colonic carcinoma cells. Cell Growth Differ. 1996;7:101–6.
30. Heerdt BG, Houston MA, Augenlicht LH. Short chain fatty acid-initiated cell cycle arrest and apoptosis of colonic epithelial cells is linked to mitochondrial function. Cell Growth Differ. 1997;8:523–32.
31. Heerdt BG, Houston MA, Anthony GM, Augenlicht LH. Mitochondrial membrane potential in the coordination of p53-independent proliferation and apoptosis pathways in human colonic carcinoma cells. Cancer Res. 1998;58:2869–75.
32. Augenlicht LH, Anthony GM, Chruch TL et al. Short chain fatty acid metabolism, apoptosis and Apc initiated tumorigenesis in the mouse gastrointestinal mucosa. Cancer Res. 1999; 59:6005–9.
33. Heerdt BG, Houston MA, Mariadason JM, Augenlicht LH. Dissociation of staurosporine-induced apoptosis from G2-M arrest in SW620 human colonic carcinoma cells: initiation of an apoptotic cascade is associated with elevation of the mitochondrial membrane potential. Cancer Res. 2000;60:6704–13.
34. Augenlicht LH, Heerdt BG. Mitochondria: integrators in tumorigenesis? Nature Genet. 2001; 28:104–5.
35. Mariadason JM, Corner GA, Augenlicht LH. Genetic reprogramming in pathways of colonic cell maturation induced by short chain fatty acids: comparison with trichostatin A, sulidac, and curcumin and implications for chemoprevention of colon cancer. Cancer Res. 2000;60:4561–72.
36. Roediger WE. Role of anaerobic bacteria in the metabolic welfare of the colonic mucosa in man. Gut. 1980;21:793–8.
37. Bordonaro M, Mariadason JM, Aslam F, Heerdt BG, Augenlicht LH. Butyrate induced cell cycle arrest and apoptotic cascade in colonic carcinoma cells: modulation of the B-catenin-Tcf pathway, and concordance with effects of sulindac and trichostatin, but not curcumin. Cell Growth Differ. 1999;10:713–20.
38. Femino AM, Fay FS, Fogarty K, Singer RH. Visualization of single RNA transcripts in situ. Science. 1998;280:585–90.
39. Wilson AJ, Velcich A, Kurland A et al. Novel detection and differential utilization of a c-myc transcriptional block in colon cancer chemoprevention. 2002 Cancer Research, in press.
40. Evan GI, Wyllie AH, Gilbert CS et al. Induction of apoptosis in fibroblasts by c-myc protein. Cell. 1992;69:119–28.
41. Arango D, Corner GA, Wadler S, Catalano PJ, Augenlicht LH. c-myc/p53 interaction determines sensitivity of human colon carcinoma cells to 5-fluorouracil in vitro and in vivo. Cancer Res. 2001;61:4910–15.
42. Giardiello FM, Hamilton SR, Knish AJ et al. Treatment of colonic and rectal adenomas with sulindac in familial adenomatous polyposis. N Engl J Med. 1993;328:1313–16.
43. Nugent KP, Farmer KC, Spigelman AD, Williams CB, Phillips RK. Randomized controlled trial of the effect of sulindac on duodenal and rectal polyposis and cell proliferation in patients with familial adenomatous polyposis. Br J Surg. 1993;80:1618–19.
44. Boolbol SK, Dannenberg AJ, Chadburn A et al. Cyclooxygenase-2 overexpression and tumor formation are blocked by sulindac in a murine model of familial adenomatous polyposis. Cancer Res. 1996;56:2556–60.
45. Rao CV, Rivenson A, Simi B et al. Chemoprevention of colon carcinogenesis by sulindac, a non-steroidal anti-inflammatory agent. Cancer Res. 1995;55:1464–72.
46. Yang WC, Velcich A, Mariadason J et al. p21WAF1/cip1 is an important determinant of intestinal cell response to sulindac in vitro and in vivo. Cancer Res. 2001;61:6297–302.
47. Goldberg Y, Nassif II, Pittas A et al. The anti-proliferative effect of sulindac and sulindac sulfide on HT-29 colon cancer cells: alterations in tumor suppressor and cell cycle-regulatory proteins. Oncogene. 1996;12:893–901.
48. Shiff SJ, Qiao L, Tsai L-L, Rigas B. Sulindac sulfide an aspirin-like compound, inhibits proliferation, causes cell cycle quiescence, and induces apoptosis in HT-29 colon adenocarcinoma cells. J Clin Invest. 1995;96:491–503.
49. El-Deiry WS, Tokino T, Waldman T et al. Topological control of p21 waf1/cip1 expression in normal and neoplastic tissues. Cancer Res. 1995;55:2910–19.
50. Deng C, Zhang P, Harper JW, Elledge SJ, Leder P. Mice lacking p21 cip1/waf1 undergo normal development, but are defective in G1 checkpoint control. Cell. 1995;82:675–84.

51. Fodde R, Edelmann W, Yang K *et al*. A targeted chain-termination mutation in the mouse Apc gene results in multiple intestinal tumors. Proc Natl Acad Sci USA. 1994;91:8969–73.
52. Yang K, Edelmann W, Fan K *et al*. A mouse model of human familial adenomatous polyposis. J Exp Zool. 1997;277:245–54.
53. Yang WC, Mathew J, Velcich A *et al*. Targeted inactivation of the p21 WAF1/cip1 gene enhances Apc initiated tumor formation and the tumor promoting activity of a Western-style high risk diet by altering cell maturation in the intestinal mucosa. Cancer Res. 2001;61:565–9.
54. Yang K, Edelmann W, Fan K *et al*. Dietary modulation of carcinoma development in a mouse model for human familial polyposis. Cancer Res. 1998;58:5713–17.
55. Pretlow TP, Siddiki B, Augenlicht LH, Pretlow TG, Kim YS. Aberrant crypt foci (ACF) – earliest recognized players or innocent bystanders in colon carcinogenesis. In: Schmiegel W, editor. Colorectal Cancer: Molecular Mechanisms, Premalignant State, and its Prevention. Lancaster: Kluwer, 1999:67–82.
56. Velcich A, Palumbo L, Jarry A, Laboisse C, Rachevskis J, Augenlicht L. Patterns of expression of lineage specific markers during the *in vitro* differentiation of HT29 colon carcinoma cells. Cell Growth Differ. 1995;6:749–57.
57. Velcich A, Palumbo L, Selleri L, Evans G, Augenlicht L. Organization and regulatory aspects of the human intestinal mucin gene (MUC2) locus. J Biol Chem. 1997;272:7968–76.
58. Aslam F, Augenlicht L, Velcich A. The Sp family of transcription factors in the regulation of the human and mouse MUC2 gene promoters. Cancer Res. 2000;61:570–6.
59. Velcich A, Yang WC, Heyer J *et al*. Colorectal cancer in mice genetically deficient in the mucin Muc2. Science. 2002;295:1726–9.
60. Itoh H, Beck PL, Inoue N, Podolsky DK. A paradoxical reduction in susceptibility to colonic injury upon targeted transgenic ablation of goblet cells. J Clin Invest. 1999;104:1539–47.

10
Patient identification and surveillance in familial adenomatous polyposis (FAP)

R. CASPARI

CLINICAL PHENOTYPE

Familial adenomatous polyposis (FAP) is an autosomal dominant precancerous condition caused by mutations in the adenomatous polyposis coli (APC) tumour suppressor gene. The prevalence of FAP is about 1:10 000 with 25% of all cases being attributable to new mutations. The penetrance of FAP is 100%, i.e. every carrier of a disease causing APC mutation will develop FAP. Accordingly, untreated FAP patients have a nearly 100% risk of developing colorectal cancer.

The hallmark of the disease is the development of hundreds to thousands of colorectal adenomas. On average, first polyps develop during the second decade, and if patients stay untreated colorectal cancer (CRC) occurs at a median age of 36 years; these patients subsequently die of CRC at a median age of 40 years[1].

In addition to colorectal adenomas a variety of extracolonic manifestations may develop. Thus, adenoma formation in FAP patients is not limited to the large bowel, but the whole gastrointestinal tract (GIT) may be affected. However, the risk of malignization is less striking in the upper GIT. In contrast to the rest of the GIT, most polyps in the stomach show not an adenomatous but a hyperplastic growth pattern; it is still debated whether these so-called fundic gland polyps confer a risk of malignization by themselves or whether the slightly elevated risk of gastric cancer in FAP patients is attributable to adenomas which occur especially in the antrum. Most authors therefore emphasize the need for regular biopsies of gastric polyps in FAP patients.

Adenomas of the duodenum, especially those located around the papilla Vateri, have the highest risk of malignization outside the colorectum. Up to 10% of FAP patients die of duodenal cancer[2]. In contrast to the decrease of CRC-related deaths due to the use of prophylactic colectomy in FAP patients the percentage of deaths from duodenal cancer is increasing over the years[3]. Thus, regular endoscopic screening is mandatory. Although ileal and jejunal adenomas also develop in most FAP patients the occurrence of cancer at these locations is relatively low. Given the obvious diagnostic and therapeutic limitations screening for ileal and jejunal polyps is not advocated.

Eldon Gardner was the first to describe the occurrence of benign skin tumours (atheromas and fibromas) and osteomas in patients with polyposis coli[4,5]. Subsequently this combination was named Gardner's syndrome. Before the genetic basis of FAP/Gardner's syndrome could be clarified it was debated whether FAP and Gardner's syndrome are distinct diseases, allelic, or just different phenotypic expressions of the same genetic defect. Following the cloning of the APC gene it has been shown that FAP/Gardner's syndrome are caused by the same APC mutations, thus, Gardner's syndrome should no longer be used as a denominator of FAP.

The occurrence of desmoid tumours in FAP patients was first reported by Gardner also[6]. Whereas skin tumours and osteomas are benign lesions desmoid tumours are potentially harmful. They occur in about 10–20% of all FAP patients, most often triggered by a surgical intervention. Like duodenal adenomas, desmoids are a leading cause of death in colectomized FAP patients with increasing tendency[2,3]. Desmoids in FAP patients develop mainly within the abdominal wall, most often in a scar after previous colectomy, and/or within the mesentery. They are histologically benign tumours built up from mature fibroblasts but may cause major problems through their locally infiltrative growth pattern. They are thus regarded as semimalignant tumours.

In 1980 Blair and Trempe[7] reported on the occurrence of congenital hypertrophies of the retinal pigment epithelium (CHRPE) in three FAP patients from one kindred. Subsequent reports confirmed that about 75% of all FAP patients develop these benign retinal pigment anomalies[8,9]. Since it could be shown that CHRPE cluster within FAP families, and the occurrence of CHRPE depends on the underlying mutation in the APC gene, indirect ophthalmoscopy can be used for predictive diagnosis in relatives of FAP patients if CHRPE are present in the patients themselves[10].

Furthermore, a number of extraintestinal malignancies may develop in FAP patients, mainly hepatoblastomas in FAP children between the ages of 2 and 5 years, adrenal adenomas and carcinomas, and thyroid carcinomas. The combination of GIT tumours and brain tumours has been designated as Turcot's syndrome. As in Gardner's syndrome, however, molecular analysis could show that brain tumours are solely a rare phenotypic manifestation in FAP as well as in the hereditary non-polyposis colorectal cancer syndrome. The name Turcot's syndrome should therefore no longer be used.

SURVEILLANCE OF PATIENTS AND PERSONS AT RISK

While screening in other inherited cancer syndromes usually leads to earlier detection of cancers, hopefully enabling curative surgery, screening in FAP aims on cancer prevention due to the fact that CRC in FAP patients develops through the well-known adenoma–dysplasia–carcinoma sequence[11]. Detection and removal of adenomas as CRC precursors therefore prevent the development of cancer. However, only in the early stages of the disease, when first polyps develop in teens or young adults, can this be accomplished by endoscopic removal of single adenomas. Later, when polyps increasingly grow in size and number and the colorectum is carpeted by adenomas, a one-by-one removal of polyps would be completely insufficient, and surgical removal of the whole colorectum, or at least the colon (see Therapy) must be performed in order to prevent malignization. Accordingly, the establishment of FAP registries and the widespread use of prophylactic surgery has led to a marked reduction in the occurrence of CRC in FAP patients, as well as patient mortality from CRC (for review see ref. 12).

An expert panel of the Leeds Castle Polyposis Group has put forward screening recommendations for at-risk persons from FAP kindreds consisting of regular endoscopic examinations, molecular genetic analysis, and indirect ophthalmoscopy.

Endoscopy

Beginning in children at ages 10–14 a rectosigmoidoscopy should be performed. This is sufficient in most cases since first polyps usually develop within the rectosigmoid.

In case of a negative result examinations should be repeated every other year; if adenomas occur, a pancolonoscopy should be performed subsequently. If symptoms such as diarrhoea or bleeding repeatedly occur in children of an FAP kindred before the age of 10 years first bowel screening should be immediately initiated. Although otherwise rare, in some children from our registry bearing the most severe APC mutation (Del 1309) even colectomies had to be performed before the age of 10 years due to otherwise untreatable bleeding complications.

Molecular genetic analysis

The objective of molecular genetic analysis is the limitation of the clinical screening examinations to those children bearing the APC mutation present in their affected parent. Children should therefore be tested at the age when endoscopic surveillance would otherwise be started. In order to be tested, however, the mutation in the given family must be known. It could be shown that the use of predictive diagnosis by means of molecular genetic analysis in FAP kindreds is even cost-effective in addition to its well-known psychosocial benefits to the non-affected members of the families[13].

Indirect ophthalmoscopy

Screening for the presence of CHRPE is of much interest in two ways: first, indirect ophthalmoscopy allows predictive diagnosis in relatives of those FAP patients in whom CHRPE are present[10]; second, knowledge concerning CHRPE status in FAP patients is helpful for molecular genetic analysis (see Genotype–phenotype correlations). Thus, most FAP centres advocate the performance of indirect ophthalmoscopy.

Osteomas are of less value for predictive diagnosis, and a general screening by orthopantomography is thus not indicated. However, if osteomas or any other extracolonic manifestation of FAP occur in a person not known to be affected by the disease a thorough examination should always be initiated, since this may lead to the detection of an FAP patient without a known family history (e.g. new mutation, adopted child).

Screening for gastroduodenal adenomas is advocated by most FAP centres, and usually initiated around the time of prophylactic surgery, although up to now no evidence on a positive effect regarding reduction of mortality or increase of life expectancy can be found in the literature. As in the case of colorectal adenomas, however, the existence of an adenoma–dysplasia–carcinoma sequence in the duodenum is generally accepted. It seems reasonable, therefore, to conclude that removal of duodenal polyps by endoscopic polypectomy, duodenotomy with polypectomy, or sometimes even a Whipple procedure in extremely severe cases, might lead to a reduction of the risk for duodenal cancers. Since up to 10% of all causes of death in colectomized FAP patients are attributable to duodenal cancers, even a reduction in overall mortality should thus be possible in the long run.

Some centres advocate screening for mesenterial desmoid tumours by magnetic resonance imaging or computerized tomography scan in colectomized FAP patients. However, given the well-known fact that desmoid tumours may slowly grow to a special size and then remain stable without causing major problems, or even resolve spontaneously, the effect of early diagnosis of asymptomatic tumours is debatable. Furthermore, intra-abdominal desmoids quite often do not grow as an encapsulated tumour mass but behave as a diffuse fibromatosis, thus causing therapeutic difficulties (see Therapy). In the case of newly developing abdominal symptoms in colectomized FAP patients, however, desmoid tumours must always be regarded as a possible explanation, and the respective diagnostic evaluation must be initiated.

DIFFERENTIAL DIAGNOSIS

In the case of 'classical' FAP the diagnosis is relatively easy; it is based on the occurrence of more than 100 colorectal polyps and the histological demonstration of an adenomatous growth pattern. In the case of an atypical FAP, however, a clear-cut diagnosis solely on the grounds of the phenotype may sometimes be impossible. Up to now a number of families with so-called attenuated adenomatous polyposis coli (AAPC) have been described[14]. AAPC are phenotypic variants of FAP due to special mutations in the APC gene (see Genotype–phenotype correlations). Clinically these patients usually develop less than 100 colorectal adenomas, on average at an older age than 'classical' FAP patients, and they tend to have no, or only a few, extracolonic manifestations. Polyps in these patients mainly develop in the right hemicolon, while polyps in classical FAP show a preponderance for the left hemicolon and usually develop in the rectum first. Kindreds with AAPC are sometimes misdiagnosed as autosomal dominant colorectal cancer families; thus, the most important differential diagnosis is the hereditary non-polyposis colorectal cancer syndrome (HNPCC). In some cases of our own series of FAP and HNPCC families at the University of Bonn the distinction between the two syndromes could be made only by the demonstration of either an APC mutation or a mutation in one of the mismatch repair genes causing HNPCC.

THERAPY

Colorectum

The objective of the treatment is the reduction of cancer occurrence and mortality in FAP patients. To achieve this the surgical removal of the colorectum or colon is necessary. At present two surgical procedures are most widely used in FAP patients: pancolectomy with ileorectal anastomosis (IRA) and pancolectomy with proctomucosectomy and ileal pouch–anal anastomosis (IAP) (for review see ref. 15). Since IRA has now been used for about 50 years there are sufficient data on the advantages and disadvantages of the procedure: in the hands of an experienced surgeon it is a safe and relatively easy procedure with low morbidity and almost no mortality, usually leading to good functional results. Since the rectal mucosa is not removed, however, patients retain the risk of rectal cancer, which necessitates a lifelong close surveillance of the remaining rectum in IRA patients. The risk of developing rectal cancer may be diminished by the use of Sulindac, a non-steroidal antiphlogistic drug leading to reversion of adenomatous polyps in FAP patients. This is therefore widely used in IRA patients, and at least over a period of about 3 years the effect of rectal adenoma clearing remains stable[16]. However, since there are reports on the development of rectal cancer under Sulindac therapy[17], the exact mechanism by which the adenoma reversion is obtained by Sulindac is still unclear, and no data on the long-time effects of Sulindac and its possible side-effects are so far available; a final judgement on the role of Sulindac in the treatment of FAP is not yet possible.

In contrast to the IRA procedure there is still limited experience with IAP in FAP patients. Due to the proctomucosectomy the remaining risk of rectal cancer in IAP patients is less than in IRA. However, a reduction to a 0% risk, which was the initial enthusiastic expectation of some surgeons, cannot be achieved. Meanwhile there are reports on cancer occurrences in IAP patients from various centres. These cancers may occur either in little islands of rectal mucosa remaining after mucosectomy[18] or in the mucosa of the 'neo-rectum', the ileal pouch[19].

Due to the limited experience with this procedure, the risk of malignization after IAP cannot yet be assessed. However, since the IAP procedure is more complicated, morbidity rates are higher than in IRA, and the functional results are inferior; the choice of surgical procedure can be made only after obtaining detailed information concerning the patient and ample discussion of the pros and cons of either procedure. As a guiding principle: in patients with early occurrence of polyps and severe rectal polyposis IAP should be performed, whereas in patients with no or little rectal polyposis an IRA might be more appropriate.

Upper GIT

In colectomized FAP patients the risk of duodenal cancer is relatively high[20]. Most centres therefore advocate endoscopic surveillance of the duodenum beginning at the time of prophylactic surgery. If duodenal polyps occur, mostly around the papilla Vateri, biopsies should be taken and larger polyps, or polyps showing higher-grade dysplasia, should be removed. If polyps are not endoscopically resectable duodenotomy with polyp excision may be necessary in some cases, usually leading to very good results with considerably low morbidity from the procedure itself. Only in very severe and rare cases has a Whipple procedure been discussed as ultima ratio, if adenoma recurrence after endoscopic or surgical excision is rapid and histological examination repeatedly shows high-grade dysplasia.

Desmoid tumours

Treatment of desmoid tumours quite often is both arduous and unsuccessful. According to the literature only about 10–20% of FAP patients develop desmoid tumours, but up to 10% of colectomized patients die of desmoid tumours[2]. For a long time surgical excision of desmoids was the treatment of choice. However, even after R0 resection the recurrence rate was very high. Furthermore, since intra-abdominal desmoids quite often appear as fibromatosis with a diffuse infiltration of the mesentery, a complete resection would necessitate removal of large parts of the small intestine, thus changing the operation into a mutilating procedure. Surgical interventions are therefore nowadays mostly restricted to encapsulated desmoids occurring in the abdominal wall, and to treatment or prevention of complications by intra-abdominal desmoids.

A number of alternative treatment options exist, all leading to stabilization, growth reduction or at best complete resolution of the tumours in only a proportion of cases. Most widely used is the hormonal treatment with anti-estrogens such as tamoxifen. The rationale for this is the preponderance of females in developing desmoids, and the presence of estrogen receptors in some of the tumours. However, even if no estrogen receptors are expressed, tumours may respond to the treatment. Other therapeutic options include a variety of nonsteroidal antiphlogistic drugs (with Sulindac being the one most often used), radiotherapy, and chemotherapy.

GENETICS

FAP is caused by mutations in the adenomatous polyposis coli (APC) tumoursuppressor gene[21,22]. APC is a relatively large gene consisting of 15 exons with a coding sequence of 8535 nucleotides, and germline mutations in FAP patients are widely spread over most parts of the coding sequence. The number of different APC mutations known so far exceeds 800.

If a mutation in the APC gene can be demonstrated in an FAP patient all of his/her relatives can be immediatly screened for the presence of this mutation. However, due to the size of the APC gene, the fact that mutations are widely spread over most parts of the coding sequence, and that only a few mutations occur in more than one unrelated FAP kindred, mutation analysis is very laborious and expensive. Furthermore, even if different techniques are combined, detection of germline mutations can be accomplished in only up to 70% of all FAP patients.

Since this kind of diagnostics is a predictive test, detailed information must be given to the patient and the relatives concerning all aspects of the testing before the analysis is started. Information concerning the disease and the underlying genetic cause, the testing procedure itself, the possible results of the genetic analysis, and the consequences of these results must be provided; furthermore, questions of possible psychosocial sequelae, or problems regarding insurance issues, should be addressed. To cope with this, counselling by an experienced geneticist seems most appropriate. In most cases the result of the molecular genetic analysis will be given to the patient in the same way.

Genotype–phenotype correlations

Although more than 800 different germline mutations in the APC gene are published, and most are unique to only one FAP family, a number of close genotype–phenotype correlations could be identified. This is mostly due to the fact that almost all APC mutations are truncating mutations; thus, it is not the mutation itself which is of relevance, but its localization within the gene, since this defines the length of the mutant APC protein.

Mutations at the 5' end, in exon 9, and at the 3' end of the gene are correlated with the development of AAPC, the attenuated form of FAP[23]. In contrast, mutations around the middle of APC's coding sequence, especially the mutation Del 1309, lead to an extremely severe course of FAP[24].

The presence of CHRPE in FAP patients is also dependent on the localization of the APC mutation: whereas CHRPE are present in patients with mutations between exon 10 and the first half of exon 15, CHRPE are lacking in patients with mutations at the 5' end of the gene[25] and in patients with mutations in the distal half of the gene[26].

Whereas the overall risk for the development of desmoid tumours in FAP patients is about 10–20%, a small subgroup of patients with mutations beyond codon 1444 tend to develop desmoid tumours with great certainty[26]. In addition, osteomas and skin lesions are also found more often in these patients.

References

1. Bülow S. Clinical features in familial polyposis coli. Results of the Danish Polyposis Register. Dis Colon Rectum. 1986;29:102–7.
2. Arvanitis ML, Jagelman DG, Fazio VW, Lavery IC, McGannon E. Mortality in patients with familial adenomatous polyposis. Dis Colon Rectum. 1990;33:639–42.
3. Belchetz LA, Berk T, Bapat BV, Cohen Z, Gallinger S. Changing causes of mortality in patients with familial adenomatous polyposis. Dis Colon Rectum. 1996;39:384–7.
4. Gardner EJ, Plenk HP. Hereditary pattern for multiple osteomas in a family group. Am J Hum Genet. 1952;4:31–6.
5. Gardner EJ, Richards RC. Multiple cutaneous and subcutaneous lesions occurring simultaneously with hereditary polyposis and osteomatosis. Am J Hum Genet. 1953;5:139–47.
6. Gardner EJ. Follow-up study of a family group exhibiting dominant inheritance for a syndrome including intestinal polyps, osteomas, fibromas and epidermal cysts. Am J Hum Genet. 1962;14:376–90.
7. Blair NP, Trempe CL. Hypertrophy of the retinal pigment epithelium associated with Gardner's syndrome. Am J Ophthalmol. 1980;90:661–7.
8. Traboulsi EI, Krush AJ, Gardner EJ et al. Prevalence and importance of pigmented ocular fundus lesions in Gardner's syndrome. N Engl J Med. 1987;316:661–7.
9. Berk T, Cohen Z, McLeod RS, Parker JA. Congenital hypertrophy of the retinal pigment epithelium as a marker for familial adenomatous polyposis. Dis Colon Rectum. 1988;31:253–7.
10. Caspari R, Friedl W, Böker T et al. Predictive diagnosis in familial adenomatous polyposis: evaluation of molecular genetic and ophthalmologic methods. Z Gastroenterol. 1993;31:646–52.
11. Fearon ER, Vogelstein B. A genetic model for colorectal tumorigenesis. Cell. 1990;61:759–67.
12. Bülow S, Bülow C, Nielsen TF, Karlsen L, Moesgaard F. Centralized registration, prophylactic examination, and treatment results in improved prognosis in familial adenomatous polyposis. Results from the Danish Polyposis Register. Scand J Gastroenterol. 1995;30:989–93.

13. Cromwell DM, Moore RD, Brensinger JD, Petersen GM, Bass EB, Giardiello FM. Cost analysis of alternative approaches to colorectal screening in familial adenomatous polyposis. Gastroenterology. 1998;114:893–901.
14. Spirio L, Olschwang S, Groden J *et al*. Alleles of the APC gene: an attenuated form of familial polyposis. Cell. 1993;75:951–7.
15. Rhodes M, Bradburn DM. Overview of screening and management of familial adenomatous polyposis. Gut. 1992;33:125–31.
16. Winde G, Schmid KW, Schlegel W, Fischer R, Osswald H, Bünte H. Complete reversion and prevention of rectal adenomas in colectomized patients with familial adenomatous polyposis by rectal low-dose Sulindac maintenance treatment. Advantages of a low-dose nonsteroidal anti-inflammatory drug regimen in reversing adenomas exceeding 33 months. Dis Colon Rectum. 1995;38:813–30.
17. Niv Y, Fraser GM. Adenocarcinoma in the rectal segment in familial polyposis coli is not prevented by Sulindac therapy. Gastroenterology. 1994;107:854–7.
18. Von Herbay A, Stern J, Herfarth C. Pouch–anal cancer after restorative proctocolectomy for familial adenomatous polyposis. Am J Surg Pathol. 1996;20:995–9.
19. Palkar VM, DeSouza LJ, Jagannath P, Naresh KN. Adenocarcinoma arising in 'J' pouch after total proctocolectomy for familial polyposis coli. Indian J Cancer. 1997;34:16–19.
20. Jagelman DG, DeCosse JJ, Bussey HJR. Upper gastrointestinal cancer in familial adenomatous polyposis. Lancet. 1988;1(8595):1149–51.
21. Groden J, Thliveris A, Samowitz W *et al*. Identification and characterization of the familial adenomatous polyposis coli gene. Cell. 1991;66:589–600.
22. Kinzler KW, Nilbert NC, Su LK *et al*. Identification of FAP locus genes from chromosome 5q21. Science. 1991;253:661–5.
23. Soravia C, Berk T, Madlensky L *et al*. Genotype–phenotype correlations in attenuated adenomatous polyposis coli. Am J Hum Genet. 1998;62:1290–301.
24. Caspari R, Friedl W, Mandl M *et al*. Familial adenomatous polyposis: mutation at codon 1309 and early onset of colon cancer. Lancet. 1994;343:629–32.
25. Olschwang S, Tiret A, Laurent-Puig P, Muleris M, Parc R, Thomas G. Restriction of ocular fundus lesions to a subgroup of APC mutations in adenomatous polyposis coli patients. Cell. 1993;75:959–68.
26. Caspari R, Olschwang S, Friedl W *et al*. Familial adenomatous polyposis: desmoid tumours and lack of ophthalmic lesions (CHRPE) associated with APC mutations beyond codon 1444. Hum Mol Genet. 1995;4:337–40.

11
Patient identification and clinical management in hereditary non-polyposis colorectal cancer

O. AL-TAIE

INTRODUCTION

First reports on hereditary non-polyposis colorectal cancer (HNPCC) families by Warthin[1] and Lynch et al.,[2] describing characteristic clinical findings in HNPCC, were published decades ago, but little attention was drawn to this tumour syndrome. Since the first characterization of genetic defects in this tumour syndrome in 1993, numerous studies on the molecular basis and clinical charac-teristics have been published (Figure 1). However, despite this increasing knowl-edge of HNPCC, many questions concerning patient identification and clinical management of HNPCC patients remain to be clarified in future studies.

CHARACTERISTICS OF HNPCC

HNPCC is an autosomal dominant-inherited disorder caused by germline muta-tions in genes involved in DNA mismatch repair (MMR) (Table 1)[3–8]. MMR-gene defects lead to microsatellite instability (MSI), characterized by a high mutation rate in repetitive DNA sequences (microsatellites) in non-coding and coding regions of the genome. MSI within the coding region of genes involved in regulation and control of cell proliferation, differentiation and apoptosis leads to their inactivation, thereby promoting cancer development (Figure 2).

The most important clinical hallmark of HNPCC is a familial clustering of colorectal cancers as well as extracolonic malignancies, especially cancer of the endometrium (Table 2). Although HNPCC patients do not present with a patho-gnomonic phenotype like colorectal polyposis in familial adenomatous polyposis (FAP), the colorectal cancers in HNPCC families present with a variety of char-acteristic clinical features (Figure 3). However, some of these, such as a tumour localization proximal to the splenic flexure, an increased frequency of cancers with poor or mucinous differentiation, and the presence of tumour infiltrating

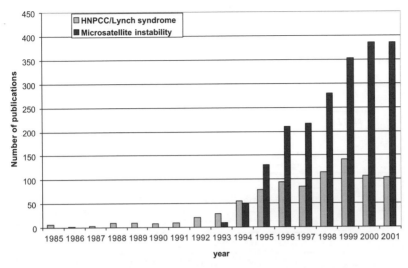

Figure 1 Number of publications registered in Medline during 1985–2001 according to the key words HNPCC/Lynch syndrome (black bars) and microsatellite instability (grey bars)

Table 1 MMR genes involved in HNPCC (kb: kilobases, aa: amino acids)

Gene	Chromosome	DNA (kb)	Protein (aa)
hMLH1	3p21	2.3	756
hMSH2	2p21–22	2.7	909
hMSH6/GTBP	2p16	4.2	1292
hPMS1	2q31–33	2.8	932
hPMS2	7p22	2.6	862

lymphocytes (TIL), are also common in sporadic MSI-positive colon cancers[9,10]. Several studies indicate that HNPCC patients have a better prognosis than patients with sporadic colorectal carcinoma[11–13]; however, most of these studies are retrospective analyses and important factors such as choice of surgical strategy and application of adjuvant or palliative chemotherapy were not assessed.

DIAGNOSIS OF HNPCC

To date the diagnosis of HNPCC is primarily based on the so-called Amsterdam Criteria I and Amsterdam Criteria II, which were proposed by the International Collaborative Group of HNPCC (ICG-HNPCC)[14,15]. In 1991 the Amsterdam Criteria I (Table 3) were established as a set of clinical selection criteria for families with HNPCC providing a basis for uniformity in collaborative studies. However, extracolonic cancers were not taken into account in these criteria. Therefore, since 1999 the Amsterdam Criteria II (Table 3), including cancers of the endometrium, small bowel, ureter and renal pelvis, are used according to the Amsterdam Criteria I to identify families that are very likely to have HNPCC.

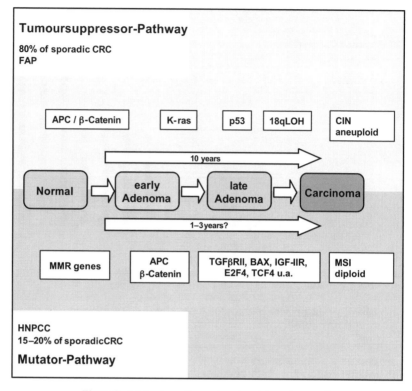

Figure 2 Molecular pathways in colorectal carcinogenesis

Table 2 Cumulative risk of cancer in HNPCC patients
(70–80 years)[46–51]

Site of cancer	Cumulative risk (%)
Colon and rectum	82–92
Endometrium	43–60
Stomach	2.1–19
Small bowel	4.5–7.2
Urinary tract	1.3–12
Ovary	3.4–12
Brain	3.7
Hepatobiliary system	2.0–18

Diagnosis of HNPCC using these criteria alone would miss a substantial number of HNPCC patients, especially in families with a small pedigree number. For the identification of these families, molecular analysis is an important tool. In 1997 the Bethesda guidelines (Table 4) were developed as selection criteria for patients whose tumours should be tested for MSI[16]. Recently, it was shown that by using only the Bethesda Criteria I–III a greater specificity and equal

94

Localisation proximal to the
splenic flexure in 50–60%

Microsatellite instability
(MSI-H)

Multiple CRC
Synchronous 18%
Metachronous 45% in 10 years

Increased frequency of
Colon cancers with
Poor differentiation
Mucinousdifferentiation
Crohn's like lesions/TIL

Lower stage at diagnosis
Better prognosis

Average age at CRC: 45 years

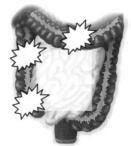

Rapid cancer development
(1–3 years)

Figure 3 Characteristical findings in colorectal cancers of HNPCC-related colorectal cancers.
(CRC: colorectal cancer, TIL: tumour-infiltrating lymphocytes)

Table 3 Amsterdam Criteria I and II

Amsterdam Criteria I[a]
There should be at least three relatives with CRC.
All the following criteria should be present:
  One should be a first-degree relative of the other two
  At least two successive generations should be affected
  At least one colorectal cancer (CRC) should be diagnosed before the age of 50

Amsterdam Criteria II[a]
There should be at least three relatives with an HNPCC-associated cancer (CRC, cancer of the
  endometrium, small bowel, or renal pelvis).
All the following criteria should be present:
  One should be a first-degree relative of the other two
  At least two successive generations should be affected
  At least one CRC should be diagnosed before the age of 50

---

[a] Familial adenomatous polyposis should be excluded and tumours should be verified by
pathological examination.

sensitivity than for using all Bethesda Criteria in the identification of HNPCC
patients is achieved[17]. In 1997, at the 'International workshop on microsatellite
instability and RER phenotypes in cancer detection and familial predisposition' a
consensus panel for MSI analysis, consisting of five microsatellite markers
(BAT16, BAT25 (both mononucleotide repeats) and D5S346, D2S123 and
D17S250 (all dinucleotide repeats)) was recommended[18]. Tumours displaying
MSI in two or more markers are defined as MSI-high and suspicious for
HNPCC (Figure 2). Previously the microsatellite marker BAT 26 was reported to
be both sensitive and specific for identification of MSI-high (MSI-H) when used
alone for MSI analysis[19,20].

In addition to HNPCC cancers, about 15% of all sporadic colorectal cancers
also show a MSI-H phenotype, mostly due to promoter methylation of hMLH1.
Therefore, MSI analysis is an important tool for the identification of tumours
with MMR defects, but it cannot be used for the diagnosis of HNPCC. In MSI-
positive cancers, immunohistochemistry of hMLH1, hMSH2 and hMSH6 is

Table 4 Bethesda Guidelines for testing of colorectal tumours for microsatellite instability

1. Individuals with cancer in families that meet the Amsterdam Criteria.
2. Individuals with two HNPCC-related cancers, including synchronous and metachronous colorectal cancers or associated extracolonic cancers[a]
3. Individuals with colorectal cancer and a first-degree relative with colorectal cancer and/or HNPCC-related extracolonic cancer and/or a colorectal adenoma; age of the cancers diagnosed at age <45 years, and the adenoma diagnosed at age <40 years
4. Individuals with colorectal cancer or endometrial cancer diagnosed at age <45 years
5. Individuals with right-sided colorectal cancer with an undifferentiated pattern (solid/cribriform) on histopathology diagnosed at age <45 years[b]
6. Individuals with signet-ring-cell-type colorectal cancer diagnosed at age <45 years[c]
7. Individuals with adenoma diagnosed at age <40 years

[a] Endometrial, ovarian, gastric, hepatobiliary, or small-bowel cancer or transitional cell carcinoma of the renal pelvis or ureter.
[b] Solid/cribriform defined as poorly differentiated or undifferentiated carcinoma composed of irregular, solid sheets of large eosinophilic cells and containing small gland-like spaces.
[c] Composed of more than 50% signet-ring cells.

used for the detection of the mutated MMR gene, that is indicated by loss of protein expression in the tumour. However, immunohistochemistry alone also cannot be used to diagnose HNPCC, because: (1) cancers with sporadic mutations in one of the three MMR genes will display MMR protein loss; (2) HNPCC can be caused by genes other than hMLH1, hMSH2 and hMSH6; (3) subtly mutated proteins may retain antigenicity while losing function; (4) cancers in some HNPCC subjects may retain DNA repair proficiency; (5) not all HNPCC kindreds develop colorectal cancer; and (6) antigen retrieval may be technically difficult in old tissue blocks[21]. In addition to immunohistochemistry, various methods such as denaturing gradient gel electrophoresis (DGGE), single-strand conformational polymorphism (SSCP) analysis, heteroduplex analysis and the protein truncation test (PTT) are used as pre-screening tests for identification of the mutated MMR gene. Mutation analysis is then usually performed by sequencing the entire coding sequence including the exon–intron junction region of the MMR genes.

Despite all these advances diagnosis of HNPCC in an individual case can still be difficult. Detection rates of pathogenic germline mutations in HNPCC families by using all methods described above range between 50% and 70%[22], and discrimination of pathogenic mutations from insignificant polymorphisms could be difficult. In addition, other types of gene defect could cause HNPCC, as indicated by reports on promoter mutations in hMSH2[23] or exonic and promoter rearrangements of hMSH2[24]. Furthermore, additional still-unknown genes might cause HNPCC. Recently, germline defects in Exo I with so-far-unknown significance have been described in HNPCC patients[25]. Furthermore, HNPCC should be considered even in atypical families, e.g. due to germline mutations in hMSH6[3,6,26]. In addition, germline mutations in hMSH2 and hMLH1[27], as well as hMSH6[28,29], have been found in patients with microsatellite-stable tumours, suggesting that the absence of MSI should not definitely preclude mutation screening. Because of these difficulties, careful interpretation of the results from mutation analyses is necessary.

Since molecular testing implies diagnostic and therapeutic as well as psychosocial consequences, comprehensive genetic and clinical counselling is a prerequisite before initiation of mutation analysis

CLINICAL MANAGEMENT IN HNPCC

In families fulfilling the Amsterdam Criteria strict surveillance is recommended for the HNPCC patients and all relatives at risk. Identification of a specific germline mutation within a clinically suspected family enables predictive genetic testing of relatives in order to limit surveillance to asymptomatic germline mutation carriers. Family members lacking the identified germline mutation are assumed to have an average cancer risk and can be excluded from specific surveillance. If genetic testing fails to identify the germline mutation within an HNPCC family, all family members at risk should be included in surveillance measures. Recommendations for surveillance in HNPCC comprise regular examinations of the colon, endometrium, ovaries, urinary tract and stomach (Table 5)[30–35]. The clinical benefit of regular colonoscopic surveillance combined with polypectomy in terms of reduction of colorectal cancer, CRC-related deaths and decrease of overall mortality has been demonstrated after 10- and 15-year periods[36,37].

In contrast to FAP, recommendations on prophylactic surgery in HNPCC are controversial. Because of their substantial risk of metachronous and synchronous colorectal cancers, in HNPCC patients presenting with colorectal cancer, subtotal colectomy instead of standard oncological resection has to be considered[38,39]. However, because of a 3% risk for cancer development in the remaining rectum within a period of 3 years after colectomy, regular endoscopic examinations of the remaining rectum are required after colectomy. Recommendations concerning prophylactic surgery in asymptomatic germline mutation carriers of an HNPCC family are also controversial. Arguments against routine prophylactic colectomy are: (1) that the colorectal cancer risk in HNPCC is only about 80% (not 100% as in FAP) and to date no clear genotype–phenotype correlation exists to predict occurrence of colorectal cancer in persons at risk in an HNPCC family, (2) HNPCC tumours can be discovered at an early stage if regular colon

Table 5 Screening recommendations in HNPCC

	Age at start of screening (years)	Interval (years)
Colonoscopy	20–25	1 (–2)
Abdominal ultrasound	30–35	1 (–2)
Gynaecological examination (including transvaginal ultrasound, CA-125)	30–35	1 (–2)
Urine analysis	30–35	1 (–2)
Gastroscopy[a]	30–35	1 (–2)

[a] Only if it runs in the family.

screening is performed, (3) prognosis of HNPCC patients is supposed to be better than for sporadic colorectal cancers and may be further improved by endoscopic screening procedures. Therefore, detailed counselling on cancer risk, necessity of a lifelong clinical surveillance programme and preventive surgical procedures is substantial. The final decision on a clinical management strategy should be based on close cooperation between surgeons, gastroenterologists, human geneticists, gynaecologists, pathologists, molecular investigators and the individual patient.

Increasing knowledge concerning tumour biology raises questions on chemotherapy strategies in MSI-positive colorectal cancers in both sporadic forms and HNPCC. The most important agents used for adjuvant and palliative chemotherapy of colorectal cancers are 5-fluorouracil (mostly in combination with leucovorin), oxaliplatin and irinotecan. In-vitro studies have shown that colorectal cell lines defective in either hMLH1 or hMSH2 display significant resistance to a variety of cytotoxic agents including cisplatin and 5-fluorouracil[40,41], but no resistance to oxaliplatin[42], and even an increased sensitivity against the topoisomerase I inhibitor camptothecin, possibly indicating a better responsiveness of MSI-positive tumours to CPT11, a camptothecin derivate[43]. However, in retrospective studies, MSI was reported as a favourable prognostic indicator in patients with colorectal cancer receiving chemotherapy[44,45]. Further randomized clinical trials are needed to clarify this important issue.

References

1. Warthin AS. Heredity with reference to carcinoma. Arch Intern Med. 1913;12:546–55.
2. Lynch HT, Shaw MW, Magnuson CW, Larsen AL, Krush AJ. Hereditary factors in cancer. Study of two large midwestern kindreds. Arch Intern Med. 1966;117:206–12.
3. Akiyama Y, Sato H, Yamada T et al. Germ-line mutation of the hMSH6/GTBP gene in an atypical hereditary nonpolyposis colorectal cancer kindred. Cancer Res. 1997;57:3920–3.
4. Bronner CE, Baker SM, Morrison PT et al. Mutation in the DNA mismatch repair gene homologue hMLH1 is associated with hereditary non-polyposis colon cancer. Nature. 1994; 368:258–61.
5. Fishel R, Lescoe MK, Rao MR et al. The human mutator gene homolog MSH2 and its association with hereditary nonpolyposis colon cancer (published erratum appears in Cell. 1994; 77:167). Cell. 1993;75:1027–38.
6. Miyaki M, Konishi M, Tanaka K et al. Germline mutation of MSH6 as the cause of hereditary nonpolyposis colorectal cancer. Nat Genet. 1997;17:271–2.
7. Nicolaides NC, Papadopoulos N, Liu B et al. Mutations of two PMS homologues in hereditary nonpolyposis colon cancer. Nature. 1994;371:75–80.
8. Papadopoulos N, Nicolaides NC, Wei YF et al. Mutation of a mutL homolog in hereditary colon cancer (See comments). Science. 1994;263:1625–9.
9. Jass JR, Smyrk TC, Stewart SM, Lane MR, Lanspa SJ, Lynch HT. Pathology of hereditary nonpolyposis colorectal cancer. Anticancer Res. 1994;14:1631–4.
10. Jass JR, Do KA, Simms LA et al. Morphology of sporadic colorectal cancer with DNA replication errors. Gut. 1998; 42:673–9.
11. Lynch HT, Bardawil WA, Harris RE, Lynch PM, Guirgis HA, Lynch JF. Multiple primary cancers and prolonged survival: familial colonic and endometrial cancers. Dis Colon Rectum. 1978; 21:165–8.
12. Sankila R, Aaltonen LA, Jarvinen HJ, Mecklin JP. Better survival rates in patients with MLH1-associated hereditary colorectal cancer (See comments). Gastroenterology. 1996;110:682–7.
13. Myrhoj T, Bisgaard ML, Bernstein I, Svendsen LB, Sondergaard JO, Bulow S. Hereditary non-polyposis colorectal cancer: clinical features and survival. Results from the Danish HNPCC register. Scand J Gastroenterol. 1997;32:572–6.

14. Vasen HF, Mecklin JP, Khan PM, Lynch HT. The International Collaborative Group on Hereditary Non-Polyposis Colorectal Cancer (ICG-HNPCC). Dis Colon Rectum. 1991;34:424–5.
15. Vasen HF, Watson P, Mecklin JP, Lynch HT. New clinical criteria for hereditary nonpolyposis colorectal cancer (HNPCC, Lynch Syndrome) proposed by the International Collaborative Group on HNPCC. Gastroenterology. 1999;116:1453–6.
16. Rodriguez-Bigas MA, Boland CR, Hamilton SR *et al*. A National Cancer Institute Workshop on hereditary nonpolyposis colorectal cancer syndrome: meeting highlights and Bethesda guidelines (See comments). J Natl Cancer Inst. 1997;89:1758–62.
17. Syngal S, Fox EA, Eng C, Kolodner RD, Garber JE. Sensitivity and specificity of clinical criteria for hereditary non-polyposis colorectal cancer associated mutations in MSH2 and MLH1. J Med Genet. 2000;37:641–5.
18. Boland CR, Thibodeau SN, Hamilton SR *et al*. A National Cancer Institute Workshop on microsatellite instability for cancer detection and familial predisposition: development of international criteria for the determination of microsatellite instability in colorectal cancer. Cancer Res. 1998;58:5248–57.
19. Loukola A, Eklin K, Laiho P *et al*. Microsatellite marker analysis in screening for hereditary nonpolyposis colorectal cancer (HNPCC). Cancer Res. 2001;61:4545–9.
20. Cravo M, Lage P, Albuquerque C *et al*. BAT-26 identifies sporadic colorectal cancers with mutator phenotype: a correlative study with clinico-pathological features and mutations in mismatch repair genes. J Pathol. 1999;188:252–7.
21. Jass JR. hMLH1 and hMSH2 immunostaining in colorectal cancer. Gut. 2000;47:315–16.
22. Giardiello FM, Brensinger JD, Petersen GM. AGA technical review on hereditary colorectal cancer and genetic testing. Gastroenterology. 2001;121:198–213.
23. Shin KH, Shin JH, Kim JH, Park JG. Mutational analysis of promoters of mismatch repair genes hMSH2 and hMLH1 in hereditary nonpolyposis colorectal cancer and early onset colorectal cancer patients: identification of three novel germ-line mutations in promoter of the hMSH2 gene. Cancer Res. 2002;62:38–42.
24. Charbonnier F, Olschwang S, Wang Q *et al*. MSH2 in contrast to MLH1 and MSH6 is frequently inactivated by exonic and promoter rearrangements in hereditary nonpolyposis colorectal cancer. Cancer Res. 2002;62:848–53.
25. Wu Y, Berends MJ, Post JG *et al*. Germline mutations of EXO1 gene in patients with hereditary nonpolyposis colorectal cancer (HNPCC) and atypical HNPCC forms. Gastroenterology. 2001;120:1580–7.
26. Shin KH, Ku JL, Park JG. Germline mutations in a polycytosine repeat of the hMSH6 gene in Korean hereditary nonpolyposis colorectal cancer. J Hum Genet. 1999;44:18–21.
27. Farrington SM, Lin-Goerke J, Ling J *et al*. Systematic analysis of hMSH2 and hMLH1 in young colon cancer patients and controls. Am J Hum Genet. 1998;63:749–59.
28. Planck M, Koul A, Fernebro E *et al*. hMLH1, hMSH2 and hMSH6 mutations in hereditary nonpolyposis colorectal cancer families from southern Sweden. Int J Cancer. 1999;83: 197–202.
29. Wang Q, Lasset C, Desseigne F *et al*. Prevalence of germline mutations of hMLH1, hMSH2, hPMS1, hPMS2, and hMSH6 genes in 75 French kindreds with nonpolyposis colorectal cancer. Hum Genet. 1999;105:79–85.
30. Winawer SJ, Fletcher RH, Miller L *et al*. Colorectal cancer screening: clinical guidelines and rationale. Gastroenterology. 1997;112:594–642.
31. Burt RW. Colon cancer screening. Gastroenterology. 2000;119:837–53.
32. Souza RF. A molecular rationale for the how, when and why of colorectal cancer screening. Aliment Pharmacol Ther. 2001;15:451–62.
33. Weber T. ICG-HNPCC. Clinical surveillance recommendations adopted for HNPCC. Lancet. 2002;348:465.
34. Burke W, Petersen G, Lynch P *et al*. Recommendations for follow-up care of individuals with an inherited predisposition to cancer. I. Hereditary nonpolyposis colon cancer. Cancer Genetics Studies Consortium. J Am Med Assoc. 1997;277:915–19.
35. Schmiegel W, Adler G, Fruhmorgen P *et al*. [Colorectal carcinoma: prevention and early detection in an asymptomatic population – prevention in patients at risk – endoscopic diagnosis, therapy and after-care of polyps and carcinomas. German Society of Digestive and Metabolic Diseases/Study Group for Gastrointestinal Oncology]. Z Gastroenterol. 2000;38:49–75.
36. Jarvinen HJ, Mecklin JP, Sistonen P. Screening reduces colorectal cancer rate in families with hereditary nonpolyposis colorectal cancer (See comments). Gastroenterology. 1995;108:1405–11.

37. Jarvinen HJ, Aarnio M, Mustonen H et al. Controlled 15-year trial on screening for colorectal cancer in families with hereditary nonpolyposis colorectal cancer. Gastroenterology. 2000;118: 829–34.
38. Box JC, Rodriguez-Bigas MA, Weber TK, Petrelli NJ. Clinical implications of multiple colorectal carcinomas in hereditary nonpolyposis colorectal carcinoma. Dis Colon Rectum. 1999;42:717–21.
39. Church JM. Prophylactic colectomy in patients with hereditary nonpolyposis colorectal cancer. Ann Med. 1996;28:479–82.
40. Fink D, Aebi S, Howell SB. The role of DNA mismatch repair in drug resistance. Clin Cancer Res. 1998;4:1–6.
41. Carethers JM, Chauhan DP, Fink D et al. Mismatch repair proficiency and in vitro response to 5-fluorouracil. Gastroenterology. 1999;117:123–31.
42. Raymond E, Faivre S, Woynarowski JM, Chaney SG. Oxaliplatin: mechanism of action and antineoplastic activity. Semin Oncol. 1998;25(2 Suppl. 5):4–12.
43. Jacob S, Aguado M, Fallik D, Praz F. The role of the DNA mismatch repair system in the cytotoxicity of the topoisomerase inhibitors camptothecin and etoposide to human colorectal cancer cells. Cancer Res. 2001;61:6555–62.
44. Hemminki A, Mecklin JP, Jarvinen H, Aaltonen LA, Joensuu H. Microsatellite instability is a favorable prognostic indicator in patients with colorectal cancer receiving chemotherapy. Gastroenterology. 2000;119:921–8.
45. Elsaleh H, Joseph D, Grieu F, Zeps N, Spry N, Iacopetta B. Association of tumour site and sex with survival benefit from adjuvant chemotherapy in colorectal cancer. Lancet. 2000;355:1745–50.
46. Watson P, Lynch HT. Extracolonic cancer in hereditary nonpolyposis colorectal cancer. Cancer. 1993;71:677–85.
47. Aarnio M, Mecklin JP, Aaltonen LA, Nystrom-Lahti M, Jarvinen HJ. Life-time risk of different cancers in hereditary non-polyposis colorectal cancer (HNPCC) syndrome. Int J Cancer. 1995;64:430–3.
48. Vasen HF, Wijnen JT, Menko FH et al. Cancer risk in families with hereditary nonpolyposis colorectal cancer diagnosed by mutation analysis. Gastroenterology. 1996;110:1020–7.
49. Aarnio M, Sankila R, Pukkala E et al. Cancer risk in mutation carriers of DNA-mismatch-repair genes. Int J Cancer. 1999;81:214–18.
50. Sijmons RH, Kiemeney LA, Witjes JA, Vasen HF. Urinary tract cancer and hereditary nonpolyposis colorectal cancer: risks and screening options. J Urol. 1998;160:466–70.
51. Vasen HF, Stormorken A, Menko FH et al. MSH2 mutation carriers are at higher risk of cancer than MLH1 mutation carriers: a study of hereditary nonpolyposis colorectal cancer families. J Clin Oncol. 2001;19:4074–80.

12
Screening strategies for sporadic colorectal cancer (CRC) in the general population

C. POX, K. SCHULMANN and W. SCHMIEGEL

INTRODUCTION

Colorectal cancer has some characteristics that make it an ideal candidate for screening programmes:

1. A high incidence with a lifetime risk of around 6% in the general population.
2. The long-term survival rate is strongly influenced by the tumour stage at the time of diagnosis. If screening results in detecting CRC at an early stage this will have a positive effect on survival.
3. About 90% of CRC develop from adenomas, and it generally takes at least 10 years for the progression to an invasive CRC. Removing adenomas by polypectomy has been shown to decrease the cancer risk by up to 90%[1]. Screening methods that are able to detect adenomas which can then be removed before becoming carcinomas should therefore have an even greater effect on survival compared to detecting CRC at an early stage.

Screening would be most cost-effective if it included only the known risk groups (e.g. familial adenomatous polyposis (FAP), hereditary non-polyposis colorectal cancer (HNPCC) or patients with a positive family history. It is estimated, however, that at least 75% of CRC are diagnosed in persons not belonging to any of the known risk groups[2]. In order to have a measurable impact on CRC-related mortality any screening programme will therefore have to include the general population with an average CRC risk.

There are several different possibilities of screening strategies for the general population:

1. faecal occult blood testing (FOBT),
2. sigmoidoscopy ± FOBT,
3. colonoscopy,
4. double-contrast barium enema (DCBE),
5. virtual colonoscopy.

Table 1 Screening guidelines published

	Gastrointestinal consortium	American College of Gastroenterology	Deutsche Gesellschaft für Verdauungs- und Stoffwechselkrankheiten
Year of publication	1997	2000	2000
FOBT	Annually after age 50	Annually after age 50	Annually after age 50
Sigmoidoscopy	Every 5 years ± annual FOBT after age 50	Every 5 years ± annual FOBT after age 50	Every 5 years + annual FOBT after age 50
Colonoscopy	Every 10 years after age 50	Every 10 years after age 50	Every 10 years after age 55

Several guidelines with recommendations on the use of these tests for screening purposes have been published[2–4] (see Table 1).

FOBT

This test method, which detects blood in the stool, relies on the fact that colorectal neoplasms tend to bleed more often than normal mucosa. Most widely used are guaiac-based tests such as Hemoccult II. If blood is present in the stool the haemoglobin with its pseudoperoxidase activity will result in a blue colour change of the test field in the presence of hydrogen peroxide. The test slides typically contain two fields to which different parts of the stool are applied. Because some colorectal neoplasms will bleed only intermittently, testing several stool samples increases the yield. It has become standard to test three consecutive stools, i.e. to use three test slides for screening purposes. A test is positive if one or more of the six test fields turns blue. A positive test should be followed up by complete colonoscopy.

The sensitivity for detecting CRC using Hemoccult ranges from 46% to 92%. The sensitivity for detecting adenomas is lower (20–40%). The sensitivity can be improved by rehydrating the test fields; this, however decreases specificity. False-positive results may be caused by non-neoplastic bleeding sources such as angiodysplasia or diet.

There have been four large prospective randomized studies addressing effectiveness of FOBT[5–8]. For three of these studies mortality data have been published (Table 2)[5–7]. Two studies from Great Britain (Nottingham study) and Denmark (Funen study) used biennial testing without rehydrating test fields. Follow-up was 7.8 and 10 years, respectively. In the Funen study any positive test was recommended to be followed up by complete colonoscopy. In the Nottingham study a positive test had to be repeated and was followed up by colonoscopy only if the repeated test was also positive. The sensitivity of detecting CRC was determined to be 46% in the Funen study and 64% in the Nottingham study. The positive predictive value for CRC in the Nottingham study was 9.9% in the first screening round and 11.9% in the second; in the Funen study it was 17.7% in the first screening round and varied between 8.4%

Table 2 Randomized studies of FOBT screening

	Minnesota study	Nottingham study	Funen study
Author	Mandel et al.[5,10]	Hardcastle et al.[7]	Kronborg et al.[6]
Screening group	Annual test 15.570, biennial test 15.587	76.466	30.967
Control group	15.394	76.384	30.966
Rehydration of test fields	Yes	No	No
Follow-up (years)	18	7.8	13
Compliance:			
With any screening round	>90%	60%	67%
With every screening round	46–60%	38	46
Sensitivity for CRC (%)	92	64	46
PPV for CRC	2.2	9.9–11.9	8.4–17.7
Relative mortality reduction (%)	Annual test 33, biennial test 21	15	15

and 16.3% for the next four screening rounds. The CRC-related mortality was reduced by 15% in the Nottingham (7.8 years follow-up) and 18% in the Funen study (10 years follow-up). After 13 years' follow-up the CRC-related mortality of the Funen study has recently been reported as 15%[9]. For persons who took part in every screening round this reduction was increased to 30%.

A third US study (Minnesota study) compared annual and biennial testing and used rehydrated Hemoccult II tests[5]. Unlike the European studies this study was performed on volunteers. The positive predictive value was 2.2%, significantly lower than in the other two studies. This is explained by the rehydration of the Hemoccult slides which is known to increase sensitivity but reduces specificity. After 13 years' follow-up the CRC-related mortality reduction was 33% for the annual group and 6% for the biennial group. After 18 years' follow-up the mortality reduction remained at 33% for the annual group compared to a 21% reduction for the biennial screening group[10]. It could be demonstrated that the CRC risk reduction using FOBT is mainly due to finding CRC at an earlier stage. For the Minnesota study, which has the longest follow-up, it could also be shown that the CRC incidence in the screening group was lower compared to the control group[11]. This decrease is thought to be due to the removal of adenomas.

Compliance rates for taking part in at least one screening round in the studies have varied between >90% for the Minnesota study and 60% and 67% in the Nottingham and Funen studies, respectively.

It can thus be concluded that there is currently strong evidence for supporting the use of FOBT as a screening test for the general population. Although both European studies started screening at age 45 only a small percentage of cancers arises before age 50. In order to save financial resources it therefore seems reasonable to start screening at age 50, as in the Minnesota study. Because the Minnesota study showed better results for the annual screening group FOBT should be performed annually. Every positive FOBT has to be followed up by complete colonoscopy. The main disadvantage of FOBT is the moderate sensitivity for detecting CRC and the low sensitivity for adenomas. This has been the rationale for looking at endoscopic methods for screening.

SIGMOIDOSCOPY

The advantage of using sigmoidoscopy as a screening method is that unlike FOBT non-bleeding carcinomas and adenomas of the rectum and sigmoid can also be detected. About 40–60% of all adenomas and carcinomas are located within the reach of the sigmoidoscope. The sensitivity of detecting neoplasms is >90%, the perforation rate is low with only one perforation occurring in more than 40 000 examinations in a recently published study[12].

Three case–control studies looking at effectiveness have been published[13–15]. In one study the screening histories of people who died of CRC were compared with age- and sex-matched controls. It was found that sigmoidoscopy was associated with a 59% reduction in mortality from cancers in the part of the colon reached by the sigmoidoscope[15]. Another study reported an 80% reduction in the risk of death from rectosigmoid cancer in patients who had undergone one or more sigmoidoscopies compared to a control group that had never done so[14]. The third study again found a 59% CRC mortality reduction[13]. In this study the benefit of endoscopy was shown to last for at least 6 years. In the study by Selby et al. the effectiveness of sigmoidoscopy was similar for people who had undergone the procedure up to 10 years earlier[15]. After an initial negative sigmoidoscopy a control sigmoidoscopy on average 3.4 years after the first examination found an adenoma in 6% but no carcinomas or large adenomas[16].

In order to further assess the effectiveness of sigmoidoscopy as a screening method in the general population prospective randomized studies in the UK and the US have been undertaken. In the US trial a 5-year screening interval is currently being assessed[17]. The UK trial is comparing the efficacy of a one-time sigmoidoscopy at age 60 compared to a control group without any screening. The baseline findings of this study, which has recruited 170 000 participants, have recently been published[12]. Compliance with sigmoidoscopy was 71%. Rectosigmoid cancers were detected in 0.3%, distal adenomas in 12.1%. First mortality data should be available in 3 years.

It is well known that patients in whom distal adenomas are found during sigmoidoscopy have an increased risk of additional proximal neoplasms. It is therefore generally recommended[2] to perform a complete colonoscopy on patients with distal adenomas >1 cm. It is controversial, however, whether every patient with a small adenoma found during sigmoidoscopy has to be followed up by complete colonoscopy. The guidelines either recommend colonoscopy follow-up for every adenoma found during sigmoidoscopy, independent of size, number and histology[3,4], or recommend considering this approach depending on the patient[2]. One study[18] found proximal neoplasias in 29% of patients with a distal adenoma <5 mm, in another study 6.4% of patients with a distal tubular adenoma <10 mm had an advanced proximal neoplasia[19]. It thus seems reasonable to offer a complete colonoscopy to anyone with an adenoma found during sigmoidoscopy independent of adenoma characteristics.

Even if every adenoma found during sigmoidoscopy is followed up by a complete colonoscopy a significant number of patients with isolated proximal neoplasms will probably be missed. In a recently published study with asymptomatic persons between 50 and 75 years, 5.4% of patients had an advanced neoplasm proximal to the sigmoid[19]. Fifty-two per cent of these patients had no distal adenomas and would thus not have been diagnosed by sigmoidoscopy.

In order to be able to detect isolated proximal neoplasms the combination of sigmoidoscopy every 5 years and annual FOBT has been advocated[2,3]. There is only one study which prospectively compares sigmoidoscopy with the combination of sigmoidoscopy and FOBT[20]. In this study patients were randomized to an annual sigmoidoscopy with or without an additional annual FOBT. Compliance was poor, and although a greater reduction of CRC-related mortality was found for the combination screening group this was of borderline significance. In a recently published study 2885 asymptomatic subjects (age range 50–75 years) had a FOBT performed[21]. They then underwent a one-time colonoscopy. Defining sigmoidoscopy as examination of the rectum and sigmoid colon during colonoscopy, sigmoidoscopy would have identified 70% of subjects with advanced neoplasia, assuming that every distal adenoma would have resulted in a complete colonoscopy. FOBT had a sensitivity of 24% and the combination of sigmoidoscopy and FOBT was slightly more sensitive at detecting advanced neoplasms (76% vs. 70%) without reaching statistical significance. However, only 19% of isolated proximal advanced neoplasms would have been detected by FOBT. Even though it is unclear how much additional benefit the annual instead of the one-time FOBT would have, this study clearly shows that even the combination of sigmoidoscopy and FOBT does not seem to greatly improve detection rates for proximal neoplasms.

COLONOSCOPY

In order to be able to detect isolated proximal neoplasms colonoscopy is an alternative screening method. It has a proven high sensitivity for detecting carcinomas and adenomas of the whole colon. Tandem colonoscopies have shown miss rates between 15% and 24% for adenomas; however, larger adenomas ≥ 1 cm were rarely missed (0–6%)[22,23]. The caecum is reached in 93–99% of all procedures, depending on the skill of the endoscopist and the quality of bowel preparation[24,25]. A colonoscopy on average takes 22 minutes if no polyps are found; if a polypectomy is performed the examination time increases to 30 minutes[24]. One disadvantage of colonoscopy is the necessary bowel cleansing before the procedure. Morbidity of the procedure is also higher compared to sigmoidoscopy. One meta-analysis found perforation rates between 0.06% and 0.2% for diagnostic colonoscopies and between 0.04% and 0.5% if polypectomies are performed. Motality varies between 0% and 0.06%[26]. Although no randomized trials evaluating the use of colonoscopy for screening of the general population have been performed several guidelines have included colonoscopy as a screening option[2,4]. One recent guideline has even recommended colonoscopy as the preferred screening strategy[3]. Reasons for this recommendation have included the data on isolated proximal neoplasia and the logical thought that data concerning the effectiveness of sigmoidoscopy should also apply to colonoscopy, i.e. mortality reduction of up to 60%. It is estimated that a negative screening colonoscopy would not have to be repeated for 10 years. After an interval of 5.5 years no cancers were detected and the incidence of adenomas with advanced pathology was

<1%[27]. In a recently published case–control study the CRC risk reduction by endoscopy was 77% after a median of 7 years and seemed to last for more than 10 years with a risk reduction of 59% after a median of 19 years[28]. However, whereas the protective effect after 7 years was valid for cancers independent of their localization, the protective effect after 19 years was significant only for cancers of the rectosigmoid. Another case–control study also showed that endoscopy seemed to protect from rectosigmoid cancer for at least 10 years[15].

OTHER POSSIBLE SCREENING PROCEDURES

Double-contrast barium enema

Double-contrast barium enemas are infrequently used for screening purposes nowadays. They have been found to be less sensitive for the detection of colorectal neoplasms compared to colonoscopies[29,30]. The procedure also requires a thorough bowel preparation, and if a polyp or neoplasm is suspected an additional colonoscopy has to be performed.

Virtual colonoscopy

Virtual colonoscopy using either computerized tomography (CT) or magnetic resonance imaging (MRI) have also been evaluated as possible CRC screening methods. In one study comparing virtual CT and conventional colonoscopy in a group at high risk for colorectal neoplasia the sensitivity for detecting large polyps ≥1 cm was found to be 91% compared to 82% for medium-sized polyps (6–9 mm) and 55% for small polyps (≤5 mm)[31]. Other studies have reported much lower sensitivities[32,33]. One major disadvantage of CT virtual colonoscopy is the high radiation exposure. This is not a problem if MRI is used. In one study the results of conventional and virtual colonoscopy using MRI were compared in 132 patients with a possible colonic mass. MRI was found to have a sensitivity of 96% for detecting large polyps (>10 mm), 61% for medium polyps (6–10 mm) but only 6% for detecting polyps <6 mm[34]. Another study with 70 patients found sensitivities of 100% for large polyps, 96% for medium polyps and 33% for small polyps[35]. It therefore looks as if virtual colonoscopy has a fairly high sensitivity for detecting large polyps but is not able to detect most of the smaller polyps. It should also be considered that, like conventional colonoscopy, virtual colonoscopy requires a thorough bowel preparation. At this time the use of virtual colonoscopy outside of studies cannot be recommended.

Genetic stool testing

Ahlquist et al. used a panel of five genetic markers for the detection of stool alterations in patients with known CRC, adenomas >1 cm or endoscopically normal colons. The sensitivity was found to be 91% for cancers and 82 for adenomas with a specificity of 93%[36]. Traverso et al. were able to detect 61% of CRC and 50% of adenomas by using a digital protein truncation test applied to stool samples[37]. However, more research is needed before genetic testing can be recommended for screening purposes.

COST-EFFECTIVENESS

Several cost-effectiveness studies have been published. An analysis by Lieberman found a one-time colonoscopy to be the most effective method for reducing CRC mortality[38]. However, FOBT was the most cost-effective screening method, and screening by colonoscopy every 10 years was not examined. A more recent study compared the effectiveness of annual FOBT, sigmoidoscopy every 5 years and colonoscopy every 10 years[39]. Compared to no screening annual FOBT yielded an increase in survival at a cost of $9700 per life-year saved. Compared to FOBT the incremental cost-effectiveness of colonoscopy was only $11.380 per life-year gained, whereas the use of sigmoidoscopy would increase costs by $65.700 per life-year gained. In another study from the same year several screening methods were found to be cost-effective, with the combination of annual FOBT and sigmoidoscopy every 5 years being most effective[40]. All these studies are limited by their theoretical design having to include several variables and assumptions. Even so they all clearly show that screening for CRC in general seems to be cost-effective. This cost-effectiveness applies to different screening methods. The studies also show that screening effectiveness is greatly influenced by compliance.

The results of these cost-effectiveness studies are difficult to transfer to the German system. The cost of endoscopic procedures is a lot higher in the US than in Germany. Whereas a colonoscopy is considered to cost about $1000 in the US[40] in Germany reimbursement is around €130, making endoscopic screening methods significantly less expensive.

Current CRC screening recommendations in Germany

In Germany, up to 2002, CRC screening consisted of an annual FOBT beginning at age 45 as part of the recommended cancer screening. Compliance with this cancer screening programme has been low, with only 14% of eligible men and 34% of eligible women taking part[41]. In 2002 a new CRC screening programme is probably going to be implemented. It consists of annual FOBT from 50 to 54 and a colonoscopy every 10 years starting at age 55. The proposed costs for this screening programme are estimated to be around €160 million yearly, assuming a compliance of 50%.

CONCLUSIONS

For any CRC screening programme to be effective the general population must be included. There are several large prospective randomized trials clearly showing that FOBT is an effective screening method. However, its sensitivity for detecting CRC is fairly low, and even lower for detecting adenomas, the removal of which has been shown to be a very effective way of preventing CRC. Sigmoidoscopy has also been shown to be effective; in case–control studies it was able to reduce CRC-related mortality by at least 60%, making it likely to be more effective than FOBT for reducing mortality of rectosigmoid cancers. Although there is no prospective study assessing the appropriateness of colonoscopy for CRC screening the fact that it has a proven high sensitivity for detecting adenomas and CRC of the whole colon, and the data from sigmoidoscopy, as well as cost-effectiveness studies, seem to justify recommending its use for CRC screening and prevention. No matter which screening method is used its impact will be greatly influenced by the compliance it is able to achieve in the general population. Even if one considers colonoscopy to be the most effective method of preventing CRC, if a patient is only willing to perform a FOBT this is certainly much better than performing no screening. Every effort should be made to improve compliance with the existing screening recommendations in the general population.

References

1. Winawer SJ, Zauber AG, Ho MN et al. Prevention of colorectal cancer by colonoscopic polypectomy. The National Polyp Study Workgroup. N Engl J Med. 1993;329:1977–81.
2. Winawer SJ, Fletcher RH, Miller L et al. Colorectal cancer screening: clinical guidelines and rationale. Gastroenterology. 1997;112:594–642.
3. Rex DK, Johnson DA, Lieberman DA, Burt RW, Sonnenberg A. Colorectal cancer prevention 2000: screening recommendations of the American College of Gastroenterology. Am J Gastroenterol. 2000;95:868–77.
4. Schmiegel W, Adler G, Frühmorgen P et al. Kolorektales Karzinom: Prävention und Früherkennung in der asynmptomatischen Bevölkerung – Vorsorge bei Risikopatienten – Endoskopische Diagnostik, Therapie und Nachsorge von Polypen und Karzinomen. Z Gastroenterol. 2000;38:49–76.
5. Mandel JS, Bond JH, Church TR et al. Reducing mortality from colorectal cancer by screening for fecal occult blood. Minnesota Colon Cancer Control Study. N Engl J Med. 1993;328:1365–71.
6. Kronborg O, Fenger C, Olsen J, Jørgensen OD, Søndergaard O. Randomised study of screening for colorectal cancer with faecal-occult-blood test. Lancet. 1996;348:1467–71.
7. Hardcastle JD, Chamberlain JO, Robinson MH et al. Randomised controlled trial of faecal-occult-blood screening for colorectal cancer. Lancet. 1996;348:1472–7.
8. Kewenter J, Bjork S, Haglind E, Smith L, Svanvik J, Ahren C. Screening and rescreening for colorectal cancer. A controlled trial of fecal occult blood testing in 27,700 subjects. Cancer. 1988;62:645–51.
9. Jørgensen OD, Kronborg O, Fenger C. A randomised study of screening for colorectal cancer using faecal occult blood testing: results after 13 years and seven biennial screening rounds. Gut. 2002;50:29–32.
10. Mandel JS, Church TR, Ederer F, Bond JH. Colorectal cancer mortality: effectiveness of biennial screening for fecal occult blood. J Natl Cancer Inst. 1999;91:434–7.
11. Mandel JS, Church TR, Bond JH et al. The effect of fecal occult-blood screening on the incidence of colorectal cancer. N Engl J Med. 2000;343:1603–7.
12. UK Flexible Sigmoidoscopy Screening Trial Investigators. Single flexible sigmoidoscopy screening to prevent colorectal cancer: baseline findings of a UK multicentre randomised trial. Lancet. 2002;359:1291–300.
13. Muller AD, Sonnenberg A. Protection by endoscopy against death from colorectal cancer. A case–control study among veterans. Arch Intern Med. 1995;155:1741–8.
14. Newcomb PA, Norfleet RG, Storer BE, Surawicz TS, Marcus PM. Screening sigmoidoscopy and colorectal cancer mortality. J Natl Cancer Inst. 1992;84:1572–5.
15. Selby JV, Friedman GD, Quesenberry CP, Weiss NS. A case–control study of screening sigmoidoscopy and mortality from colorectal cancer. N Engl J Med. 1992;326:653–7.
16. Rex DK, Lehman GA, Ulbright TM, Smith JJ, Hawes RH. The yield of a second screening flexible sigmoidoscopy in average-risk persons after one negative examination. Gastroenterology. 1994;106:593–5.
17. Prorok PC, Andriole GL, Bresalier RS et al. Design of the prostate, lung, colorectal and ovarian (PLCO) cancer screening trial. Control Clin Trials. 2000;21:273–309S.
18. Read TE, Read JD, Butterly LF. Importance of adenomas 5 mm or less in diameter that are detected by sigmoidoscopy. N Engl J Med. 1997;336:8–12.

19. Lieberman DA, Weiss DG, Bond JH, Ahnen DJ, Garewal H, Chejfec G. Use of colonoscopy to screen asymptomatic adults for colorectal cancer. N Engl J Med. 2000;343:162–8.
20. Winawer SJ, Flehinger BJ, Schottenfeld D, Miller DG. Screening for colorectal cancer with fecal occult blood testing and sigmoidoscopy. J Natl Cancer Inst. 1993;85:1311–18.
21. Lieberman DA, Weiss DG. One-time screening for colorectal cancer with combined fecal occult-blood testing and examination of the distal colon. N Engl J Med. 2001;345:555–60.
22. Hixson LJ, Fennerty MB, Sampliner RE, McGee D, Garewal H. Prospective study of the frequency and size distribution of polyps missed by colonoscopy. J Natl Cancer Inst. 1990;82:1769–72.
23. Rex DK, Cutler CS, Lemmel GT et al. Colonoscopic miss rates of adenomas determined by back-to-back colonoscopies. Gastroenterology. 1997;112:24–8.
24. Lieberman DA, Smith FW. Screening for colon malignancy with colonoscopy. Am J Gastroenterol. 1991;86:946–51.
25. Rogge JD, Elmore MF, Mahoney SJ et al. Low-cost, office-based, screening colonoscopy. Am J Gastroenterol. 1994;86:946–51.
26. Froehlich F, Gonvers J-J, Vader J-P, Dubois RW, Burnand B. Appropriateness of gastrointestinal endoscopy: risk of complications. Endoscopy. 1999;31:684–6.
27. Rex DK, Cummings OW, Helper DJ et al. 5-year incidence of adenomas after negative colonoscopy in asymptomatic average-risk persons. Gastroenterology. 1996;111:1178–81.
28. Brenner H, Arndt V, Stürmer T, Stegmaier C, Ziegler H, Dhrm G. Long-lasting reduction of risk of colorectal cancer following screening endoscopy. Br J Cancer. 2001;85:972–6.
29. Winawer SJ, Stewart ET, Zauber AG et al. A comparison of colonoscopy and double-contrast barium enema for surveillance after polypectomy. N Engl J Med. 2000;342:1766–72.
30. Rex DK, Rahmani EY, Haseman JH, Lemmel GT, Kaster S, Buckley JS. Relative sensitivity of colonoscopy and barium enema for detection of colorectal cancer in clinical practice. Gastroenterology. 1997;112:17–23.
31. Fenlon HM, Nunes DP, Schroy III PC, Barish MA, Clarke PD, Ferrucci JT. A comparison of virtual and conventional colonoscopy for the detection of colorectal polyps. N Engl J Med. 1999;341:1496–503.
32. Pescatore P, Glücker T, Delarive J et al. Diagnostic accuracy and interobserver agreement of CT colonography (virtual colonoscopy). Gut. 2000;47:126–30.
33. Spinzi G, Belloni G, Martegani A, Sangiovani A, Del Favero C, Minoli G. Computed tomographic colonography and conventional colonoscopy for colon diseases: a prospective blinded study. Am J Gastroenterol. 2001;96:394–400.
34. Luboldt W, Bauerfeind P, Wildermuth S, Marincek B, Fried M, Debatin JF. Colonic masses: detection with MR colonography. Radiology. 2000;216:383–8.
35. Pappalardo G, Polettini E, Frattaroli FM et al. Magnetic resonance colonography versus conventional colonoscopy for the detection of colonic endoluminal lesions. Gastroenterology. 2000;119:300–4.
36. Ahlquist DA, Skoletsky JE, Boynton KA et al. Colorectal cancer screening by detection of altered human DNA in stool: feasibility of a multitarget assay panel. Gastroenterology. 2000;119:1219–27.
37. Traverso G, Shuber A, Levin B et al. Detection of APC mutations in fecal DNA from patients with colorectal tumors. N Engl J Med. 2002;346:311–20.
38. Lieberman DA. Cost-effectiveness model for colon cancer screening. Gastroenterology. 1995;109:1781–90.
39. Sonnenberg A, Delcó F, Inadomi JM. Cost-effectiveness of colonoscopy in screening for colorectal cancer. Ann Intern Med. 2000;133:573–84.
40. Frazier AL, Colditz GA, Fuchs CS, Kuntz KM. Cost-effectiveness of screening for colorectal cancer in the general population. J Am Med Assoc. 2000;284:1954–61.
41. Gesetzliche Krankheitsfrüherkennungsmaßnahmen. Dokumentation der Untersuchungsergebnisse – Männer und Frauen – Krebs 1989 und 1990. Kassenärztliche Bundesvereinigung und Spitzenverbände der Krankenkassen.

Section IV
Noxious dietary compounds

13
Red meat: a dietary risk factor for colorectal cancer?

H. BOEING, E. RIBOLI and T. NORAT

In the past, the coincidence of Western lifestyle with high rates of colorectal cancer has led to the idea that specific components of the Western diet might be linked with this disease. Ecological studies comparing country-specific food balance information on various food items with the observed rates of colorectal cancer identified meat as one of the promising dietary candidates affecting disease risk. The correlation of meat intake in a country with mortality rates from colorectal cancer was one of the strongest, and for example Armstrong and Doll, 1975, decided to show a graph on this issue in their well-known publication[1]. Thus, meat was in the minds of many oncologists since the early days of research into nutrition and cancer, and was considered a hot candidate for a causal link between dietary habits and risk of colorectal cancer.

Thereafter epidemiological methodology proceeded and individual-based study designs became more important. Individual-based study designs generate stronger evidence regarding a causal link between a factor and disease risk than ecological studies because exposure and disease endpoints are directly studied in human subjects. In the past, case-control and recently cohort studies have investigated whether meat consumption is associated with an increased risk of colorectal cancer. Other areas of research were opened up in the field of toxicological evaluation of meat and meat products, especially when being prepared. Several compounds of meat were found to be carcinogenic in experimental studies, including animal models. Most of these compounds are particularly formed during meat preparation and include, among others, heterocyclic aromatic amines, polycyclic hydrocarbons, and N-nitroso compounds. Carcinogenic or mutagenic compounds of meat and meat products and the underlying carcinogenic mechanisms are discussed separately in this book (Chapter 7, this volume).

However, there are more substances in meat and meat products than the typical carcinogens which are worthwhile to be considered as possible causal links between meat consumption and risk of colorectal cancer. Since ancient times, meat has been considered to be an excellent source of energy and energy-providing nutrients and of some of the essential nutrients, such as iron. The contribution of meat to fat and energy intake is high in some human dietary regimens. Obesity, as a consequence of a positive energy balance that might be partly caused by high fat intake, is a well established risk factor for colon cancer[2]. There is also some evidence that saturated fat in particular increases the risk of colon cancer independently of energy (Chapter 14, this volume). A high protein intake through meat and meat products may increase the risk of colorectal cancer by raising the intraluminal pH level and/or the production of ammonia in the colon lumen[3]. However, during the last four decades, the dietary composition of meat has changed. Nowadays the fat content of meat is much lower than in previous times. Whether this change in the dietary composition of meat is meaningful in terms of risk remains a study area of the future.

Meat is an excellent source of iron. In fresh meat, iron is bound mostly to myoglobin and only to a lesser extent to haemoglobin. Myoglobin and haemoglobin are part of the haeme-iron fraction, whereas plant sources of iron form the non-haeme fraction. The haeme-iron in its reduced form as Fe^{2+} is preferentially absorbed in the human gut. The oxidized form of iron needs to be reduced in the gut before absorption and therefore usually has a low absorption rate. High levels of iron stores are indicated by high transferrin saturation and increased ferritin levels in peripheral blood and are often associated with a meat-rich diet. However, the exact availability of iron from meat depends on the actual meat handling procedures. After slaughtering myoglobin is partly oxidized to oxymyoglobin (Fe^{3+}) that changes the colour of meat from red to brown. Today the treatment of meat is directed to increase the amount of myoglobin in meat compared with other forms. Another mode of preserving the colour and protecting meat from harmful bacterial growth is to cure meat with nitrite and salt. Curing of meat results in the formation of nitrosomyoglobin, also a Fe^{2+} product. If cured meat is heated, nitrosohaemochrome develops, also having the Fe^{2+} loading preferentially absorbed. However the fate of the different myoglobin products in the gastrointestinal tract of humans is still unknown in quantitative terms[4].

There is a lack of good survey data about the quantitative amounts to fresh meat being consumed, and the various forms of meat being preserved by nitrite. About 90% of the processed meat in Germany is cured. It seems that the curing of meat is higher in Europe than in the US, and in the North of Europe higher than in the South of Europe. In the near future the situation in the European cohorts of EPIC (European Prospective Investigation into Cancer and Nutrition) on meat preparation methods is going to be published[5].

A major hypothesis on the harmful role of iron concerns augmenting oxygen radical synthesis by the Haber-Weis or Fenton reaction. This hypothesis is derived from results of *in vitro* and *in vivo* animal studies. Thus, it might be useful to review the studies that looked at the effect of iron intake and iron status on risk of colorectal cancer. A summary of the results of case–control and cohort studies that investigated the role of iron on risk for colorectal cancer and colorectal adenomas in humans is already available in the literature[6]. A focus will be given on the results of cohort studies due to its high-quality design, with colorectal cancer as the endpoint. Iron exposure was defined as intake of dietary iron, iron stores, and hereditary haemochromatosis. The latter is a genetic disorder due to a polymorphism (C282Y mutation) in the haemochromatosis gene that

Table 1 Cohort studies on dietary iron and iron status and risk of colorectal cancer

Study population (cases/cohort size)	Study results[a]	Study reference
Dietary iron		
136/8876	+	NHANES I-Follow up, USA[b]
105/15 785	0	NY Women's Health, USA[c]
Iron load		
126/8345	+	NHANES I-Follow up, USA[b]
441/38 600	−	Kaiser Permanente, USA[d]
173/41 300	0	Mobile Health Clinic, Finland[e]
11/1200	+	Mobile Health Clinic, Finland subjects with transferrin saturation >60%[e]
105/15 785	0	NY Women's Health[c]

[a] +, positive relationship; −, inverse relationship; 0, no significant relationship;
[b] Wurzelmann et al. 1996[14]; [c] Kato et al. 1999[15]; [d] Herrington et al. 1995[16]; [e] Knekt et al. 1994[17].

generates a protein regulating iron storage and absorption. Carriers of this polymorphism often experience high iron loads in their bodies.

A high dietary iron intake will lead to a high availability of iron in the gut lumen and thus test whether iron plays particularly an intraluminal role. A high iron store tests whether the effect of iron is due to its increased concentration in body fluids and/or specific compartments. Two prospective cohort studies have tested the dietary hypothesis so far and five the latter iron load hypothesis (Table 1). For both hypotheses, no consistent results exist and even inverse relationships could be observed. However, the two studies on dietary iron do agree in that a non-significant increase in risk in the proximal part of the colon was observed. Markers of iron load, such as serum ferritin levels and transferrin saturation, are liable to be influenced by inflammation status and are probably not very sensitive to iron overload. This might be one reason that the current cohort studies are not consistent in their results. In case-control studies, the subjects who were homo- or heterozygous carriers of the polymorphism predisposing for hereditary haemochromatosis did not experience a higher risk of colorectal cancer across studies so far[7–9].

Although the evidence is weak, we cannot refute the idea that iron is directly linked to risk of colorectal cancer. Interactions may also exist between the mechanism of oxygen radical generation by iron and other food substances. In general, antioxidative compounds interplay with radical formation and dietary fibre and its phytic acid forms phytate with iron and other minerals[10]. Another mechanism by which iron may interfere with colorectal cancer is constipation, occasionally a consequence of high iron provision.

Subsequently, we investigate the evidence that the consumption of meat and meat products is linked with risk of colorectal cancer. The individual-based cohort and case–control studies conducted so far on this question are taken as the source of information. Ninety-nine studies of this type were identified up to 1999, which, in addition, present quantitative data on meat consumption and relative risk estimates.

These studies were first analysed regarding their published relative risk estimates[11]. Here we display the results separately for total meat (Table 2), red meat

Table 2 Summary of study results on total meat up to 1999 (adapted from Norat and Riboli 2001[11])

	Relative risk				
	<1 S[a]	<1.5 NS[b]	>1.5 NS[c]	>1 S[d]	Number of studies
Case–control studies	3	22	6	5	36
Cohort studies	—	6	3	1	10

[a] Significant inverse relationships; [b] non-significant studies with relative risk estimates less than 1.5; [c] non-significant studies with relative risk estimates higher than 1.5; [d] studies with a significant positive association.

Table 3 Summary of study results on red meat up to 1999 (adapted from Norat and Riboli 2001[11])

	Relative risk				
	<1 S[a]	<1.5 NS[b]	>1.5 NS[c]	>1 S[d]	Number of studies
Case–control studies	1	15	2	8	26
Cohort studies	—	7	1	2	10

[a] Significant inverse relationships; [b] non-significant studies with relative risk estimates less than 1.5; [c] non-significant studies with relative risk estimates higher than 1.5; [d] studies with a significant positive association.

Table 4 Summary of study results on processed meat up to 1999 (adapted from Norat and Riboli 2001[11])

	Relative risk				
	<1 S[a]	<1.5 NS[b]	>1.5 NS[c]	>1 S[d]	Number of studies
Case–control studies	1	18	1	13	33
Cohort studies	—	3	1	2	6

[a] Significant inverse relationships; [b] non-significant studies with relative risk estimates less than 1.5; [c] non-significant studies with relative risk estimates higher than 1.5; [d] studies with a significant positive association.

(Table 3) and processed meat (Table 4). The studies were categorized into those with significant inverse relationships, non-significant studies with relative risk estimates less than 1.5, non-significant studies with relative risk estimates higher than 1.5 and studies with a significant positive association. From the 36 case–control studies on total meat, the majority fell into the category of non-significant studies with relative risk less than 1.5. The same was observed for the cohort studies. With respect to red meat (Table 3), more studies now exist than those of total meat that were significantly positive. This picture of an increasing percentage of studies with a positive link with risk of colorectal cancer was further extended when processed meat is considered (Table 4). The last table highlights the fact

Table 5   Dose–response analysis between intake of total meat (120 g/day) and risk of colorectal cancer (adapted from Norat and Riboli 2001[12])

	Relative risk (95% CI)	Number of studies
All studies	1.12 (0.98–1.30)	18
Case–control	1.10 (0.94–1.29)	13
Cohort	0.99 (0.71–1.39)	5
Males	1.07 (0.85–1.34)	6
Females	0.87 (0.72–1.09)	6
Europe	1.26 (1.05–1.51)	9
USA	1.04 (0.75–1.45)	5

CI, confidence interval.

Table 6   Dose–response analysis between intake of red meat (120 g/day) and risk of colorectal cancer (adapted from Norat and Riboli 2001[12])

	Relative risk (95% CI) Number of studies	
All studies	1.24 (1.08–1.41)	17
Case–control	1.26 (1.02–1.55)	8
Cohort	1.22 (1.05–1.41)	9
Males	1.36 (1.18–1.55)	9
Females	1.11 (0.78–1.56)	8
Europe	1.56 (1.07–2.26)	5
USA	1.22 (1.05–1.41)	10

CI, confidence interval.

that, if there is any link of meat with colorectal cancer, the risk will probably be due mostly to processed meat and, to a lesser extent, to red meat consumption rather than to total meat consumption.

In a second recent publication, the quantitative effect of meat consumption on risk of colorectal cancer, taking the studies published in the period between 1973 and 1999, was estimated[12]. The most important results of the dose–response analysis, including selected subgroup analyses, are listed in Tables 5–7. This quantitative meta-analysis gave a non-significant result for total meat considering the 18 eligible studies on this topic (Table 5). Subgroup analysis identified the 9 European studies showing a significant increased relative risk of the order of 1.26 (95% confidence interval 1.05–1.51) for each increment of intake of total meat by 120 g/day. All other presented subgroup analyses were non-significant. Red meat consumption was evaluated in 17 studies showing a significant increase in relative risk of 1.24 (95% confidence interval 1.08–1.41) for each increment of intake of red meat by 120 g/day (Table 6). Subgroup analyses were also significantly positive for all categories except for fresh meat. The effect of processed meat on risk of colorectal cancer was evaluated in 16 studies (Table 7). The summary figure revealed an increase in relative risk of 1.36 (95% confidence interval 1.15–1.61) per 30 g of intake. The smaller amount was taken because of the traditionally lower amount of intake of processed meat compared with fresh meat.

Table 7 Dose–response analysis between intake of processed meat (30 g/day) and risk of colorectal cancer (adapted from Norat and Riboli 2001[12])

	Relative risk (95% CI)	Number of studies
All studies	1.36 (1.15–1.61)	16
Case–control	1.37 (1.13–1.66)	9
Cohort	1.54 (1.10–2.17)	7
Males	1.48 (1.08–2.04)	6
Females	1.44 (1.10–1.89)	4
Europe	1.39 (1.09–1.77)	8
USA	1.54 (1.32–1.78)	6

CI, confidence interval.

The meta-analysis clearly identified processed meat as one of the dietary components associated with a modest increase in risk. The relative risk associated with consumption of processed meat stands out compared with total meat and red meat. Total meat, including poultry and fish, was not related to risk of colorectal cancer except for European countries. In these countries, it is probable that a higher proportion of total meat is eaten as processed meat than in other countries. Red meat, in particular if eaten partly as processed meat, could also be linked with a moderate increase in relative risk for colorectal cancer.

In the future there will be several research directions trying to shed more light on this issue. First, more epidemiological studies will be published which provide a broader basis for subsequent quantitative meta-analyses. It would be useful if the investigators of future studies describe meat consumption in a comparable way. Second, we need to learn more about meat and processed meat and the carcinogenic mechanisms behind this food group. This may especially revive the research into N-nitroso compounds and their role in colorectal carcinogenesis[13]. Third, we may use the progress made in genetics of xenobiotic metabolisms to identify those substances in meat and meat preparation which are causally linked to colorectal cancer. This strategy will identify pathways in which genetic variants play a functional role and lead to investigations on interactions between genotype and exposure in the epidemiological studies.

References

1. Armstrong B, Doll R. Environmental factors and cancer incidence and mortality in different countries, with special reference to dietary practices. Int J Cancer. 1975;15:617–31.
2. IARC Handbooks of cancer prevention No 6. Weight control and physical activity. Lyon: IARC Press, 2002.
3. West DW, Slattery ML, Robison LM et al. Dietary intake and colon cancer: Sex- and anatomic site-specific associations. Am J Epidemiol. 1989;130:883–94.
4. Sakata R, Honikel KO. Untersuchungen zu physikalisch-chemischen Eigenschaften roter Pigmente in Fleischerzeugnissen. Fleischwirtschaft. 2001;5:182–90.
5. Rohrmann S, Linseisen J, Becker N et al. Cooking of meat and fish in Europe – Results from the European Prospective Investigation into Cancer and Nutrition (EPIC). Eur J Clin Nutr. 2002.
6. Nelson RL. Iron and colorectal cancer risk: Human studies. Nutr Rev. 2001;59:140–8.
7. Beckmann LE, Van Landeghem GF, Sikstrom C et al. Interaction between haemochromatosis and transferrin receptor genes in different neoplastic disorders. Carcinogenesis. 1999;20:1231–3.

8. Altes A, Gimferrer E, Capella G, Barcelo MJ, Baiget M. Colorectal cancer and HFE gene mutations. Haematologica. 1999;84:479–80.

9. Macdonald GA, Tarish J, Whitehall VJ *et al.* No evidence of increased risk of colorectal cancer in individuals heterozygous for the Cys282Tyr haemochromatosis mutation. J Gastroenterol Hepatol. 1999;14:1188–91.

10. Graf E, Eaton JW. Dietary suppression of colonic cancer: fiber or phytate? Cancer. 1985; 56:717–18.

11. Norat T, Riboli E. Meat consumption and colorectal cancer: A review of epidemiologic evidence. Nutr Rev. 2001;59:37–47.

12. Norat T, Lukanova A, Ferrari P, Riboli E. Meat consumption and colorectal cancer risk: Dose-response meta-analysis of epidemiological studies. Int J Cancer. 2002;98:241–56.

13. Hughes R, Cross AJ, Pollock JR, Bingham S. Dose-dependent effect of dietary meat on endogenous colonic N-nitrosation. Carcinogenesis. 2001;22:199–202.

14. Wurzelmann JI, Silver A, Schreinemachers DM, Sandler RS, Everson RB. Iron intake and the risk of colorectal cancer. Cancer Epidem Biomar. 1996;5:503–7.

15. Kato I, Dnistrian AM, Schwartz M *et al.* Iron intake body stores and colorectal cancer risk in women: A nested case-control study. Int J Cancer. 1999;80:693–8.

16. Herrington L, Friedman GD, Baer D, Selby JV. Transferrin saturation and risk of cancer. Am J Epidemiol. 1995;142:692–8.

17. Knekt P, Reunanen A, Takkunen H, Aromaa A, Heliövaara M, Hakulinen T. Body iron stores and risk of cancer. Int J Cancer. 1994;56:379–82.

14
Types of dietary fat and colon cancer risk

B. S. REDDY, Y. HIROSE and C. V. RAO

INTRODUCTION

Cancer of the large bowel is one of the leading causes of cancer deaths in both men and women in Western countries, including the United States where about 150 000 new cases of this cancer and 56 000 related deaths were reported for the year 2000[1]. Marked international differences in the incidence and mortality of colon cancer and increase of risk in populations migrating from low- to high-risk areas suggest that environmental factors, specifically dietary habits, play an important role in the aetiology of this cancer. Importantly, nutritional epidemiological studies conducted in Japan point to the fact that the increase in colon cancer in Japan has been attributed to Westernization of Japanese food habits[2]. Diet, especially fat intake, has received considerable interest as a possible risk factor in the aetiology of colorectal cancer. The purpose of this chapter is to provide a brief overview of epidemiological evidence on the association between dietary fat and colon cancer risk, and to discuss the results of preclinical (laboratory animal model) studies conducted in our laboratory on the relationship between the types of dietary fat and colon cancer.

EPIDEMIOLOGIC EVIDENCE

Based on comparative date and case–control studies in Japan and the United States in the late 1960s, Wynder *et al.*[3] suggested that colon cancer risk is mainly associated with dietary fat. This pioneering study led to several ecological and case–control studies on the relationship between dietary fat and colon cancer[4-6]. Since then several epidemiological studies have been conducted to understand the relationship between dietary factors and colon cancer risk, but the conduct and interpretation of some of these well-designed studies have been complicated by inherent problems in testing dietary hypotheses because of the lack of an accurate method of measurement of types of dietary fat in populations being studied. The importance of types of dietary fat differing in fatty acid composition rather than total fat cannot be discounted, because several preclinical studies strongly supported the notion that the colon tumour-promoting effect of dietary fat depends on the types of dietary fat[7]. A recent report by the AICR/WCRF expert panel came to a scientific consensus that evidence for an association between the intake of saturated fat and/or animal fat and colon cancer risk is very strong[6]. A recent ecological study suggests that mortality data for colorectal cancer in 22 European countries, the United States, and Canada, correlate with the consumption of animal fat[8]. That eating a diet with high polyunsaturated fat rich in omega-3 fatty acids may decrease the risk of colorectal cancer has been hypothesized in relation to fish and fish oil[8]. Caygill and Hill[9] reported an inverse correlation between fish and fish oil consumption and colorectal cancer. On the basis of epidemiological evidence it is reasonable to suggest that diets high in saturated fat increase the risk of colorectal cancers, whereas diets high in fish and fish oil reduce the risk.

PRECLINICAL STUDIES

Laboratory animal studies have provided convincing evidence that not only the amount but also types of dietary fat differing in fatty acid composition are important factors in determining the modulating effect of this nutrient in colon tumour development[7,10–12]. Investigations were carried out in our laboratory to evaluate the effect of diets containing 5% and 20% beef fat on colon carcinogenesis by a variety of colon-specific carcinogens including 1,2-dimethylhydrazine, methylazoxymethanol acetate, 3,2'-dimethyl-4-aminobiphenyl or methylnitrosourea[13]. In these studies semipurified diets containing 5% and 20% beef fat were fed to male F344 rats before, during, and after carcinogen treatment, to study the effect of animal fat on the initiation and post-initiation stages of colon carcinogenesis. These studies indicate that, irrespective of colon carcinogens used to induce colon tumours, diet containing a high amount of beef fat had a greater colon tumour-promoting effect than the diet low in such fat. Additional studies conducted in our laboratory also demonstrate that male F344 rats fed the diets containing 20% lard or 20% corn oil were more susceptible to 1,2-dimethylhydrazine-induced colon carcinogenesis compared with those fed the diets containing 5% lard or 5% corn oil[14]. These studies provided evidence that diet containing high amounts of beef fat or lard, saturated fat of animal origin or corn oil, high in omega-6 polyunsaturated fatty acids had a greater colon tumour-enhancing effect than the diet low in fat.

Further studies in our laboratory have evaluated the modulating effects of high dietary safflower oil and corn oil rich in polyunsaturated fatty acid linoleic acid, olive oil high in monounsaturated fatty acid oleic acid, coconut oil high in medium-chain fatty acids such as lauric acid, and fish oil rich in omega-3 fatty acids such as docosahexaenoic acid and eicosapentaenoic acid during the post-initiation stage of azoxymethane-induced colon carcinogenesis in male F344 rats[11]. Animals fed the diets containing high corn oil or high safflower oil (23.5%) had a higher incidence of colon tumours than did those fed the diets low in fat (5%). By contrast, diets high in coconut oil, olive oil or menhaden fish oil had no such colon tumour-enhancing effect (Table 1). The varied effects of different types of fat on colon carcinogenesis during the post-initiation stage suggest that fatty acid composition is one of the determining factors in colon tumour promotion by a dietary fat, and that the influence of type and amount of dietary fat is exerted during the post-initiation phase of carcinogenesis[11,15,16]. In a phase II clinical trial of patients with colonic polyps, dietary fish oil supplements have inhibited cell proliferation in the colonic mucosa[17].

Thus far, progress has been made with regard to the relationship between dietary fat intake and colon cancer risk, in that we know of the tumour-promoting effects of diets rich in omega-6 fatty acids and saturated fatty acids, and the lack of such effects by omega-3 fatty acid-rich diets. However, it should be recognized that, among the sources of dietary fat, animal fat with its high saturated fatty acid content is by far the most important contributor, amounting to about 60% of the Western diet. Importantly, dietary fat intake in the United States and Canada, and other Western countries where colon cancer rates are high, consists predominantly of a mixture of saturated, monounsaturated, and polyunsaturated fats[6,18]. A recent study in mice demonstrated that high dietary fat simulating mixed lipid composition of the average Western-style diet produced dysplastic lesions in the colon, indicative of tumorigenesis[19].

In view of the significance of mixed lipids in colon cancer, and because of potential tumour-inhibitory properties of omega-3 fatty acids, we have conducted a study to examine the effects of high-fat diets that contain mixed lipids

Table 1 Effect of types and amount of dietary fat on azoxymethane(AOM)-induced colon carcinogenesis in F344 rats

Experiment no.	Reference no.	Dietary treatment		Male (M) or female (F)	Percentage of animals with colon tumours
1	11	5% corn oil	AOM, 20 mg/kg body weight, once, s.c.	F	17*
		23.5% corn oil	AOM, 20 mg/kg body weight, once, s.c.	F	46
		5% safflower oil	AOM, 20 mg/kg body weight, once, s.c.	F	13*
		23.5% safflower oil	AOM, 20 mg/kg body weight, once, s.c.	F	36
		5% olive oil	AOM, 20 mg/kg body weight, once, s.c.	F	10
		23.5% olive oil	AOM, 20 mg/kg body weight, once, s.c.	F	13
		23.5% coconut oil	AOM, 20 mg/kg body weight, once, s.c.	F	13
2	13	5% corn oil	AOM, 50 mg/kg body weight, once, s.c.	M	54
		23.5% corn oil	AOM, 50 mg/kg body weight, once, s.c.	M	92
		4% fish oil + 1% corn oil	AOM, 50 mg/kg body weight, once, s.c.	M	50†
		22.5% fish oil + 1% corn oil	AOM, 50 mg/kg body weight, once, s.c.	M	33†

* Significantly different from their respective high-fat diet ($p < 0.05$).
† Significantly different from high-fat corn oil diet ($p < 0.05$).
s.c. = Subcutaneously.

Table 2 Effect of type and amount of dietary fat on azoxymethane-induced colon tumour incidence and multiplicity during different stages of carcinogenesis

Dietary treatment	Tumour incidence (percentage of animals with tumours)			Tumour multiplicity (no. of tumours/rat)[b]		
	23 weeks	38 weeks		23 weeks	38 weeks	
	Total[a]	Total[a]	Adenocarcinomas	Total[a]	Total	Adenocarcinomas
LFCO	50	63	57.8	0.75 ± 0.12	1.31 ± 0.22	1.18 ± 0.18
HFML	80[c]	100[d]	100[d]	1.50 ± 0.20[c]	5.14 ± 0.34[e]	4.70 ± 0.31[e]
HFFO	50	69	62	0.62 ± 0.10	1.67 ± 0.26	1.43 ± 0.27

[a] Includes adenomas and adenocarcinomas.
[b] Values are mean ± SE.
[c] Significantly different from LFCO and HFFO diet groups, $p < 0.01$.
[d] Significantly different from LFCO and HFFO diet groups, $p < 0.0001$–0.0002.
[e] Significantly different from LFCO and HFFO diet groups, $p < 0.001$.
(Data from ref. 20).

rich in saturated fatty acids, and to compare them with the effects of fish oil during the different stages of colon carcinogenesis in male F344 rats[20]. Colonic aberrant crypt foci (ACF) were assessed in animals fed the experimental diets for weeks 8, 23 and 38. ACF were predominantly observed in the distal colons of carcinogen-treated rats. Rats fed the high-fat, mixed lipids (HFML) diet showed a significantly greater (77%) number of ACF per colon compared with those fed the low-fat corn oil (LFCO) or high-fat fish oil (HFFO) diet at all time points. The incidence of multicrypt aberrant foci was also higher in the HFML diet group than in the HFFO or LFCO diet groups, suggesting that administration of the HFFO diet significantly inhibits the formation and growth of preneoplastic lesions in the colon, whereas the HFML diet promotes the growth of such lesions. Also, dietary HFML significantly increased colon tumour incidence and multiplicity when compared with the HFFO or LFCO diets (Table 2). Importantly, rats fed the HFML diet showed 100% incidence of colonic adenocarcinomas compared with incidences of 63% and 69% in rats fed the LFCO and HFFO diets, respectively (Table 2). The multiplicity of adenocarcinomas was also significantly higher in animals fed the HFML diet (about 4-fold increase) as compared to those fed the LFCO diet. Equally important, the HFFO diet containing 20% fat (mostly in the form of fish oil) induced fewer tumours than the HFML diet containing the same amount of total fat mostly from mixed lipids. This reinforces the theory that both the type and the amount of dietary fatty acids in the diets play a critical role in colon carcinogenesis. In general, overall evidence from preclinical studies is consistent with the epidemiological data.

POSSIBLE MODE OF ACTION OF TYPES OF DIETARY FAT IN COLON CARCINOGENESIS

With regard to the mode of action of saturated fats, omega-6 polyunsaturated fatty acids (PUFA) and omega-3 PUFA in colon carcinogenesis, several studies indicate that diets high in saturated fatty acids (beef tallow and lard) and omega-6 PUFA (corn oil or safflower oil) increase the concentration of colonic luminal secondary bile acids including deoxycholic acid and lithocholic acid, whereas dietary fish oil high in omega-3 PUFA had no such enhancing effect[21-25]. Secondary bile acids have been shown to induce cell proliferation and to act as promoters in colon carcinogenesis[26]. There are studies to indicate that inducible nitric oxide synthase (iNOS), which is regulated primarily at the transcriptional levels, is over-expressed in human colon adenomas[27] and in chemically induced colon tumours of laboratory animal models[28]. Accumulating data also indicate that the overproduction of NO by iNOS induces deaminated DNA lesions, thus resulting in DNA damage[29]. Both NO and peroxynitrate produced in the tissues by NO also activate cyclooxygenase (COX)-2. Studies conducted in our laboratory indicate that deoxycholic acid induces iNOS activity in intestinal cells, suggesting one of the mechanisms by which tumour promoters, including secondary bile acids, may involve an increase in expression of iNOS that enhances colon carcinogenesis[30].

There are studies to indicate that overexpression of COX-2 plays an important role in colon carcinogenesis[31]. Tsujii and DuBois[32], who have implicated COX-2 activity in the regulation of apoptosis of rat intestinal epithelial cells, have shown that overexpression of COX-2 can lead to the suppression of apoptosis. Additionally, the high intake of saturated fat and omega-6 PUFA alters membrane phospholipid turnover, releasing membrane arachidonic acid from phospholipids, and affecting prostaglandin synthesis via COX enzyme[24,25]. Elevated levels of COX-2 have been observed in human colon tumours and chemically induced colon tumours in rodents[33,34]. Recent studies conducted in our laboratory have provided convincing evidence that a HFML diet enhances AOM-induced expression of COX-2 and eicosanoid formation from arachidonic acid in colon tumours of rats, whereas the omega-3 PUFA in the HFFO diet inhibit the levels of COX-2[20]. In this study administration of the HFML diet produced 472 ± 33 pmol/min (mean $\pm$ SE) of eicosanoids, significantly higher levels than the LFCO diet (380 ± 29 pmol/min) or HFFO diet (348 ± 28 pmol/min) indicating higher COX activity. The results of these studies, which indicate that overexpression of COX-2 in the tumours of animals fed the HFML diet increases COX-2 activity and inhibits apoptosis and the consequent tumour burden, support the contention that overexpression of COX-2 can lead to the suppression of apoptosis.

Recent studies from our laboratory have shown that the HFCO diet enhances activities of diverse enzymes including protein kinases that have been implicated directly or indirectly in colon tumour promotion, whereas the HFFO diet appears to suppress the activities of these enzymes[25,35]. It is interesting that several kinases have been shown to participate in ras-mediated growth-promoting signal transduction pathways[36]. The ras-p21, a guanine nucleotide-binding 21 kDa protein product of ras genes that is anchored to the cytoplasmic face of plasma membrane, functions in the regulation of cell proliferation. Mutational versions of ras-p21 are implicated in the aetiology of human colon cancer[37]. It is also known that trafficking of pro-ras from cytosol to plasma membrane is facilitated by a series of closely linked post-tranlational modifications including farnesylation, which is catalysed by farnesyl protein transferase. It appears that inhibition

Table 3 Effect of types and amount of dietary fat on expression levels of *ras*-p21 in azoxymethane-induced colon tumours in F344 rats

	Dietary regimen		
	LFCO	HFCO	HFFO
Colon mucosa			
Cytosolic	0.7 ± 4[a]	0.6 ± 2	3.1 ± 1.2
Membrane-bound	11.9 ± 3.0	17.2 ± 4.5[b]	5.9 ± 2.3
Total	12.3 ± 4.5	17.5 ± 3.8[b]	9.2 ± 1.5
Colon tumours			
Cytosolic	0.8 ± 5	0.9 ± 4	6.2 ± 2.2
Membrane-bound	24.0 ± 5.2	33.1 ± 8.0[b]	12.3 ± 3.8
Total	25.0 ± 6.0	34.5 ± 7.5[b]	17.9 ± 6.2

[a] Results are expressed as nanograms of *ras*-p21/mg protein; values are mean ± SD.
[b] Significantly different from LFCO and HFFO diets, $p < 0.01–0.001$.
(Data from ref. 38).

of *ras* farnesylation blocks membrane association of *ras*-p21 and prevents neoplastic transformation of cells. Studies conducted in our laboratory have provided data to indicate that dietary HFCO increases *ras*-p21 expression in colonic tumours, whereas the HFFO diet appears to exert antitumour activity by interfering with post-translational modification and membrane localization of *ras*-p21 through the modulation of farnesyl protein transferase activity, thus inhibiting *ras*-p21 function[38] (Table 3).

Additional studies conducted in our laboratory have demonstrated that docosahexaenoic acid (DHA) inhibits growth of Caco-2 colon cancer cells *in vitro* and induces apoptosis[39]. Using Caco-2 cells we also examined the effects of DHA on the genetic precursors of human colon cancer at the transcription level using DNA oligonucleotide arrays[39]. Alterations in gene expression due to DHA treatment were observed to be in the multiple signalling pathways involved in the regulation of cell cycle regulatory genes, COX-2 target genes, lipoxygenases and peroxisome proliferators. Effects of DHA on cell cycle progression and induction of apoptosis were directly paralleled by an increase in the activation of several proapoptotic caspases and genes such as *p21*, *waf1/cip1* and *p27*. Comprehensive evaluation of several of these precursor genes and transcription factors will facilitate determination of the chemopreventive efficacy of DHA and other important omega-3 fatty acids present in fish oil, and thus prevent colon cancer. Also, comprehensive evaluation of these precursor genes and transcription factors provided several simultaneously expressed biological activities, many of which suggest themselves as molecular targets for effective intervention by nutritional factors.

SUMMARY AND CONCLUSION

In conclusion, on the basis of epidemiological evidence from ecological and case–control studies it is reasonable to suggest that diets high in total fat, especially in saturated fat, increase the risk of colorectal cancer, whereas diets high in fish and fish oil reduce the risk. Preclinical model studies have provided evidence that the colon tumour-promoting effect of dietary fat depends on the type of fat, suggesting that the composition of ingested dietary fatty acids is more critical to colon cancer risk than is the total amount of fat. Preclinical model studies indicate that a Western-style diet high in mixed lipids has a higher potential to promote colon tumorigenesis than ingestion of a diet with an equivalent amount of fat containing fish oil rich in omega-3 PUFA. Although the mechanisms by which diets high in saturated fats (such as those in Western diets) promote colon carcinogenesis are not fully known, the studies conducted thus far indicate that the modulation of *ras*-p21 activity, eicosanoid production via the influence on COX activity, and the expression of apoptosis by the types of dietary fat may play a key role in colon carcinogenesis.

Acknowledgements

This work was supported by USPHS grants CA 37663 and CA 17613 from the National Cancer Institute. The authors gratefully acknowledge that the preparation of this manuscript was, in part, supported by the Foundation for Promotion of Cancer Research Fellowship Program, Japan, to Bandaru S. Reddy. The host institution for the Fellowship Program was Aichi Cancer Center Research Institute, Nagoya, Japan.

References

1. Greenlee RT, Murray T, Bolen S, Wingo PA. Cancer statistics, 2000. CA Cancer J Clin. 2000;50:7–33.
2. Kakizoe T, Yamaguchi N, Mitsuhashi F, Koshiji M, Oshima A, Ohtaka M. Cancer statistics in Japan-2001. Foundation for Promotion of Cancer Research in Japan, 2001.
3. Wynder EL, Kajitani T, Ishikawa S, Dodo H, Takano A. Environmental factors of cancer of colon and rectum. Cancer (Phila.) 1969;23:1210–20.
4. Miller AB, Howe GR, Jain M. Food items and food groups as risk factors in a case–control study of diet and colon cancer. Int J Cancer. 1983;32:155–62.
5. Giovannucci E, Willett WC. Dietary factors and risk of colon cancer. Ann Med. 1994;26:443–52.
6. Panel on Food. Nutrition and the Prevention of Cancer. Washington, DC: American Institute for Cancer Research, 1997.
7. Reddy BS. Diet and Colon Cancer: Evidence from Human and Animal Model Studies. Boca Raton, FL: CRC Press, 1986.
8. Caygill CPJ, Charland SL, Lippin JA. Fat, fish, fish oil, and cancer. Br J Cancer. 1996;74:159–64.
9. Caygill CP, Hill MJ. Fish, n-3 fatty acids and human colorectal and breast cancer mortality. Eur J Cancer Prev. 1995;4:329–32.
10. Bull AW, Soullier BK, Wilson PS, Hayden MT, Nigro ND. Promotion of azoxymethane-induced intestinal cancer by high fat diets in rats. Cancer Res. 1979;39:4956–9.
11. Reddy BS, Maeura Y. Tumor promotion by dietary fat in azoxymethane-induced colon carcinogenesis in female F344 rats: influence of amount and sources of dietary fat. J Natl Cancer Inst. 1984;72:745–50.
12. Reddy BS, Maruyama H. Effect of different levels of dietary corn oil and lard during the initiation phase of colon carcinogenesis in male F344 rats. J Natl Cancer Inst. 1986;77:815–22.
13. Reddy BS. Nutritional factors and colon cancer. Crit Rev Food Sci Nutr. 1995;35:175–90.
14. Reddy BS, Narisawa T, Vukusich D, Weisburger JH, Wynder EL. Effect of quality and quantity of dietary fat and dimethylhydrazine in colon carcinogenesis in rats. Proc Soc Exp Biol Med. 1976;151:237.

15. Reddy BS, Burill C, Rigotty J. Effect of diets high in ω-3 and ω-6 fatty acids on initiation and postinitiation stages of colon carcinogenesis. Cancer Res. 1991;51:487–91.
16. Reddy BS, Sugie S. Effect of different levels of ω-3 and ω-6 fatty acids on azoxymethane-induced colon carcinogenesis in F344 rats. Cancer Res. 1988;48:6642–7.
17. Anti M, Armelao F, Marra G. Effect of different doses of fish oil on rectal cell proliferation in patients with sporadic colonic adenomas. Gastroenterology. 1994;107:1709–18.
18. Yang K, Fan K, Newmark H et al. Cytokeratin, lectin, and acidic mucin modulation in differentiating colonic epithelial cells of mice after feeding Western-style diets. Cancer Res. 1996;56:4644–8.
19. Risio M, Lipkin M, Newmark H et al. Apoptosis, cell proliferation, and Western-style diet-induced tumorigenesis in mouse colon. Cancer Res. 1996;56:4910–16.
20. Rao CV, Hirose Y, Indranie C, Reddy BS. Modulation of experimental colon tumorigenesis by types and amounts of dietary fatty acids. Cancer Res. 2001;61:1927–33.
21. Reddy BS, Watanabe K, Weisburger JH, Wynder EL. Promoting effect of bile acids in colon carcinogenesis in germ-free and conventional F344 rats. Cancer Res. 1977;37:3238–42.
22. Craven RA, Pfanstial J, DeRubertis FR. Role of activation of protein kinase C in the stimulation of colonic epithelial proliferation and reactive oxygen formation by bile acids. J Clin Invest. 1987;79:532–41.
23. Davidson LA, Jiang YH, Derr JN, Aukema HM, Lupton JR, Chapkin RS. Protein kinase isoforms in human and rat colonic mucosa. Arch Biochem Biophys. 1994;312:547–53.
24. Rao CV, Reddy BS. Modulating effect of amount and types of dietary fat on ornithine decarboxylase, tyrosine protein kinase, and prostaglandins production during colon carcinogenesis. Carcinogenesis. 1993;14:1327–33.
25. Rao CV, Simi B, Wynn T-T, Garr K, Reddy BS. Modulating effect of amount and types of dietary fat on colonic mucosal phospholipase A2, phosphatidylinositol-specific phospholipase C activities, and cyclooxygenase metabolite formation during different stages of colon tumor promotion in male F344 rats. Cancer Res. 1996;56:532–7.
26. Bull AW, Marnett LJ, Dawe EJ, Nigro ND. Stimulation of deoxythymidine incorporation in the colon of rats treated intrarectally with bile acids and fats. Carcinogenesis. 1993;4:207–10.
27. Ambs S, Merriam WG, Bennett WP et al. Frequent nitric oxide synthase-2 expression in human colon adenomas: implication for tumor angiogenesis and colon cancer progression. Cancer Res. 1998;58:334–41.
28. Takahashi M, Fukuda K, Ohata T, Sugimura T, Wakabayashi K. Increased expression of inducible and endothelial constitutive nitric oxide synthase in rat colon tumors induced by azoxymethane. Cancer Res. 1997;57:1233–7.
29. De Rojas-Walker T, Tamir S, Ji H, Wishnok JS, Tannenbaum SR. Nitric oxide induces oxidative damage in addition to deamination in macrophage DNA. Chem Res Toxicol. 1995;8:473–7.
30. Hirose Y, Rao CV, Reddy BS. Modulation of inducible nitric oxide synthase expression in rat intestinal cells by colon tumor promoters. Int J Oncol. 2001;18:141–6.
31. Eberhart CE, Coffey RJ, Radhika A, Giardiello FM, Ferrenbach S, DuBois RN. Up-regulation of cyclooxygenase-2 gene expression in human colorectal adenomas and adenocarcinomas. Gastroenterology. 1994;107:1183–8.
32. Tsujii M, DuBois RN. Alterations in cellular adhesion and apoptosis in epithelial cells overexpressing prostaglandin endoperoxide synthase 2. Cell. 1995;83:493–501.
33. Kargman SL, O'Neill GP, Vickers PJ, Evens JF, Mancini JA, Jothy S. Expression of prostaglandin G/H-1 and -2 protein in human colon cancer. Cancer Res. 1995;55:2556–9.
34. DuBois RN, Radhika A, Reddy BS, Entingh AJ. Increased cyclooxygenase-2 levels in carcinogen-induced rat colonic tumors. Gastroenterology. 1996;110:1259–62.
35. Reddy BS, Simi B, Patel N, Aliaga C, Rao CV. Effect of amount and types of dietary fat on intestinal bacterial 7-dehydroxylase and phosphatidylinositol-specific phospholipase C and colonic mucosal diacylglycerol kinase and PKC activities during different stages of colon tumor promotion. Cancer Res. 1996;56:2314–20.
36. Egan SE, Weinberg RA. The pathway to signal achievement. Nature (Lond). 1993;365:781–3.
37. Barbacid M. Ras oncogenes: their role in neoplasia. Eur J Clin. Invest. 1990;20:225–35.
38. Singh J, Hamid R, Reddy BS. Modulating effect of types and amount of dietary fat on ras-p21 function during promotion and progression stages of colon cancer. Cancer Res. 1997;57:253–8.
39. Narayanan BA, Narayanan NK, Reddy BS. Docosahexaenoic acid regulated genes and transcription factor inducing apoptosis in human colon cancer cells. Int J Oncol. 2001;19:1255–62.

15
Alcohol and colorectal cancer

H. K. SEITZ, G. PÖSCHL and F. STICKEL

EPIDEMIOLOGY

In 1974 Breslow and Enstrom were the first to consider the possibility of an association between beer drinking and the occurrence of rectal cancer[1]. To date seven correlational studies, more than 40 case–control studies, and 17 prospective cohort studies have been performed to elucidate the role of alcohol in the development of colorectal cancer[2,3]. An association was found in five of the seven correlational studies and in more than half of the case–control studies. In the majority of the case–control studies using community controls, such a correlation was detected, suggesting that the absence of an asociation when hospital controls were used is due to the high prevalence of alcohol consumption and alcohol-related diseases in hospital controls. Eleven of the 17 cohort studies also demonstrated a positive correlation with alcohol. A positive trend with respect to dose–response was found in five of the 10 case–control studies and in all prospective cohort studies in which this factor has been taken into consideration.

Six studies have investigated the effect of chronic ethanol consumption on the occurrence of adenomatous polyps of the large bowel[2,3]. In five of these such a correlation was observed. In addition, an RR increase of hyperplastic polyps of the distal colon and rectum was also observed by increasing amounts of alcohol[4]. When more than 30 g alcohol per day were consumed, the RR for men was 1.8 and for women 2.5.

Finally, alcohol may influence the adenoma–carcinoma sequence at different early steps, as reported recently by Boutron et al.[5]. Excessive alcohol consumption also favours high-risk polyp or colorectal cancer occurrence among patients with adenomas[6]. In addition it was reported that a comprehensive reduction in ethanol intake for individuals with genetic predisposition for colorectal cancer may have a large beneficial effect on tumour incidence[7]. Most recently the epidemiological data on alcohol and colorectal cancer have been reviewed by a panel of experts at a World Health Organization (WHO) Consensus Conference on Nutrition and Colorectal Cancer, and it was concluded that, although the data are still somewhat controversial, chronic alcohol ingestion even at low daily intake (10–40 g), especially consumed as beer, results in a 1.5–3.5-fold risk of rectal cancer and to a lesser extent of colonic cancer in both sexes, but predominantly in males[8]. Epidemiological studies also underline the importance of the lack of dietary factors such as methionine and folate which modulate the ethanol-associated colorectal cancer risk[9].

ANIMAL EXPERIMENTS

The results of animal experiments on alcohol and colorectal cancer depend on the experimental design; the type of carcinogen used; and the route, time, duration, and dosage of carcinogen and alcohol administration. Chronic alcohol administration alone, without the application of a primary or secondary carcinogen, does not produce tumours. Table 1 summarizes the effect of chronic alcohol consumption on colorectal cancer. In two of the eight studies ethanol was given in the drinking water, and the results of these experiments therefore have to be questioned[10,11]. When the two procarcinogens dimethylhydrazine (DMH) and azoxymethane (AOM) were used to induce colorectal tumours, different results were reported, depending on the experimental conditions[12-15]. In these studies it is important to note that both compounds need metabolic activation by cytochrome P-450-dependent microsomal enzymes to become carcinogenic. The results of these studies depend on the ethanol dose used and on the timing of ethanol administration. The conclusions derived from these experiments are as follows:

1. The modulation of experimental colonic tumorigenesis by chronic dietary beer and ethanol consumption is because of alcohol rather than being due to other beverage constituents.
2. The tumorigenesis in the right and left colorectum is affected differently by alcohol and may depend on the levels of alcohol consumption. Thus, high alcohol intake (18–33% of total calories) inhibits carcinogenesis in the right colon and has no effect on the left colon, while lower ethanol consumption (9–12% of total calories) enhances tumour development in the left colon without effect on the right colon.
3. Ethanol effects carcinogenesis during the preinduction and/or induction phase, including carcinogen metabolism, but not in the postinduction phase (promotion).
4. An interaction between ethanol and procarcinogen metabolism does occur, and this may influence tumour incidences.

It must be emphasized that, in one experiment with DMH, ethanol ingestion enhanced tumour development only in the rectum, but not in the remaining large intestine[12]. In this study ethanol was given during acclimatization and initiation, but at the time of procarcinogen application ethanol was not present in the body of the animal. In a similar study by McGarrity and co-workers, these results could not be confirmed[13]. In addition, in two other animal experiments the primary carcinogen acetoxymethylmethylnitrosamine (AMMN) was used to induce rectal tumours[16,17]. This carcinogen does not need metabolic activation to exert its carcinogenic effect. It was applied locally to the rectal mucosa of rats and the animals were endoscoped regularly. Since chronic ethanol administration, either as liquid diets or intragastrically, accelerates the appearance of rectal tumours

Table 1 Effect of ethanol on chemically induced colorectal carcinogenesis in rats

Carcinogen	Ethanol administration	Ethanol effect	Ref.
DMH, s.c.	6% LD (36% total calories), preinduction	Increased rectal but not colonic tumours	12
DMH, s.c.	5% DW, induction	No effect	10
DMH, s.c.	5% DW, preinduction/induction	No effect	11
DMH, s.c.	6% LD (36% total calories), preinduction	No effect	13
AMMN, i.r.	6% LD (36% total calories), preinduction/induction	Increased rectal tumours	16
AOM, s.c.	LD (11%, 22%, 33% total calories), preinduction/induction, postinduction	Inhibition of tumour development in the left but less than in the right colon. Higher ethanol intake has a stronger inhibitory effect. No effect when ethanol is given in the postinduction phase	14
AOM, s.c.	LD (9% total calories ethanol) (12%, 23% total calories beer), preinduction/induction	High ethanol inhibits tumours in the right colon, but not in the left colon, while low ethanol enhances tumours in the left colon, but not in the right colon. No effect of beer	15
AMMN, i.r.	i.g. (4.8 g/kg body weight per day), preinduction/induction	Increased rectal tumours. Carcinogenesis was further stimulated when cyanamide, an acetaldehyde dehydrogenase inhibitor, was administered additionally	17

LD = liquid diet, DW = drinking water, DMH = dimethylhydrazine, AOM = azoxymethane, AMMN = azoxymethylmethylnitrosamine, s.c. = subcutaneously, i.r. = intrarectally, i.g. = intragastrically.

induced by AMMN, it seems most likely that alcohol enhances carcinogenesis, at least in part, by local mechanisms in the rectal mucosa and not only by increasing the activation of procarcinogens. Furthermore, in these experiments acetaldehyde (AA) concentrations were experimentally increased by the administration of cyanamide, an AA-dehydrogenase (ALDH) inhibitor, and this led to a stimulation of colorectal carcinogenesis induced by AMMN, emphasizing the pathogenetic role of AA.

MECHANISMS BY WHICH ALCOHOL STIMULATES COLORECTAL CARCINOGENESIS

Acetaldehyde

Recent research has identified AA as a highly toxic, mutagenic and carcinogenic substance. AA interferes at many sites with DNA synthesis and repair, and consequently tumour development[18]. Numerous *in-vitro* and *in-vivo* experiments in prokaryotic and eukaryotic cell cultures and in animal models have shown that AA has direct mutagenic and carcinogenic effects. It causes point mutations in certain genes and induces sister chromatid exchanges and gross chromosomal aberrations[19–21]. It induces inflammation and metaplasia of tracheal epithelium, delays cell cycle progression, stimulates apoptosis, and enhances cell injury associated with hyperregeneration[22]. It has also been shown that AA interferes with the DNA repair machinery. AA directly inhibits O6-methylguanyltransferase, an enzyme important for the repair of adducts caused by alkylating agents[23]. Moreover, when inhaled, AA causes nasopharyngeal and laryngeal carcinoma[24]. According to the International Agency for Research on Cancer there is sufficient evidence to identify AA as a carcinogen in animals[18].

AA also binds rapidly to cellular protein and DNA, which results in morphological and functional impairment of the cell. The covalent binding to DNA and the formation of stable adducts represents one mechanism by which AA could trigger the occurrence of replication errors and/or mutations in oncogenes or tumour-suppressor genes[25]. The occurrence of stable DNA adducts has been shown in different organs of alcohol-fed rodents and in leukocytes of alcoholics[26]. Moreover, it has recently been shown that the major stable DNA adduct, N2-ethyldeoxyguanosine, can indeed be used efficiently by eukariotic DNA polymerase[27].

In addition, AA adducts represent neoantigens that lead to the production of specific antibodies and to the stimulation of the immune system, which probably leads to a cytotoxic immune response. AA also destroys folate[28], which has striking consequences on methyl-transfer, especially DNA methylation, which will be discussed below.

Recent and striking evidence for the causal role of AA in ethanol-associated carcinogenesis derives from genetic linkage studies in alcoholics. Individuals who accumulate AA due to polymorphism and/or mutation in the genes coding for enzymes responsible for AA generation and detoxification have been shown to have an increased cancer risk[22]. ADH2 and ADH3 are polymorphic and the ADH2*2 and ADH3*1 alleles code for an enzyme which produces 40 and

2.5 times more AA compared with the corresponding ADH2*1 and ADH3*2 alleles[29]. While the ADH2*2 allele is rare in the Caucasian population, and seems to be protective against the consumption of alcohol in Asia[22], the ADH3*1 allele was found in some studies to be associated with an increased risk for cancer of the oropharynx, larynx, oesophagus, liver and breast in alcoholics[30–34]. However, other studies could not find such an effect[35–36].

With respect to colorectal cancer a recent study did show the ADH3 genotype not to be a predictive factor for colorectal cancer[37]. In contrast, preliminary data from our laboratory found an increased frequency of AD3*1 allele in alcoholics with colorectal cancer as compared to age-matched alcoholics without cancer[22].

In addition, individuals with a mutation of ALDH2, who accumulate AA when they consume alcohol (approximately 40% of the Japanese population) exhibit an increased risk for colorectal cancer[38].

Clinically, it was found that alcoholics revealed a disturbed morphology in rectal biopsies with crypt destruction and inflammation, which completely returned to normal after 3 weeks of withdrawal[39]. We showed that chronic alcohol consumption resulted in an increased crypt cell production rate and an extension of the proliferative compartment of the crypt in rodents. This was associated with a decrease of the functional compartment[40]. The mucosal hyperproliferation was paralleled by a significant increase in rectal mucosal ornithine decarboxylase (ODC) activity, a marker for high risk with respect to colorectal cancer[12].

Furthermore, when we extended our studies to humans, we again found that chronic alcoholics had an increased proliferation in their crypts with extension of their proliferative compartment, a condition associated with an increased cancer risk[41]. In contrast, cell differentiation regarding cytokeratin expression pattern was found to be unchanged, as well as regulatory factors involved in carcinogenesis and/or apoptosis.

There is some evidence that AA is involved in these observed morphological alterations as precursors for colorectal cancer:

1. Crypt cell production rate correlated significantly with AA levels in the colonic mucosa[42].
2. Animal experiments showed an increased occurrence of colorectal tumours induced by the specific locally acting carcinogen acetoxymethylmethylnitrosamine, when cyanamide, an ALDH inhibitor, was applied and AA levels were increased[17].
3. High AA levels occur in the colon due to bacterial production from ethanol[43].
4. Colonic AA levels show a significant inverse correlation with mucosal folate concentrations, which supports in-vitro data showing a destruction of folate by AA[44].
5. Individuals with the inactive form of ALDH2 exhibit an increased risk for colorectal cancer when they consume alcohol, as discussed above[38].

The role of AA in ethanol-associated carcinogenesis is illustrated in Figure 1.

Cytochrome P-4502E1 induction

Chronic ethanol consumption results in an induction of cytochrome P-4502E1 (CYP2E1) in the liver and other organs, inluding the mucosa of the gastrointestinal

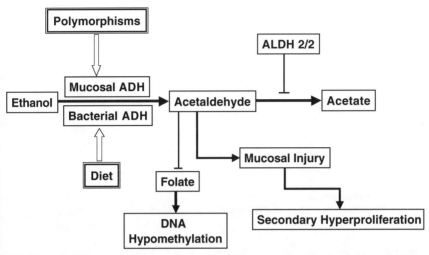

Figure 1 Acetaldehyde is the pivotal toxin generated from ethanol and its disposal is mediated by aldehyde dehydrogenases. The extent of acetaldehyde burden in tissues is dependent on the activity of enzymes involved in its generation and disposal. Several genotypes of alcohol dehydrogenase (ADH) and aldehyde dehydrogenase (ALDH) with different enzymatic activities are terminants of acetaldehyde exposure

tract[3]. CYP2E1 metabolizes ethanol to AA, but is also involved in the activation of various procarcinogens to their ultimate carcinogenic metabolites[45]. CYP2E1 induction also leads to the generation of reactive oxygen species (ROS)[3]. An induction of CYP2E1 occurs at a relatively low ethanol intake. We recently demonstrated a significant induction of CYP2E1 after only 2 weeks of consumption of 30 g ethanol daily[46]. CYP2E1 is also induced by ethanol in the colorectal mucosa of rodents[47] and in humans (H. K. Seitz, personal communication).

The effect of chronic ethanol ingestion on the induction of CYP2E1 and the activation of a procarcinogen has been elegantly demonstrated by various animal experiments using AOM as an inducing procarcinogen for colorectal cancer[48]. Hamilton et al. demonstrated that the metabolism of AOM is inhibited in the presence of ethanol, but significantly enhanced when ethanol is withdrawn in a condition where CYP2E1 is induced and is completely available for the activation of AOM[48]. Thus, the induction of CYP2E1 in the colorectal mucosa can result in an enhanced activation of nitrosamines or polycyclic hydrocarbons ubiquitously present in diets, and thus also in the faeces, and may therefore be one mechanism by which chronic alcohol ingestion stimulates colorectal cancer development.

CYP2E1 induction also leads to ROS generation. The role of ROS in upper alimentary tract cancer has been demonstrated by Eskelson et al.[49]. They reported that chronic ethanol consumption increases the carcinogenesis induced by N-nitrosomethylbenzylamine (NMBA) in the oesophagus, which was associated with an increased production of ROS, and which was inhibited by the administration of the scavenger α-tocopherol. We have investigated the effect of

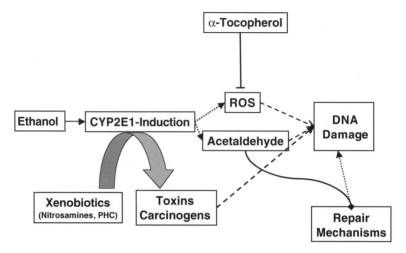

Figure 2 Induction of cytochrome P4502E1 by its principal substrate ethanol leads to formation of toxic acetaldehyde and reactive oxygen species (ROS). In addition, increased amounts of toxins and carcinogens from previously innocuous compounds are generated. Antioxidants such as tocopherol may counteract increased oxidative stress along with alcohol metabolism, but not DNA damage induced by mutagens (e.g. alkylating substances generated by CYP2E1). PHC – polycyclic hydrocarbons

α-tocopherol on alcohol-induced mucosal hyperregeneration in the colorectum of rodents, and found a significant inhibition by vitamin E[50], which may support the hypothesis that ROS are involved in the pathogenesis of alcohol-associated colorectal hyperproliferation.

The role of CYP2E1 in ethanol-associated carcinogenesis is illustrated in Figure 2.

Interaction between ethanol and retinoids

The complex interaction between the metabolism of retinoids and ethanol has been reported for a long time. Clinically, chronic ethanol consumption leads to vitamin A deficiency but also enhanced toxicity of vitamin A and β-carotene when supplemented. Changes in retinol metabolism due to alcohol may have a pathophysiological impact in alcohol-associated cancer as retinoic acid (RA), the most active form of vitamin A, is an important regulator of normal epithelial cell growth, function and differentiation. Under normal conditions ingested retinol is metabolized to retinaldehyde via cytosolic ADH, microsomal dehydrogenases, and several types of cytosolic retinol dehydrogenase, and retinaldehyde is further oxidized to RA via ALDH. RA binds to retinoic acid receptors (RAR), initiating intracellular signal transduction leading to a cascade of events and finally to a decrease in cell regeneration. It is not surprising the interaction between ethanol and retinoid metabolism is complex as the two substrates share common pathways, namely: (a) ADH, (b) ALDH, and (c) CYP2E1 (Figure 3).

It has been shown that chronic alcohol consumption decreases hepatic retinol and RA concentrations due to various mechanisms, including increased mobilization of

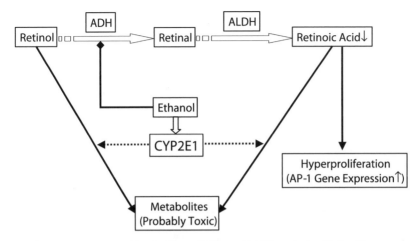

Figure 3 Ethanol interacts with retinoid metabolism and inhibits retinol oxidation. Tissue concentrations of retinoic acid are decreased, thereby leading to hyperproliferation via activation of downstream kinases, e.g. c-jun/c-fos (activator protein-1 [AP-1]) CYP2E1 is capable of metabolizing retinol and retinoic acid, thereby producing toxic apo-retinoids

retinyl esters to extrahepatic tissues and an enhanced hepatic metabolism of retinol and RA to polar metabolites, predominantly via induced CYP2E1[51–53]. These metabolites include 18-OH-RA, 4-OXO-RA, and some unidentified metabolites, possibly with fibrogenic and toxic properties. Decreased hepatic RA concentrations are associated with a functional down-regulation of RAR, enhanced expression of AP-1 gene (c-jun and c-fos), and increased hepatic cell regeneration, all of which return to normal following RA supplementation[54,55].

In contrast, retinol concentrations in extrahepatic tissues such as the oesophagus and the colonic mucosa were found to be increased rather than decreased following chronic ethanol consumption[52]. This was also confirmed in alcoholics with oropharyngeal cancer, in whom normal retinol concentrations were found in normal oral mucosa adjacent to cancerous tissue[56]. It was believed that one mechanism for this observation was increased mobilization of retinyl esters from the liver to the gastrointestinal mucosa. It has also been shown that ethanol in concentrations frequently observed after social drinking inhibits retinol oxidation in the intestine[57]. This effect was due to an inhibition of low K_m and high K_m ADH, and seems especially relevant in the colon[57]. This may explain the accumulation of retinol in the colonic mucosa, and may lead to reduction of RA.

In humans it has been shown that retinol is a physiological substrate for ADH3 in the gastrointestinal mucosa. ADH3 has a low K_m for ethanol (1–2 mM) and is the only class I ADH gene that contains an RAR element in the promoter region. It has been suggested that RA activation of ADH constitutes a positive feedback loop regulating RA synthesis[58]. Ethanol was found to be a competitive inhibitor of retinol for class I ADH, but also for class II and IV ADH[59,60]. It has been shown that class IV ADH (present only in the mucosa of the upper gastrointestinal tract) has a low K_m for all-*trans*-retinol of 15–60 μM and has the highest catalytic efficiency of 3800–4500 mmol/min[60,61]. *In-vitro* studies using class IV ADH enzyme preparations have shown strong inhibition of metabolism of all-*trans*-retinol and 9-*cis*-retinol by ethanol with a K_i of 6–10 mM[60]. Oxidation of retinol to retinaldehyde is probably the rate-limiting step in the generation of RA, and an inhibition of RA generation by acetaldehyde has been reported in the oesophageal mucosa[62]. In addition, it is most likely that an enhanced RA degradation also occurs through induction of CYP2E1 in the colonic mucosa.

It is interesting that class IV, in contrast with class I, ADH is not expressed in the human colorectal mucosa. However, it was found recently that, in a number of biopsies from colorectal polyps of alcoholics, class IV ADH was expressed[22]. One explanation for such a *de-novo* expression of class IV ADH could be RA deficiency in a critical premalignant condition to guarantee increased generation of RA to suppress mucosal hyperregeneration.

Thus, the observed mucosal hyperregeneration following chronic ethanol ingestion may be due not only to the direct toxic action of AA, but also to RA deficiency, and AA may contribute by preventing its generation.

DNA hypomethylation in the colonic mucosa

Chronic ethanol consumption increases the requirement for methyl groups[63] and dietary methyl deficiency enhances hepatocarcinogenesis[64]. Methionine obtained from the diet and synthesized by several reactions is the sole precursor of *S*-adenosylmethionine (SAM), the primary methyl donor in the body. Disruption in methionine metabolism and methylation reaction may be involved in the cancer process. SAM is involved in the methylation of a small percentage of cytosine bases of the DNA. Findings suggest that enzymatic DNA methylation is an important component of gene control and may serve as a silencing mechanism for gene function (Figure 4). Some carcinogens interfere with enzymatic DNA

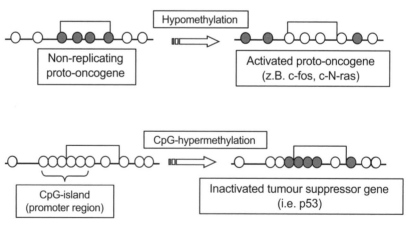

Figure 4 Hypomethylation of genes leads to activation of transcription whereas hypermethylation has a silencing effect on genes. In proto-oncogenes (c-fos, c-ras) hypomethylation may lead to the initiation of tumorigenesis, while hypermethylation of tumour-suppressor genes (e.g. p53) may lead to loss of their protective action

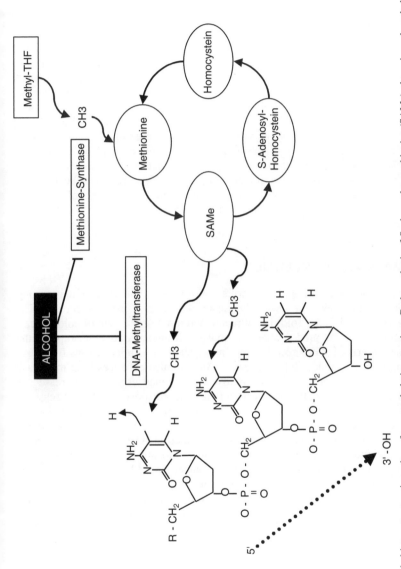

Figure 5 Alcohol interacts at various sites of transmethylation reactions. Both synthesis of *S*-adenosyl-L-methionine (SAMe), the universal methyl donor in one-carbon metabolism, and the final methyl transfer to DNA sequences may be inhibited by alcohol through inhibition of crucial enzymes

137

methylation, and thus may allow oncogene activation. DNA hypomethylation has been observed in many cancer cells and tumours[65]. Chronic ethanol consumption decreases intake of methionine and its conversion to SAM[66,67] (Figure 5).

Folate deficiency, which is common in the alcoholic[68], may additionally contribute to an inhibition of transmethylation, since it is an important factor in one-carbon transport[69] (Figure 5). Decreased folate levels after alcohol intake are caused by, among other factors, a decreased ability to retain folate in the liver or to an increased breakdown of folate[68]. Most recently it has been demonstrated that vitamin B_6 deficiency, which also occurs following chronic ethanol consumption, also leads to a decrease of SAM[70]. Another factor for DNA hypomethylation is the AA-mediated inhibition of methyltransferase activity[71].

In the colon of chronically ethanol-fed rats a significant reduction of folate associated with increased AA levels has been reported[44]. This may explain, at least in part, the genomic DNA hypomethylation observed in the colonic mucosa following chronic alcohol ingestion[72]. However, no effect of alcohol consumption was found when the region of the p53 gene that is most closely linked to colonic carcinogenesis was examined[72]. Epidemiologically it has been shown that individuals with low folate and methionine intake and an alcohol consumption of more than 20 g per day have a more than 7-fold increased risk for distal colorectal cancer[9].

SUMMARY AND CONCLUSION

Epidemiological data are still somewhat controversial, but it seems that chronic alcohol ingestion, even at low daily intake (10–40 g), especially consumed as beer, results in a 1.5–3.5-fold risk of rectal, and to a lesser extent of colonic, cancer in both sexes, but predominantly in males. Chronic alcohol consumption also increases the risk for colorectal polyps and speeds up carcinogenesis from low-risk polyp to high-risk polyp and cancer. Alcohol also enhances liver metastasis in colorectal carcinoma patients. Finally, alcohol may especially increase colorectal cancer risk in individuals with a familial predisposition to the disease.

Mechanisms involved in ethanol-associated colorectal carcinogenesis include the action of acetaldehyde, the first and most toxic metabolite of ethanol. AA is generated mainly by faecal bacteria and by mucosal ADH, which shows polymorphism. Individuals with ALDH mutation who are incapable of removing AA have an increased risk for colorectal cancer. In addition, the induction of CYP2E1 by chronic ethanol consumption may lead to the generation of ROS and to that of other compounds involved in carcinogenesis. Radical scavengers such as α-tocopherol may be beneficial. Finally, low RA levels associated with mucosal hyperregeneration and low folate levels associated with DNA hypomethylation due to chronic alcohol ingestion may affect carcinogenesis at an early stage.

Thus, as a consequence, chronic heavy drinkers should be colonoscoped earlier than the general population for early detection of colorectal polyps and cancer. This is especially important for individuals with an additional positive family history and other risk factors for colorectal cancer.

References

1. Breslow NE, Enstrom JE. Geographic correlations between mortality rates and alcohol, tobacco consumption in the United States. J Natl Cancer Inst. 1974;53:631–9.
2. Kune GA, Vitetta L. Alcohol consumption and the etiology of colorectal cancer: a review of the scientific evidence from 1957 to 1991. Nutr Cancer. 1992;18:97–111.
3. Seitz HK, Pöschl G, Simanowski UA. Alcohol and cancer. Recent Dev Alcohol. 1998;14:7–95.
4. Kearney J, Giavannucci E, Rim EB et al. Diet, alcohol and smoking and the occurrence of hyperplastic polyps of the colon and rectum. Cancer Causes Control. 1995;6:45–56.
5. Boutron MC, Faivre J, Dop MC et al. Tobacco, alcohol and colorectal tumors: a multistep process. Am J Epidemiol. 1995;141:1038–46.
6. Bardou M, Montembault S, Giraud V et al. Excessive alcohol consumption favors high risk polyp or colorectal cancer occurrence among patients with adenomas: a case control study. Gut. 2002;50:38–42.
7. Le Marchand L, Wilkens LR, Hankin JH et al. Independent and joint effects of family history and lifestyle on colorectal cancer risk: implications for prevention. Cancer Epidemiol Biomarkers Prev. 1999;8:45–51.
8. Scheppach W, Bingham S, Boutron-Ruault MC et al. WHO consensus statement on the role of nutrition in colorectal cancer. Eur J Cancer Prev. 1990;8:57–62.
9. Giovannucci E, Rimm EB, Ascherio A, Stampfer MJ, Colditz GA, Willett WC. Alcohol, low methionine–low folate diets, and risk of colon cancer in men. J Natl Cancer Inst. 1995; 87:265–73.
10. Howarth AE, Phil E. High fat diet promotes and causes distal shift of experimental rat colonic cancer – beer and alcohol do not. Nutr Cancer. 1985;6:229–35.
11. Nelson RL, Samelson SL. Neither dietary ethanol nor beer augments experimental colon carcinogenesis in rats. Dis Col Rectum. 1985;28:460–2.
12. Seitz HK, Czygan P, Waldherr R et al. Enhancement of 1,2-dimethylhydrazine induced rectal carcinogenesis following chronic ethanol consumption in the rat. Gastroenterology. 1984;86:886–91.
13. McGarrity TJ, Via EA, Colony PC. Changes in tissue sialic acid content and staining in dimethylhydrazine (DMH)-induced colorectal cancer: effects of ethanol. Gastroenterology. 1986;90:A1543.
14. Hamilton SR, Sohn OS, Fiala ES. Effects of timing and quantity of chronic dietary ethanol consumption on azoxymethane induced colonic carcinogenesis and azoxymethane metabolism in Fischer 344 rats. Cancer Res. 1987;47:4305–11.
15. Hamilton SR, Hyland J, McAvinchey D et al. Effects of chronic dietary beer and ethanol consumption on experimental colonic carcinogenesis by azoxymethane in rats. Cancer Res. 1987; 47:1551–9.
16. Garzon FZ, Simanowski UA, Berger MR et al. Acetoxymethyl-methylnitrosamine (AMMN)-induced colorectal carcinogenesis is stimulated by chronic alcohol consumption. Alcohol Alcohol Suppl. 1987;1:501–2.
17. Seitz HK, Simanowski UA, Garzon FZ et al. Possible role of acetaldehyde in ethanol related rectal carcinogenesis in the rat. Gastroenterology. 1990;98:1–8.
18. Anonymous. Acetaldehyde. IARC Monogr Eval Carcinog Risk. Chem Hum. Vol. 36, 1985.
19. Dellarco VL. A mutagenicity assessment of acetaldehyde. Mutat Res. 1988;195:1–20.
20. Helander A, Lindahl-Kiessling K. Increased frequency of acetaldehyde-induced sister-chromatid exchanges in human lymphocytes treated with an aldehyde dehydrogenase inhibitor. Mutat Res. 1991;264:103–7.
21. Obe G, Jonas R, Schmidt S. Metabolism of ethanol in vitro produces a compound which induces sister-chromatid exchanges in human peripheral lymphocytes in vitro: acetaldehyde not ethanol is mutagenic. Mutat Res. 1986;174:47–51.
22. Seitz HK, Matsuzaki S, Yokoyama A et al. Alcohol and cancer. Alcohol Clin Exp Res. 2001; 25(Suppl):137–43S.
23. Espina N, Lima V, Lieber CS, Garro AJ. In vitro and in vivo inhibitory effect of ethanol and acetaldehyde on O6-methylguanine transferase. Carcinogenesis. 1998;9:761–6.
24. Woutersen RA, Appelmann LM, Van Garderen-Hoetmer A, Feron VJ. Inhalation toxicity of acetaldehyde in rats: III. Carcinogenicity study. Toxicology. 1986;41:213–31.

25. Fang JL, Vaca CE. Development of a ^{32}P-postlabelling method for the analysis of adducts arising through the reaction of acetaldehyde with 2'-deoxyguanosine-3'-monophosphate and DNA. Carcinogenesis. 1995;16:2177–85.
26. Fang JL, Vaca CE. Detection of DNA adducts of acetaldehyde in peripheral white blood cells of alcohol abusers. Carcinogenesis. 1997;18:627–32.
27. Matsuda T, Terashima I, Matsumoto Y, Yabushita H, Matsui S, Shibutani S. Effective utilization of N2-ethyl-2'-deoxyguanosine triphosphate during DNA synthesis catalyzed by mammalian replicative DNA polymerases. Biochemistry. 1999;38:929–35.
28. Shaw S, Jayatilleke E, Herbert V, Colman N. Cleavage of folates during ethanol metabolism. Biochem J. 1989;257:277–80.
29. Borras E, Coutelle C, Rosell A et al. Genetic polymorphism of alcohol dehydrogenase in Europeans: the ADH2*2 allele decreases the risk for alcoholism and is associated with ADH3*1. Hepatology. 2000;31:984–9.
30. Harty IC, Caporaso NE, Hayes RB et al. Alcohol dehydrogenase 3 genotype and risk of oral cavity and pharyngeal cancers. J Natl Cancer Inst. 1997;89:1698–705.
31. Coutelle C, Ward PJ, Fleury B et al. Laryngeal and oropharyngeal cancer and alcohol dehydrogenase 3 and glutathione-S-transferase M1 polymorphism. Hum Genet. 1997;99:319–25.
32. Ji J, Bensova M, Götte K et al. Enhanced risk of upper alimentary tract cancer in patients with alcohol dehydrogenase 3*1 allele due to increased salivary acetaldehyde following ethanol ingestion. Gastroenterology. 2001;120:A160.
33. Stickel F, Benesova M, Schuppan D et al. Alcohol dehydrogenase 3*1 genotype is associated with alcohol-related hepatocellular carcinoma. J Hepatol. 2002;36(Suppl. 1):A84.
34. Freudenheim J, Ambrosone CB, Moysich KB et al. Alcohol dehydrogenase 3 genotype modification of the association of alcohol consumption with breast cancer risk. Cancer Causes Control. 1999;10:369–77.
35. Olshan AF, Weissler MC, Watson MA et al. Risk of head and neck cancer and the alcohol dehydrogenase 3 genotype. Carcinogenesis. 2001;22:57–61.
36. Bouchardy C, Hirvonen A, Coutelle C. Role of alcohol dehydrogenase 3 and cytochrome P4502E1 genotypes in susceptibility to cancer of the upper aerodigestive tract. Int J Cancer. 2000;87:734–40.
37. Chen J, Ma J, Stampfer MJ et al. Alcohol dehydrogenase 3 genotype is not predictive for risk of colorectal cancer. Cancer Epidemiol Biomarkers Prev. 2001;10:133–4.
38. Yokoyama A, Muramatsu T, Ohmori T et al. Alcohol-related cancers and aldehydrogenase-2 in Japanese alcoholics. Carcinogenesis. 1998;19:1383–7.
39. Brozinski S, Fami K, Grosberg JJ. Alcohol ingestion-induced changes in the human rectal mucosa: light and electronmicroscopic studies. Dis Colon Rectum. 1979;21:329–35.
40. Simanowski UA, Seitz HK, Baier B, Kommerell B, Schmidt-Gayk H, Wright NA. Chronic ethanol consumption selectively stimulates rectal cell proliferation in the rat. Gut. 1986; 27:278–82.
41. Simanowski UA, Homann N, Knühl M. Increased rectal cell proliferation following alcohol abuse. Gut. 2001;49:418–22.
42. Simanowski UA, Suter P, Russell RM et al. Enhancement of ethanol induced rectal mucosal hyperregeneration with age in F344 rats. Gut. 1994;35:1102–6.
43. Jokelainen K, Matysiak-Budnik T, Mäkisalo H, Höckerstedt K, Salaspuro M. High intracolonic acetaldehyde levels produced by a bacteriocolonic pathway for ethanol oxidation in piglets. Gut. 1996;39:100–4.
44. Homann N, Tillonen J, Salaspuro M. Heavy alcohol intake leads to local colonic folate deficiency in rats: evidence of microbial acetaldehyde production from ethanol as the pathogenic substance. Int J Cancer. 2000;86:169–73.
45. Seitz HK, Osswald BR. Effect of ethanol on procarcinogen activation. In: Watson RR, editor. Alcohol and Cancer. Boca Raton, FL: CRC Press, 1992;55–72.
46. Oneta CM, Lieber CS, Li JJ et al. Dynamics of cytochrome P4502E1 in man: induction by ethanol and disappearance during withdrawal phase. J Hepatol. 2002; 36:47–52.
47. Hakkak R, Korourian S, Ronis MJ et al. The effects of diet and ethanol on the expression and localisation of cytochromes P450 E1 and P450 2C7 in the colon of male rats. Biochem Pharmacol. 1996; 51:61–9.
48. Sohn OA, Fiala ES, Puz C et al. Enhancement of rat liver microsomal metabolism of azoxymethane to methylazoxymethanol by chronic ethanol administration: similarity to the microsomal metabolism of N-nitrosomethylamine. Cancer Res. 1987;47:3123–9.

49. Eskelson CD, Odelely OE, Watson RR et al. Modulation of cancer growth by vitamin E and alcohol. Alcohol Alcohol. 1993;28:117–26.

50. Vincon P, Wunderer J, Simanowski UA et al. Inhibition of alcohol-associated hyperregeneration in the rat colon by alpha-tocopherol. Alcohol Clin Exp Res. 2000;24:213A.

51. Leo MA, Lieber CS. Hepatic vitamin A depletion in alcoholic liver injury. N Engl J Med. 1982;304:597–600.

52. Mobarhan S, Seitz HK, Russell RM et al. Age-related effects of chronic ethanol intake on vitamin A status in Fisher 344 rats. J Nutr. 1991;121:510–17.

53. Liu C, Russell RM, Seitz HK, Wang XD. Ethanol enhances retinoic acid metabolism into polar metabolites in rat liver via induction of cytochrome P4502E1. Gastroenterology. 2001; 120:179–89.

54. Wang X-D, Liu C, Chung J, Stickel F, Seitz HK, Russell RM. Chronic alcohol intake reduces retinoic acid concentration and enhances AP1 (c-Jun and c-Fos) expression in rat liver. Hepatology. 1998;28:744–50.

55. Seitz HK. Ethanol and retinoid metabolism. Gut. 2000;47:748–50.

56. Leo MA, Seitz HK, Maier H. Carotinoid, retinoid and vitamin E status of the oropharyngeal mucosa in the alcoholic. Alcohol Alcohol. 1995;30:163–70.

57. Parlesak A, Menzl I, Feuchter A et al. Inhibition of retinol oxidation by ethanol in the rat liver and colon. Gut. 2000;47:825–31.

58. Duester G, Shean ML, McBride MS et al. Retinoic response element in the human alcohol dehydrogenase gene ADH3: implication for regulation of retinoic acid synthesis. Mol Cell Biol. 1991;11:1638–45.

59. Han CL, Liao CS, Wu CW et al. Contribution to first pass metabolism of ethanol and inhibition by ethanol for retinol oxidation in human alcohol dehydrogenase family: implications for etiology of fetal alcohol syndrome and alcohol related diseases. Eur J Biochem. 1998;254:25–31.

60. Allali-Hassani A, Peralba JM, Martras S et al. Retinoids, omega-hydroxy fatty acids and cytotoxic aldehydes as physiological substrates, and H2-receptor antagonists as pharmacological inhibitors of human class IV alcohol dehydrogenase. FEBS Lett. 1998;426:362–6.

61. Kedishvili NY, Gough WH, Davis WI et al. Effect of cellular retinol binding protein on retinol oxidation by human class IV retinol/alcohol dehydrogenase and inhibition by ethanol. Biochem Biophys Res Commun. 1998;249:191–6.

62. Shirashi H, Yokoyama H, Matsumoto M et al. Characterization of oxidation pathway from retinal to retinoid acid in esophageal mucosa. Alcohol Clin Exp Res. 2000;24(Suppl):A168.

63. Trimble KC, Molloy AM, Scott JM et al. The effect of ethanol on one-carbon metabolism: increased methionine catabolism and lipotrope methyl group wastage. Hepatology. 1993; 18:984–9.

64. Stickel F, Schuppan D, Hahn EG et al. Cocarcinogenic effects of alcohol in hepatocarcinogenesis. Gut. 2002;51:132–9.

65. Feinberg AP, Vogelstein B. Hypomethylation distinguishes genes of some human cancers from their normal counterparts. Nature (Lond). 1983;301:98–102.

66. Lieber CS, Casini A, DeCarli LM et al. S-adenosyl-L-methionine attenuates alcohol-induced liver injury in the baboon. Hepatology. 1990;11:165–72.

67. Halsted CH, Villanueva J, Chandler CJ et al. Ethanol feeding of micropigs alters methionine metabolism and increased hepatocellular apoptosis and proliferation. Hepatology. 1996; 23:497–505.

68. Seitz HK, Suter PM. Ethanol toxicity and nutritional status. In: Kotsonis FN, Mackey MA, editors. Nutritional Toxicology, 2nd edn. London: Taylor & Francis, 2002:122–54.

69. Glynn SA, Albanez D. Folate and cancer: a review of the literature. Nutr Cancer. 1994; 22:101–19.

70. Stickel F, Choi SW, Kim YI et al. Effect of chronic alcohol consumption on total plasma homocysteine level in rats. Alcoholism Clin Exp Res. 2000;24:259–64.

71. Garro AJ, McBeth DL, Lima V et al. Ethanol consumption inhibits fetal DNA methylation in mice: implications for the fetal alcohol syndrome. Alcoholism Clin Exp Res. 1991;15:395–8.

72. Choi SW, Stickel F, Baik HW et al. Chronic alcohol consumption induces genomic but not p53-specific DNA hypomethylation in rat colon. J Nutr. 1999;129:1945–50.

141

16
Potential link between sphingomyelin metabolism and colonic tumorigenesis

R.-D. DUAN

INTRODUCTION

Sphingomyelin (SM) is a sphingolipid that comprises a phosphocholine head-group, a long-chain sphingosine backbone and a fatty acid in amide linkage to the sphingosine. In eukaryotic cells SM is mainly located in the outer leaflet of plasma membrane, due to the positive charges of the headgroup of the molecule. The historic concept that SM is an inert membrane constituent that influences the fluidity of membrane has been revolutionized by the finding that the metabolism of SM is rapidly changed in response to various extracellular stimuli[1]. Recent studies from several authors indicate that the metabolism of SM may have implications in colonic tumorigenesis. This chapter aims to summarize the progress, and special attention will be paid to an enzyme located specifically in the intestinal mucosa, which may have preventive effects on the development of colorectal cancer.

METABOLISM OF SPHINGOMYELIN

A simplified SM metabolism pathway and the enzymes responsible to these reactions are shown in Figure 1. Along the pathway three enzymes are thought to be important. The first is sphingomyelinase (SMase), which triggers the degradation of SM and generates ceramide. Several SMases have been identified and the classification of the enzymes is commonly based on their optimal pH values. Acid SMase is a lysosomal enzyme with optimal pH around 4–5, whereas neutral SMase is membrane-bound Mg^{2+}-dependent with optimal pH being about 7–7.5. Several other types of neutral SMase have also been identified. Both acid- and membrane-bound neutral SMases have been cloned and are considered common enzymes in many cell types[2-4]. In the intestinal tract there is a SMase that prefers alkaline pH and was called alkaline SMase[5,6]. We will

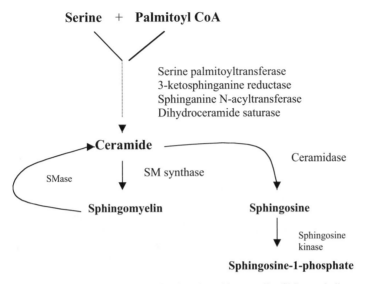

Figure 1 A simplified schematic picture showing the sphingomyelin (SM) metabolism pathway. The major products are in bold and the enzymes responsible for the reactions are shown on the right

discuss this enzyme in detail later in this chapter. The second enzyme that is important for SM metabolism is ceramidase, which catalyses ceramide degradation and also ceramide synthesis. Based on optimal pH, several types of ceramidase have also been identified, purified and cloned[7–10]. The third important enzyme for SM metabolism is serine palmitoyltransferase, which catalyses the first reaction of biosynthesis of ceramide and SM. This enzyme is located in membrane fractions specifically of the endoplasmic reticulum. Previous studies found that serine palmitoyltransferase is present in many tissues including the intestine, and that the activity of the enzyme correlates with cellular SM levels[11].

The products such as ceramide, sphingosine, and sphingosine-1-phosphate generated from metabolism SM are important lipid messengers with multiple biological functions. The biological effects of ceramide have been intensively studied during the 1990s and diverse functions have been identified, including inhibition of cell proliferation, induction of cell differentiation and apoptosis, regulation of immunological response, and modification of inflammatory process[12–15]. Sphingosine is an endogenous inhibitor of protein kinase C and has also been found to have antiproliferative effects in many cells[16]. Sphingosine-1-phosphate is an activator of phospholipase D and mitogen-activated protein (MAP) kinase, and can mobilize intracellular Ca^{2+} (see refs 17–20). Generally speaking, SM metabolism generates both antiproliferative and proliferative molecules, whose balance is of importance in initiation and progress of tumorigenesis. A detailed description of signalling effects of these lipid messengers is not the theme of this chapter, and readers who are interested in this field should refer to several excellent reviews[12,13,21].

SPHINGOMYELIN HYDROLYSIS IN THE GUT

In the intestinal tract there are both endogenous and exogenous SM. The exogenous SM is derived from dietary products, particularly milk, egg, meat and fish[22–24]. The daily SM intake in humans who eat a Western diet is estimated to be about 200–250 mg. The endogenous SM comes from the slough of the intestinal mucosal cells and from bile.

In the intestinal tract a SMase with alkaline pH optimum was first identified by Nilsson in 1969 in humans, pigs, and rats[5]. Different from acid and neutral SMase, which are commonly present in many tissues, the activity of alkaline SMase was found only in the intestinal mucosa of many species except guinea pig, and in the bile of humans but not the bile of many other species including the baboon[25–27]. The activity of the enzyme is absent in the duodenum, increased in the middle of the small intestine, peaked at the end of jejunum and decreased in the ileum and colon[25]. We have purified the enzymes from the intestinal mucosa of rat and from the intestinal content and bile of humans[28,29]. In contrast to neutral and/or acid SMase, alkaline SMase is not Mg^{2+}-dependent, not inhibited by glutathione, and not inactivated by trypsin digestion. The activity is dependent on

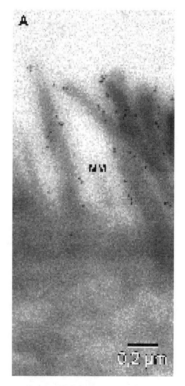

Figure 2 Electron microscopy showing the localization of intestinal alkaline sphingomyelinase in human ileum by immunogold labelling using rabbit anti-human intestinal alkaline sphingomyelinase. MM: microvillar membrane

taurocholate and taurochenodeoxycholate, two major taurine-conjugated primary bile salts, but inhibited by other commonly used detergents such as Triton X100 and CHAPS. Western blot demonstrated that, in the rat, the enzyme is expressed in the intestine but not in other organs including brain, heart, spleen, pancreas and liver[28]. Immunohistochemical studies show that human alkaline SMase is located in the microvillar membrane and synthesized in enterocytes (Figure 2).

The alkaline SMase is responsible for digestion of dietary SM. Animal studies have demonstrated that hydrolysis of dietary SM occurred in the part of the small intestine where alkaline SMase is abundant[30,31]. Studies have provided clear evidence that digestion of dietary SM in the gut is slow and incomplete[30,31], resulting in a considerable amount of undigested SM and unabsorbed ceramide reaching the colon. Human studies found that, after feeding 250 mg of SM, about 14% of intact SM and 9% of generated ceramide can be recovered in the colon within the first 8 hours[32]. The amount of SM and ceramide in the colon is proportional to the amount of SM intake.

A neutral ceramidase activity has been identified in the intestinal mucosa and the lumen[30,33,34]. The enzyme is bile salt-dependent and is distributed in a way parallel to that of alkaline SMase, indicating cooperation between the two enzymes in digestion of SM in the gut.

SPHINGOMYELIN METABOLISM AND COLON CANCER

Indications that sphingomyelin metabolism in the gut affects colonic carcinogenesis

It is well known that both genetic mutations and environmental factors play important roles in colonic carcinogenesis. Dietary factors such as fat, red meat, fibre, and physical activity and lifestyle have been reported to be related to colon cancer development. Recent studies indicate that metabolism of SM may be another potentially important factor that affects carcinogenesis in the colon. The first indication was provided by Dudeja et al., who demonstrated that, in rats, administration of 1,2-dimethylhydrazine (DMH) caused a reduction of neutral SMase activity and an accumulation of SM in colonic plasma membrane[35]. Recently Dillehay et al. and Schmelz et al. reported that administration of SM reduced the development of colonic aberrant crypt foci and reduced the proportion of malignant carcinoma to benign adenoma, induced by DMH in CF1 mice[36,37]. The inhibitory effects of dietary SM are proposed to be mediated by its breakdown product ceramide, as administration of ceramide analogues gives similar results[38]. One study reported that incubation of colon cancer cells with sphingosine reduced cytosolic and nuclear β-catenin, indicating that the APC/β-catenin system might be a target of SM breakdown product[39].

Intestinal alkaline SMase may play important roles in inhibition of colonic tumorigenesis

Although dietary experiments indicate a link of SM metabolism with colonic carcinogenesis, the biochemical mechanisms or factors that are responsible for these events are still not clear. As alkaline SMase is an enzyme specifically present in the intestinal tract, and is probably the key enzyme responsible for SM digestion, we have performed a series of experiments on the changes and functions of the enzyme in colonic tumorigenesis. Our findings point to a potential link between the enzyme and colon cancer, as summarized below.

The activity and expression of alkaline SMase are significantly decreased in colon adenocarcinoma tissues

We first demonstrated that the activity of the enzyme is significantly reduced by 50% in the tissues of human colorectal adenoma, by 75% in carcinoma and by 90% in the mucosa of familial adenomatous polyposis (FAP)[40,41]. Western blot using rabbit anti-human alkaline SMase demonstrated that the enzyme protein was significantly decreased in human cancer tissues compared with the surrounding tissues of the same patient (Figure 3). Acid and neutral SMase activities are also decreased in colorectal cancer and in the flat mucosa of FAP patients, but the extents of the changes are much smaller than that of alkaline SMase. In sporadic adenomas the activity reduction occurs only in alkaline SMase[41].

The reduction of alkaline SMase occurs prior to tumorigenesis. In mice injected with DMH a 20% reduction of enzyme activity was found as early as 5 weeks after the first injection (unpublished data). Human chronic colitis is associated with a high risk of colorectal cancer. As reported recently by Sjöqvist et al., who measured enzyme activity in biopsies from colitis patients with and without dysplasia, enzyme activity was decreased by 20% in no-dysplasia samples and by 36% in dysplasia samples[42].

APC is one of the most important genes in colonic tumorigenesis. Germline mutation of APC is the genetic reason for FAP, and somatic mutation of APC was found in at least 60% of colorectal cancer and in 63% of colorectal benign tumours. However, in human colorectal cancer patients the reduction of alkaline SMase appears not to be a direct downstream target of the APC gene, as similar activities were obtained in colon cancer tissues with or without APC mutations[32]. This may indicate that the changes of alkaline SMase are more closely affected by environmental factors, particularly dietary factors.

Purified intestinal alkaline SMase from rat and humans inhibit proliferation and DNA synthesis of HT29 cells

As shown in Figure 4, human alkaline SMase, when incubated with HT29 cells, inhibited cell proliferation and DNA synthesis. At the equivalent hydrolytic capacity, neutral SMase failed to show any effects on cell proliferation. However, in this experiment both alkaline SMase from rat and human failed to induce apoptosis when added in the medium of cell culture. This has been confirmed by determinations of the formation of histone DNA complex, and by flow cytometry. Because the results above were obtained from an *in-vitro* experiment where the enzyme was present in the medium of cell culture, the possibility that the enzyme *in situ* may induce apoptosis cannot be excluded. To study the changes in transfected cells overexpressed the enzyme should be very informative. At least one previous report showed that the activity of alkaline SMase, but not neutral or acid SMase, in colonic mucosa was well correlated to caspase-3 activity[43].

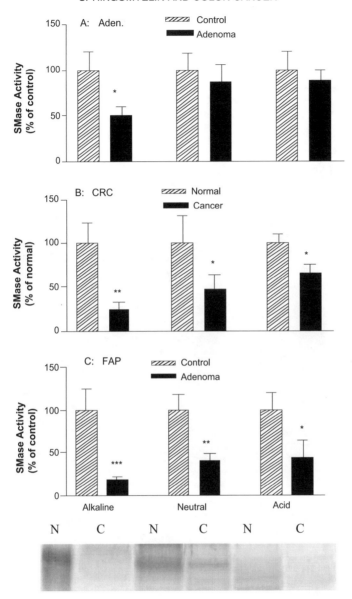

Figure 3 Changes of acid, neutral and alkaline sphingomyelinase activities in human colonic sporadic adenomas (panel A), colorectal carcinomas (panel B) and in the adenomas of FAP patients
(panel C) compared with either normal individuals or with the adjacent normal mucosa. The bottom
panel is a Western blot comparing expression of intestinal alkaline SMase in cancer tissues (C)
with the surrounding normal tissues (N) from three patients. * $p < 0.05$, ** $p < 0.01$, *** $p < 0.001$
compared with control or normal tissue

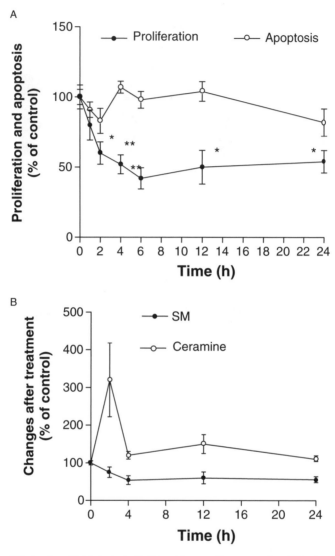

Figure 4 Effects of purified intestinal alkaline sphingomyelinase on cell proliferation and apoptosis after incubation with HT29 cells (upper panel). * p < 0.05, ** p < 0.01 compared with that at zero time. The lower panel shows the changes of sphingomyelin (SM) and ceramide in the cells after incubation with the enzyme

Experiments with anticancer agents and dietary factors point to a role of alkaline SMase in colonic tumorigenesis

We studied the effects of some anticancer agents and dietary factors on intestinal alkaline SMase activity. Ursodeoxycholic acid (UDCA) has been shown to have anticarcinogenic effects on colon cancer in animals[44–46]. We found that, in rats, administration of UDCA increased dose-dependently the levels of alkaline

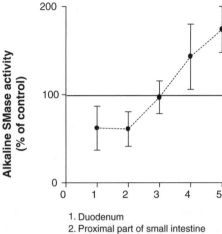

1. Duodenum
2. Proximal part of small intestine
3. Middle of small intestine
4. Distal part of small intestine
5. Colon

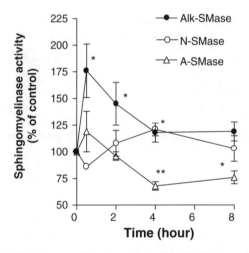

Figure 5 Effects of 5-ASA (upper panel) *in vivo* and boswellic acids (lower panel) *in vitro* on the activities of sphingomyelinase (SMase). In the upper panel, rats were fed with 5-ASA at dose of 100 mg/kg per day by gavage for 10 days. The control rats were fed same amount of saline. The mucosa of duodenum (1), proximal part of small intestine (2), middle of small intestine (3), distal part of small intestine (4), and colon (5) were scraped and homogenised. Alkaline SMase activities in each part were determined. The activities in each part of intestine in 5-ASA treated rats were compared with those in control rats and expressed as percentages of the control values. In the lower panel the HT29 cells were incubated with acetyl-β-keto-bowsellic acid (100 μM) or without (control) for the time indicated. The cells were then washed, scrapped, lysed and the SMase activity determined. The activities were expressed as percentage of control. * $p < 0.05$, ** $p < 0.01$, compared with control

SMase in the colon, accompanied by a correlated increase in caspase-3 activity[43]. 5-Acetylsalicylic acid (5-ASA) is an anti-inflammatory drug that has been found to have chemopreventive effects against colon cancer. We found that administration of 5-ASA in rats selectively increased alkaline SMase in rat colon (Figure 5). Boswellic acids, another type of anti-inflammatory drug, which inhibits 5-lipoxygenase[47], induced apoptosis and inhibited cell proliferation in HT29 cells, and the effects were accompanied by a rapid increase in alkaline SMase activity (Figure 5). The stimulatory effect occurs rapidly and lasts for at least 24 hours. Boswellic acids also increased neutral SMase activity less effectively, but significantly decreased acid SMase activity.

Epidemiological and experimental studies suggest that a high-fat diet increases and high-fibre diet decreases the risk of colorectal cancer. In animal studies we found that a high-fat (50% of energy intake) diet decreased the alkaline SMase activity in the colon by 65% and the reduction was partially reversed by supplement of water-soluble fibre psyllium but not water-insoluble fibre cellulose. A diet containing 10% of psyllium significantly increased alkaline SMase activity by 61%, slightly increased neutral SMase by 16%, but reduced acid SMase by 31%. A diet containing 10% of cellulose only mildly increased neutral and acid SMase activity but had no effect on alkaline SMase (Table 1). The response of ceramidase to dietary factors is a matter of controversy, due to the lack of a simple and good method to assay ceramidase activity. Using a synthetic radiolabelled short-chain ceramide (C_8-ceramide) as substrate, we found that a high-fat diet had no significant effect on ceramidase activity, and psyllium reduced ceramidase activity significantly by 50% (Table 1). Psyllium might thus be an important dietary factor that increases the levels of ceramide in the colonic cells by the activation of alkaline SMase and the inhibition of ceramidase. Although the molecular mechanism underlying the effects shown above remains elusive, the results interestingly indicate that SM metabolism in the colon is changed in response to extracellular stimuli. SMase, particularly alkaline SMase, can be up-regulated by both medications and dietary factors.

Apart from a long-term *in-vivo* effect of a high-fat diet on the levels of SMases, we found that the presence of triglycerides, cholesterol and phospholipids can strongly inhibit the catalytic activity of alkaline SMase in test tubes.

Table 1 Changes of sphingomyelinase (SMase) in the colon after various diets

Diet	Sphingomyelinase activity (pmol/h per mg)		
	Alk-SMase	N-SMase	A-SMase
Control	112.5 ± 18.1	98.9 ± 5.2	644.7 ± 18.6
High psyllium	178.7 ± 21.5*	112.1 ± 6.3	427.8 ± 44.9**
High fat	40.1 ± 6.1 **	98.9 ± 4.8	718.0 ± 29.3*
High fat + psyllium	65.0 ± 15.9*	106.8 ± 5.2	565.9 ± 28.9

Mice were fed semisynthetic diets based on AIN-93G for 4 weeks. In all diets the percentages of energy for protein were kept constant. The percentage of energy of carbohydrates for control and high psyllium was 62.9% and that for high fat and high fat plus psyllium was 26.2%. The percentage of energy of fat for control and high psyllium was 16.3% and that for high fat and high fat plus psyllium was 52.9%.
*$p < 0.05$; **$p < 0.01$ compared with control diet.

The results may indicate that a high-fat and high-cholesterol diet in the intestinal lumen may reduce the production of ceramide in the gut[48,49]. This can be another factor which links to the noxious effects of fat on colon tumorigenesis.

SUMMARY

SM metabolism represents a novel signal transduction pathway that has close implications in tumorigenesis. In the intestinal tract there are both endogenous and exogenous SM, and both SMase and ceramidase that catalyse SM hydrolysis. Alkaline SMase is a specific enzyme expressed in the intestinal mucosa. The activity and expression of the enzyme is decreased in colonic adenomas, carcinomas, and in the colonic mucosa of FAP patients. Purified human alkaline SMase inhibited the proliferation of colon cancer cells. Several drugs with anti-cancer and anti-inflammatory effects, such as ursodeoxycholic acid, Boswellic acid, and 5-ASA, increase enzyme activity. High psyllium significantly increased alkaline SMase levels in the colon, whereas a high-fat diet significantly reduced alkaline SMase activity in the colon and also hydrolytic activity in the lumen. These data indicate that SM metabolism triggered by SMase, most likely alkaline SMase in the gut, has implications in tumorigenesis of colon.

Acknowledgements

I gratefully acknowledge the contributions of numerous co-workers including Drs Å. Nilsson, E. Hertervig, Y. Cheng, J.-J. Liu, L. Nyberg, L. Yang, G. Hanssen, P. Lundgren, and L. Ohlsson. The data in this paper derived from our laboratory were supported by grants from the Swedish Cancer Foundation, Swedish Science Research Council, Albert Påhlsson Foundation, Swedish Association of Medicine, Swedish Gastroenterology Association, and Dr Falk Pharma Foundation.

References

1. Hannun YA, Bell RM. Functions of sphingolipids and sphingolipid breakdown products in cellular regulation. Science. 1989;243:500–7.
2. Chatterjee S, Han H, Rollins S, Cleveland T. Molecular cloning, characterization, and expression of a novel human neutral sphingomyelinase. J Biol Chem. 1999;274:37407–12.
3. Quintern LE, Schuchman EH, Levran O et al. Isolation of cDNA clones encoding human acid sphingomyelinase: occurrence of alternatively processed transcripts. EMBO J. 1989;8:2469–73.
4. Tomiuk S, Hofmann K, Nix M, Zumbansen M, Stoffel W. Cloned mammalian neutral sphingomyelinase: functions in sphingolipid signaling? Proc Natl Acad Sci USA. 1998;95:3638–43.
5. Nilsson Å. The presence of sphingomyelin- and ceramide-cleaving enzymes in the small intestinal tract. Biochim Biophys Acta. 1969;176:339–47.
6. Duan R-D, Nyberg L, Nilsson Å. Alkaline sphingomyelinase activity in rat gastrointestinal tract: distribution and characterization. Biochim Biophys Acta. 1995;1259:49–55.
7. Hong SB, Li CM, Rhee HJ et al. Molecular cloning and characterization of a human cDNA and gene encoding a novel acid ceramidase-like protein. Genomics. 1999;62:232–41.
8. El Bawab S, Roddy P, Qian T, Bielawska A, Lemasters JJ, Hannun YA. Molecular cloning and characterization of a human mitochondrial ceramidase. J Biol Chem. 2000;275:21508–13.
9. Mitsutake S, Tani M, Okino N et al. Purification, characterization, molecular cloning, and subcellular distribution of neutral ceramidase of rat kidney. J Biol Chem. 2001;276:26249–59.
10. Mao C, Xu R, Szulc ZM et al. Cloning and characterization of a novel human alkaline ceramidase. A mammalian enzyme that hydrolyzes phytoceramide. J Biol Chem. 2001;276:26577–88.

11. Merrill AH Jr, Nixon DW, Williams RD. Activities of serine palmitoyltransferase (3-ketosphinganine synthase) in microsomes from different rat tissues. J Lipid Res. 1985;26:617–22.
12. Hannun YA, Linardic CM. Sphingolipid breakdown products: anti-proliferative and tumor-suppressor lipids. Biochim Biophys Acta. 1993;1154:223–36.
13. Kolesnick RN. Sphingomyelin and derivatives as cellular signals. Prog Lipid Res. 1991;30:1–38.
14. Merrill AH, Lingrell S, Wang E, Nikolova-Karakashian M, Vales TR, Vance DE. Sphingolipid biosynthesis de novo by rat hepatocytes in culture. Ceramide and sphingomyelin are associated with, but not required for, very low density lipoprotein. J Biol Chem. 1995;270:13834–41.
15. Hannun YA, Obeid LM. Ceramide: an intracellular signal for apoptosis. Trends Biochem Sci. 1995;20:73–7.
16. Hannun YA, Loomis CR, Merrill AH, Bell RM. Sphingosine inhibition of protein kinase C activity and of phorbol dibutyrate binding in vitro and in human platelets. J Biol Chem. 1986; 261:12604–9.
17. Natarajan V, Jayaram HN, Scribner WM, Garcia JG. Activation of endothelial cell phospholipase D by sphingosine and sphingosine-1-phosphate. Am J Respir Cell Mol Biol. 1994;11:221–9.
18. Olivera A, Spiegel S. Sphingosine-1-phosphate as second messenger in cell proliferation and FCS mitogens. Nature. 1993;365:557–60.
19. Spiegel S, Olivera A, Zhang H, Thompson EW, Su Y, Berger A. Sphingosine-1-phosphate, a novel second messenger involved in cell growth regulation and signal transduction, affects growth and invasiveness of human breast cancer cells. Breast Cancer Res Treat. 1994; 31:337–48.
20. Wu J, Spiegel S, Sturgill TW. Sphingosine-1-phosphate rapidly activates mitogen-activated protein kinase pathway by a G protein-dependent mechanism. J Biol Chem. 1995;270:11484–8.
21. Merrill AH Jr, Schmelz EM, Dillehay DL et al. Sphingolipids – the enigmatic lipid class: biochemistry, physiology, and pathophysiology. Toxicol Appl Pharmacol. 1997;142:208–25.
22. Zeisel SH, Char D, Sheard NF. Choline phosphatidylcholine and sphingomyelin in human and bovine milk and infant formulas. J Nutr. 1986;116:50–8.
23. Holmes-McNary MQ, Cheng WL, Mar MH, Fussell S, Zeisel SH. Choline and choline esters in human and rat milk and in infant formulas. Am J Clin Nutr. 1996;64:572–6.
24. Blank M, Cress EA, Smith ZL, Snyder F. Meats and fish consumed in the American diet contain substantial amounts of ether-linked phospholipids. J Nutr. 1992;122:1656–61.
25. Duan R-D, Hertervig E, Nyberg L et al. Distribution of alkaline sphingomyelinase activity in human beings and animals. Dig Dis Sci. 1996;41:1801–6.
26. Duan R-D. Hydrolysis of sphingomyelin in the gut and clinical implications in colorectal tumorigenesis and other gastrointestinal diseases. Scand J Gastroenterol. 1998;33:673–83.
27. Nyberg L, Duan R-D, Axelsson J, Nilsson Å. Identification of an alkaline sphingomyelinase activity in human bile. Biochim Biophys Acta. 1996;1300:42–8.
28. Cheng Y, Nilsson Å, Tömquist E, Duan RD. Purification, characterization and expression of rat intestinal alkaline sphingomyelinase. J Lipid Res. 2002;43:316–24.
29. Duan R-D, Nilsson Å. Purification of a newly identified alkaline sphingomyelinase in human bile and effects of bile salts and phosphatidylcholine on enzyme activity. Hepatology. 1997;26:823–30.
30. Nilsson Å. Metabolism of sphingomyelin in the intestinal tract of the rat. Biochim Biophys Acta. 1968;164:575–84.
31. Nyberg L, Nilsson Å, Lundgren P, Duan R-D. Localization and capacity of sphingomyelin digestion in the rat intestinal tract. J Nutr Biochem. 1997;8:112–18.
32. Hertervig E. Alkaline Sphingomyelinase: a potential inhibitor in colorectal carcinogenesis. Lund: Rahms Lund AB, 2000.
33. Duan R-D, Cheng Y, Yang L, Ohlsson L, Nilsson A. Evidence for specific ceramidase present in the intestinal contents of rats and humans. Lipids. 2001;36:807–12.
34. Lundgren P, Nilsson Å, Duan R-D. Distribution and properties of neutral ceramidase activity in rat intestinal tract. Dig Dis Sci. 2001;46:765–72.
35. Dudeja PK, Dahiya R, Brasitus TA. The role of sphingomyelin and sphingomyelinase in 1,2-dimethylhydrazine-induced lipid alterations of rat colonic plasma membranes. Biochim Biophys Acta. 1986;863:309–12.
36. Dillehay DL, Webb SK, Schmelz E-M, Merrill AH. Dietary sphingomyelin inhibits 1,2-dimethylhydrazine-induced colon cancer in CF1 mice. J Nutr. 1994;124:615–20.

37. Schmelz EM, Dillehay DL, Webb SK, Reiter A, Adams J, Merrill AH Jr. Sphingomyelin consumption suppresses aberrant colonic crypt foci and increases the proportion of adenomas versus adenocarcinomas in CF1 mice treated with 1,2-dimethylhydrazine: implications for dietary sphingolipids and colon carcinogenesis. Cancer Res. 1996;56:4936–41.

38. Schmelz E, Bushnev A, Dillehan DL, Sullards M, Liotta D, Merrill AH. Ceramide-beta-D-glucuronide: synthesis, digestion, and suppression of early markers of colon carcinogenesis. Cancer Res. 1999;59:5768–72.

39. Schmelz EM, Roberts PC, Kustin EM *et al*. Modulation of intracellular beta-catenin localization and intestinal tumorigenesis *in vivo* and *in vitro* by sphingolipids. Cancer Res. 2001;61:6723–9.

40. Hertervig E, Nilsson Å, Nyberg L, Duan R-D. Alkaline sphingomyelinase activity is decreased in human colorectal carcinoma. Cancer. 1996;79:448–53.

41. Hertervig E, Nilsson Å, Björk J, Hultkrantz R, Duan R-D. Familial adenomatous polyposis is associated with a marked decrease in alkaline sphingomyelinase activity: a key factor to the unrestrained cell proliferation. Br J Cancer. 1999;81:232–6.

42. Sjöqvist U, Hertervig E, Nilsson Å *et al*. Chronic colitis is associated with a reduction of mucosal alkaline sphingomyelinase activity. Inflam Bowel Dis. 2002;8:258–63.

43. Cheng Y, Tauschel H-T, Nilsson Å, Duan R-D. Administration of ursodeoxycholic acid increases the activities of alkaline sphingomyelinase and caspase-3 in rat colon. Scand J Gastroenterol. 1999;34:915–20.

44. Brasitus TA. Primary chemoprevention strategies for colorectal cancer: ursodeoxycholic acid and other agents. Gastroenterology. 1995;109:2036–8.

45. Earnest DL, Holubec H, Wali RK *et al*. Chemoprevention of azoxymethane-induced colonic carcinogenesis by supplemental dietary ursodeoxycholic acid. Cancer Res. 1994;54:5071–4.

46. Suh H, Jung EJ, Kim TH, Lee HY, Park YH, Kim KW. Anti-angiogenic activity of ursodeoxycholic acid and its derivatives. Cancer Lett. 1997;113:117–22.

47. Safayhi H, Mack T, Sabieraj J, Anazodo MI, Subramanian LR, Ammon HP. Boswellic acids: novel, specific, nonredox inhibitors of 5-lipoxygenase. J Pharmacol Exp Ther. 1992;261:1143–6.

48. Liu J-J, Nilsson Å, Duan R-D. Effects of phospholipids on sphingomyelin hydrolysis induced by intestinal alkaline sphingomyelinase: an *in vitro* study. J Nutr Biochem. 2000;11:192–7.

49. Liu J-J, Nilsson Å, Duan R-D. *In vitro* effects of fat, fatty acids, and cholesterol on sphingomyelin hydrolysis induced by rat intestinal alkaline sphingomyelinase. Lipids. 2002;37:469–74.

Section V
Lifestyle factors and CRC risk

17
Energy balance and obesity

R. W. HART

Energy balance can be viewed as a complex set of biochemical reactions and metabolic compartments the concentration and reaction rate and fluxes of which vary over the course of differentiation and aging. Each of these reactions is under gene control and influenced by a plethora of external factors including both the quantity and quality of nutrients consumed.

From an evolutionary perspective energy balance may be viewed as the optimal intake of nutrients and resources required to produce and nurture progeny while having the least deleterious impact on a species niche, with the allocation of energy being distributed between somatic activities such as growth, defense, repair and maintenance and reproduction. In homeotherms, significant under-nutrition without malnutrition results in a slowing of growth and decrease in reproduction, with an increase in defence, repair and maintenance, thus optimizing the ultimate successful production of progeny by the individual once more food is available. Relative to carcinogenesis, under-nutrition without malnutrition has, regardless of species or sex studied, been demonstrated to significantly slow the rate of occurrence of most spontaneous, chemically, physically or virally induced tumours. Concurrent with this change is the up-regulation of a number of physiological functions related to the ability of an organism to maintain homeostasis including body temperature, rates of renal clearance, free radical formation/inactivation, xenobiotic metabolism, DNA repair, fidelity of DNA replication, gene expression, apoptosis, cell–cell communication and immune competency. Over-nutrition without malnutrition has been associated with an increase of certain but not all cancers, also across species and sexes, and a relative decrease in the aforementioned homeostatic processes.

Unfortunately, only recently has the examination of either under- or over-nutrition included caloric utilization. In these recent studies increased caloric utilization through exercise has led to mixed results. The complexity of these results appear to relate in part to the varying effects of exercise duration and intensity on a number of physiological functions including the immune system, elevated prolactin levels, sensitivity of the hypothalamic–pituitary axis, altered energy metabolism, free-radical formation and cell death. Thus, while it is well established that changes in energy balance can significantly influence tumour formation and that individual dietary components can modulate the rate and frequency of occurrence of specific types of tumours, we still do not understand the complex interaction of exercise, nutrition and malnutrition on tumour occurrence.

18
Physical activity and colorectal cancer: independent and interactive effects

M. L. SLATTERY

INTRODUCTION

Physical activity has been one of the most consistently identified factors associated with reduced risk of colon, although not rectal, cancer[1,2]. The data from both case–control and cohort studies are in agreement with these findings. Physical activity is associated with reduced risk of colon cancer in men and women, and in younger and older people. Early studies detected reduced risk of colon cancer among people who were occupationally active; more recent studies conducted in the United States suggest that the best indicator of reduced risk is long-term involvement in vigorous physical activities[1–6].

To put the association between physical activity and colon cancer in perspective, a comparison with heart disease, a disease for which we have long acknowledged the importance of physical activity, can be made. People who are sedentary have a 30–40% increased risk of developing heart disease; people who are sedentary have a 60% to two-fold increased risk of developing colon cancer. While 5% of heart disease can be attributed to a sedentary lifestyle, it has been estimated that 13% of colon cancer can be attributed to a sedentary lifestyle[7]. Comparing physical inactivity with other risk factors for colon cancer, we have estimated that 13% of colon cancer in the population can be attributed to physical inactivity, 12% of colon cancer can be attributed to not using aspirin or NSAID, 12% can be attributed to eating to a Western dietary pattern, and 8% can be attributed to having a family history of colorectal cancer. Physical activity also influences the magnitude of colon cancer risk of other factors, e.g. diet and lifestyle factors[7].

Given the important association between physical activity and colon cancer, why does rectal cancer appear not to be associated with physical activity? It is unknown whether differences in association between colon and rectal cancer are real; are the result of small samples of rectal cases; stem from different techniques used to collect and analyze physical activity data; are the result of uncontrolled confounding; are the result of differences in effect based on underlying characteristics in the population; or whether different biological mechanisms account for differences in association. It is possible that physical activity questionnaires capture different components of physical activity and, even in studies of colorectal cancer, ability to detect associations with colon cancer may be different from those for rectal cancer if biological mechanisms differ. These issues are explored and discussed in this chapter.

METHODS

Recent studies of colon and rectal cancer are reviewed to evaluate associations. To further explore the associations between physical activity and colon and rectal cancer, data were used from two multicentre studies, one of colon cancer and one of rectal cancer[8]. These data were collected and analysed in the same manner; the physical activity questionnaire obtained details of activity performed at moderate and vigorous effort and for a 20-year time period prior to diagnosis of cancer.

Data were collected at both the Northern California Kaiser Permanente Medical Care Program (KPMCP) and an eight-county area in Utah (Davis, Salt Lake, Utah, Weber, Wasatch, Tooele, Morgan and Summit counties) for the colon cancer study which included cases diagnosed with first-primary incident colon cancer (ICD-O, 2nd edition codes 18.0, 18.2 to 18.9) between 1 October 1991 and 30 September 1994, between 30 and 79 years of age at the time of diagnosis, and mentally competent to complete the interview. To make the data more comparable with those collected in the rectal study, participants from the Minnesota portion of the colon cancer study were not included in these analyses, leaving 1327 cases and 1521 controls for analysis. Between 1 June 1997 and 30 May 2001, first-primary incident cases with adenocarcinoma or carcinoma of the rectosigmoid junction or rectum (defined as the first 15 cm from the anal opening) were studied. Preliminary data from the rectal portion of the study are included (813 cases and 983 controls). Cases with known familial adenomatous polyposis, ulcerative colitis or Crohn's disease were not eligible for either study. Controls, in addition to the eligibility criteria for cases, had no history of colorectal cancer. Controls were selected from eligibility lists for KPMCP and driver's licence lists, or Health Care Finance Administration (HCFA) lists for Utah. Controls were matched to cases by 5-year age groups and gender. Methods of control selection have been described in detail[9].

The associations

In the literature the consistency of the association between physical activity is much less for rectal cancer than it is for colon cancer[5–12]. While some more recent studies that have assessed the association for physical activity for colon and rectal cancers separately have found significant inverse associations of the same order of magnitude for both cancers, others have not detected associations for rectal cancer but have observed reduced risk for colon cancer[2,10–12].

From data collected as part of a multicentre study of colorectal cancer, it appears that associations between long-term vigorous physical activity and colon and rectal cancer are the same (Table 1). Among men there is a significant halving of risk for both colon and rectal cancers. Among women the associations also are very similar, although those women reporting the highest level of activity had a lower risk for rectal cancer (OR 0.45, 95% CI 0.29–0.70) than for colon cancer (OR 0.57, 95% CI 0.40–0.82).

Confounding

The association between physical activity and colon cancer does not appear to be confounded by body size, cigarette smoking status, regular use of aspirin/NSAID, family history of colorectal cancer, alcohol use, or multivitamin use (Table 2). Estimates of association are similar regardless of adjustment factors. The association between physical activity and colon cancer is estimated

Table 1 Associations[a] between long-term vigorous physical activity with colon and rectal cancer in Utah and northern California

Level of physical activity	Colon cancer		Rectal cancer[b]	
	No. cases/controls	OR (95% CI)	No. cases/controls	OR (95% CI)
Men				
1 (low)	162/142	1.00	96/74	1.00
2	259/256	0.90 (0.68–1.20)	138/154	0.65 (0.44–0.96)
3	231/259	0.82 (0.60–1.09)	143/182	0.57 (0.39–0.84)
4 (high)	100/179	0.53 (0.37–0.74)	88/129	0.52 (0.34–0.79)
Women				
1 (low)	214/185	1.00	100/85	1.00
2	152/197	0.67 (0.50–0.89)	87/118	0.61 (0.41–0.92)
3	126/180	0.60 (0.44–0.82)	100/130	0.62 (0.41–0.93)
4 (high)	83/123	0.57 (0.40–0.82)	61/111	0.45 (0.29–0.70)

[a] Adjusted for age, BMI, energy intake, dietary calcium and fibre.
[b] Data for the rectal study are preliminary data for 813 cases and 983 controls.

Table 2 Effects of confounding on associations between physical activity and colorectal cancer

Adjusted for	Colon cancer OR (95% CI)	Rectal cancer[a] OR (95% CI)
BMI	0.6 (0.5–0.7)	0.5 (0.4–0.7)
Cigarette smoking	0.6 (0.5–0.7)	0.5 (0.4–0.7)
Aspirin/NSAID	0.6 (0.5–0.7)	0.5 (0.4–0.7)
Family history	0.6 (0.5–0.7)	0.5 (0.4–0.7)
Alcohol	0.6 (0.5–0.7)	0.5 (0.4–0.7)
Energy intake	0.6 (0.4–0.7)	0.5 (0.4–0.7)
Vegetable intake	0.6 (0.5–0.7)	0.6 (0.4–0.7)
Fibre intake	0.6 (0.5–0.7)	0.5 (0.4–0.7)

[a] Data for the rectal study are preliminary data for 813 cases and 983 controls.

at 0.6 (95% CI 0.5–0.7) for participating in long-term vigorous physical activity. Similarly, the association between physical activity and rectal cancer is not confounded by any of the factors evaluated, with a consistent point estimate of 0.5 (95% CI 0.3–0.7).

Biological mechanisms

One possible reason for differences in association observed for colon and rectal cancer in some studies may relate to biological mechanisms. We are beginning to understand disease pathways whereby physical activity may exert action on risk of cancer. Three proposed mechanisms, energy balance, modulation of insulin-related factors, and altered transit time, can be crudely explored by looking at combined associations between physical activity, and body mass index (BMI),

Table 3 Combined effects[a] of physical activity, BMI, dietary fibre, and glycaemic index (GI) on risk of colon and rectal cancers in Utah and Northern California (USA)

| | Physical activity | | |
	High OR (95% CI)	Intermediate OR (95% CI)	Low OR (95% CI)
Colon			
BMI			
<22	1.0	1.0 (0.6–1.7)	1.2 (0.6–2.4)
23–24	1.0 (0.5–1.8)	1.1 (0.6–1.9)	2.1 (1.1–3.9)
25–29	1.1 (0.6–1.8)	1.3 (0.8–2.1)	1.5 (0.9–2.6)
≥30	1.0 (0.6–1.8)	1.7 (1.04–2.9)	2.1 (1.2–3.6)
Fibre			
High	1.0	1.3 (0.9–1.9)	1.7 (1.03–2.7)
Intermediate	1.3 (0.9–2.0)	1.8 (1.3–2.6)	2.4 (1.6–3.6)
Low	2.0 (1.1–3.6)	1.9 (1.3–3.0)	2.4 (1.5–3.9)
GI/fibre			
Low	1.0	1.3 (0.9–2.1)	1.5 (0.9–2.5)
Intermediate	1.2 (0.8–1.9)	1.4 (0.9–2.1)	2.2 (1.4–3.3)
High	0.9 (0.6–1.6)	1.9 (1.2–2.9)	1.9 (1.4–3.1)
Rectum[b]			
BMI			
<22	1.0	1.9 (1.0–3.9)	6.9 (2.8–17.0)
23–24	1.1 (0.5–2.6)	2.1 (1.1–4.1)	2.2 (1.0–4.9)
25–29	1.8 (1.0–3.4)	1.5 (0.8–2.7)	2.5 (1.3–5.0)
≥30	1.6 (0.8–3.1)	2.2 (1.2–4.1)	3.2 (1.6–6.4)
Fibre			
High	1.0	1.1 (0.7–1.6)	1.2 (0.6–2.3)
Intermediate	1.5 (0.9–2.3)	1.7 (1.1–2.5)	2.9 (1.8–4.7)
Low	1.9 (1.0–3.5)	2.6 (1.6–4.4)	4.7 (2.6–8.6)
GI/fibre			
Low	1.0	1.0 (0.6–1.7)	2.2 (1.1–4.5)
Intermediate	1.0 (0.6–1.7)	1.3 (0.8–2.1)	1.9 (1.1–3.2)
High	1.2 (0.7–2.2)	1.5 (0.9–2.4)	2.8 (1.5–5.1)

[a] Adjusted for age, sex, BMI, energy intake, calcium, and dietary fibre.
[b] Data for the rectal study are preliminary data for 813 cases and 983 controls.

diet and lifestyle factors[13-15]. Thus, evaluation of effect modification can potentially provide clues to reasons for inconsistencies observed in the literature for physical activity and cancers of the colon and rectum. Unlike confounding, that distorts associations and is something to identify and control, effect modification is a data characteristic to identify and understand. An understanding of effect modification may provide clues to aetiology and relevant biological mechanisms.

BMI, an indicator of energy balance, dietary fibre, a dietary factor that may influence transit time, and the ratio of dietary glycaemic load to dietary fibre intake, an indicator of insulin-related factors, were evaluated with physical activity for both colon and rectal cancers (Table 3). The combined effect of physical inactivity and a large BMI was greater than either factor alone for both colon and rectal cancers. The adjusted risk associated with physical inactivity and a BMI of 30 or more compared with physical activity and a BMI of 22 or less was 2.1 (95% CI 1.2–3.6) for colon cancer and 3.2 (95% CI 1.6–6.4) for rectal cancer. The adjusted risk associated with being physically inactive and having a low intake of dietary fibre and a high ratio of glycaemic load to dietary fibre also was greater for rectal cancer than for colon cancer.

DISCUSSION

Although studies have consistently identified physical activity as an important factor in the aetiology of colon cancer, these data suggest that a similar level of importance may exist for rectal cancer. Because detailed physical activity data were consistently collected for both colon and rectal cancer, it is possible that changing levels of other factors in the population may be attributing to the current observed risk.

These data hint at ways in which physical activity may be operating: perhaps facilitating transit time through the colon, given the modification effect of dietary fibre; influencing body weight, given the modifying effects of BMI; influencing insulin which in turn influences IGF levels, given the modification effects of glycaemic index and dietary fibre. The relative importance of physical activity in the population may be influenced by the prevalence of obesity and dietary composition. Thus, the underlying characteristics of the population may influence our ability to see associations with physical activity.

In summary, a high level of physical activity has been consistently related to lower risk of colon cancer; in our preliminary data available on rectal cancer, it appears that similar inverse associations exist. From the data presented here the associations do not appear to be confounded by other measured risk factors. However, physical activity appears to have importance beyond its independent association with colorectal cancer by its ability to influence the relative importance of other risk factors for colorectal cancer. Similarly, the relative importance of physical activity may be influenced by diet and lifestyle factors.

Acknowledgements

This work was funded by a grant from the National Cancer Institute No. CA48998. This research was supported by the Utah Cancer Registry, which is funded by Contract No. N01-PC-67000 from the National Cancer Institute, with additional support from the State of Utah Department of Health, the Northern California Cancer Registry, and the Sacramento Tumor Registry. Contributors to this work include collaborators at the Kaiser Permanente Medical Care Program, Donna Schaffer and Dr Bette Caan, and collaborators at the University of Utah, Sandra Edwards, Roger Edwards, Karen Curtin, and Khe Ni Ma. The contents of this chapter are solely the responsibility of the authors and do not necessarily represent the official view of the National Cancer Institute.

References

1. IARC Handbooks on Cancer Prevention, Weight Control and Physical Activity. International Agency for Research on Cancer, World Health Organization, Vol. 6, Lyon, 2002.
2. Potter JD, Slattery ML, Bostick RM, Gapstur SM. Colon cancer: a review of the epidemiology. Epidemiol Rev. 1993;15:499–545.
3. Le Marchand L, Wilkens LR, Kolonel LN, Hankin JH, Lyu LC. Associations of sedentary lifestyle, obesity, smoking, alcohol use, and diabetes with the risk of colorectal cancer. Cancer Res. 1997;57:4787–94.
4. Colbert LH, Hartman TJ, Malila N et al. Physical activity in relation to cancer of the colon and rectum in a cohort of male smokers. Cancer Epidemiol Biomarkers Prev. 2001;10:265–8.
5. Slattery ML, Edwards SL, M KN, Friedman GF, Potter JD. Physical activity and colon cancer: a public health perspective. Ann Epidemiol. 1997;7:137–45.
6. Lee I-M, Paffenbarger RS Jr, Hsieh C. Physical activity and risk of developing colorectal cancer among college alumni. J Natl Cancer Inst. 1991;83:1324–19.
7. Slattery ML, Potter JD. Physical activity and colon cancer: confounding, effect modification, and biological mechanism. Med Sci Sports Exercise. 2002;34:913–9.
8. Slattery ML, Potter JD, Caan BJ et al. Energy balance and colon cancer – beyond physical activity. Cancer Res. 1997;57:75–80.
9. Slattery ML, Edwards SL, Caan BJ, Kerber RA, Potter JD. Response rates among control subjects in case–control studies. Ann Epidemiol. 1995;5:245–9.
10. Longnecker MP, Gerhardsson le Verdier M, Frumkin H, Carpenter C. A case–control study of physical activity in relation to risk of cancer of the right colon and rectum in men. Int J Epidemiol. 1995;24:42–50.
11. Tavani A, Braga C, La Vecchia C et al. Physical activity and risk of cancers of the colon and rectum: an Italian case–control study. Br J Cancer. 1999;79:1912–16.
12. Nilsen TI, Vatten LJ. Prospective study of colorectal cancer risk and physical activity, diabetes, blood glucose and BMI: exploring the hyperinsulinaemia hypothesis. Br J Cancer. 2001;84:417–22.
13. Bingham SA, Cummings JH. Effect of exercise and physical fitness on large intestinal function. Gastroenterology. 1989;97:1389–99.
14. Rissanen A, Fogelholm M. Physical activity in the prevention and treatment of other morbid conditions and impairments associated with obesity: current evidence and research issues. Med Sci Sports Exercise. 1999;31:S635–45.
15. McCarty MF. Up-regulation of IGF binding protein-1 as an anticarcinogenic strategy: relevance to caloric restriction, exercise, and insulin sensitivity. Med Hypoth. 1997;48:297–308.

19
Smoking and colorectal cancer

A. CHAO, M. J. THUN and S. J. HENLEY

INTRODUCTION

Over one billion people use tobacco worldwide[1]. Tobacco use currently causes over 400 000 deaths annually in the United States (US), where about 25% of US adults and 36% of high-school students are current cigarette smokers, and 23% of adults are former smokers[2,3]. Tobacco use is now considered the single most important and preventable cause of disease in the US and Western Europe[4-7], and is expected to become so in the world by the 2020s[5]. Eight cancers have been designated to be smoking-related by the US Surgeon General[7] and the International Agency for Research on Cancer[8]. These include cancers of the lung, mouth, pharynx, larynx, oesophagus, pancreas, kidney, and bladder[7-9], but not colorectal cancer.

Colorectal cancers are the third most common incident cancer and cancer cause of death among men and women in the US; the American Cancer Society (ACS) estimates that 148 300 new cases and 56 600 deaths due to colorectal cancer will occur in the US in 2002[10]. Worldwide, colorectal cancer incidence and mortality rates are the highest in Western Europe, North America, Australia/New Zealand, and Japan[11,12].

In the epidemiological literature cigarette smoking has consistently been associated with colorectal adenomas but inconsistently with colorectal cancer. Possible explanations for this difference have included different study methodology or potential adenoma detection bias in smokers compared to non-smokers. The modestly elevated risk in some studies has also been thought to reflect uncontrolled confounding by factors associated with both smoking and colorectal cancer[13]. However, recent studies that have examined smoking timing and duration consistently show increased risk of colorectal cancer with long-duration smoking. Giovannucci et al. hypothesized that carcinogens in cigarette smoke may initiate tumours in the colon and rectum, so that a period of 35–40 years may be necessary between initiation of tobacco smoking and clinical disease[14-17]. If this is true, then earlier studies may have missed an association due

165

to insufficient follow-up time for the necessary tumour growth, particularly studies conducted among women since the smoking epidemic began later in women than in men[17,18].

Clarifying the relationship between cigarette smoking and colorectal cancer has both public health and clinical implications. If long-term smoking begun during youth is aetiologically important in colorectal cancer, then this relationship could influence past and future trends of colorectal cancer incidence and mortality. Clinically, current and former smokers may be considered a high-risk group to be targeted for colorectal cancer screening. If a causal relationship is established, then colorectal cancer should be appropriately classified as a tobacco-related cancer, thus increasing estimates of smoking-attributable cancers substantially.

We review published epidemiological studies of cigarette smoking in relation to colorectal adenoma and cancer, focusing on studies that examined current smokers separately from former smokers and never smokers. We also present results from a published study[19] conducted in the US in the American Cancer Society Cancer Prevention Study II (CPS II) prospective cohort.

REVIEW OF THE LITERATURE

The relationship of cigarette smoking to colorectal adenoma and cancer has been evaluated in a number of prospective and case–control studies. Figure 1 presents studies of colorectal adenomatous polyps in relation to current cigarette smoking status. With only one exception[21], current cigarette smoking status is consistently associated with increased risk of colorectal adenomas in men and women, with odds ratio estimates ranging between 1.5 and 3.8 after adjustment for age and multiple covariates[23–32]. Current smokers are generally at higher risk than former smokers[20,22,23,25,26,29–32]. Former smoking is associated with significantly increased risk of colorectal adenomas in five studies[24,25,28,29,31], two of which found greater increased risk in former compared to current smokers[20,24]. One Japanese study[21] found no increased risk of adenomas associated with current or former smoking. A randomized clinical trial[22] of antioxidant vitamins in polyp prevention found no association between smoking and recurrence of colorectal adenomas. Of two studies[20,32] that compared adenoma cases to both hospital controls and population controls, one[20] found increased risk only when comparing cases to hospital controls, while the other[32] found comparably increased risk of adenomas when comparing cases to either hospital or population controls.

The majority of studies examining risk of adenomas in relation to cigarette smoking duration or pack-years have found a significantly positive association[14,15,22–26,28–33]. Three prospective studies have found a significant increase in risk of proximal and distal colorectal adenomas with total duration and pack-years of smoking in men and women[14,15,25]. Both the Health Professionals Follow-up Study[14] and the Nurses' Health Study[15] found an association between pack-years of cigarettes smoked more than 20 years in the past and prevalence of large distal adenomas. Pack-years smoked within the past 20 years were associated with small distal adenomas. Case–control studies have reported significant

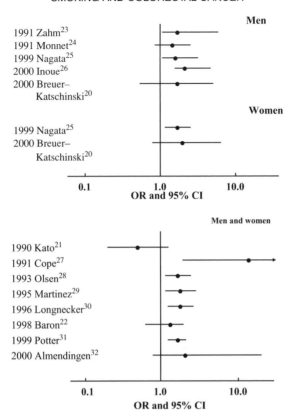

Figure 1 Studies of current cigarette smoking and colorectal adenoma, by year of publication and last name of first author

dose–response with pack-years[22,29–31,33] and duration of smoking[28,32] in studies of men and women combined. When examined separately by sex, there is consistently a significant dose–response observed with pack-years and smoking duration among men[23,24,26,34,35], but a non-significant trend among women[34,35]. One case–control study reported no association between adenoma risk and pack-years in men or women[36].

Prospective cohort studies of colon (Figure 2) and rectal (Figure 3) cancer incidence and mortality among US men have generally reported increased risk associated with current cigarette smoking status, with relative risks ranging between 1.2 and 1.4 for colon cancer, and 1.4 and 2.0 for rectal cancer, regardless of the number or type of covariates adjusted for[37–40]. Two Norwegian studies also reported risk estimates within this range[41,42], but a study of Swedish male construction workers found no increased risk with current or former smoking[43]. Over half of the Swedish cohort was younger than age 40 years at cohort entry, substantially younger than other cohorts in which increased risk was observed. Current smoking was associated with increased mortality from colon (RR 1.36) and rectal (RR 2.30) cancer in the 40-year follow-up of the British Doctors' Study[44].

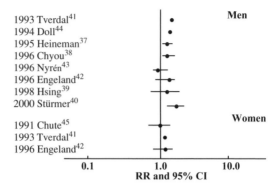

Figure 2 Prospective cohort studies of current cigarette smoking and colon cancer, by year of publication and last name of first author

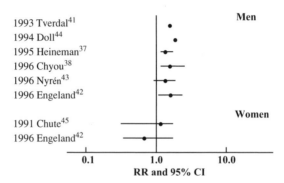

Figure 3 Prospective cohort studies of current cigarette smoking and rectal cancer, by year of publication and last name of first author

No increased risk of colorectal cancer incidence or mortality was found among current smokers in two Norwegian cohort studies of women[41,42], or in the 8-year follow-up report of the Nurses' Health Study[45]. Two of these studies[41,45] included women aged 30–55 at cohort enrollment. Two other cohort studies of men and women combined found no increased risk of colon or rectal cancer incidence with cigarette smoking[46,47]. The relative risk estimates associated with former smoking among men and women are generally between 1.0 and 1.5 and, with some exceptions[37,39,42,43,45], are intermediate between the risk observed among current smokers and lifelong non-smokers.

Case–control studies (Figure 4) of colon and rectal cancer incidence by current cigarette smoking status generally have shown no increased risk in men[48–50], and have been inconsistent in studies of women, or women and men combined[48–52]. One study[51] of US women found a significant increase in risk associated with current smoking: odds ratio (OR) = 1.3 for colon cancer and OR = 1.7 for rectal cancer. When examined by cigarette smoking duration the OR estimates increased with the number of years smoked. The OR among

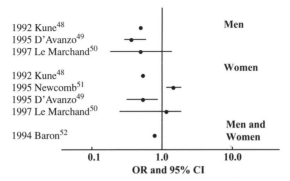

Figure 4 Case–control studies of current cigarette smoking and colon cancer, by year of publication and last name of first author

women who had smoked 31–40 years was 1.7 for colon and 1.5 for rectal cancers[51]. This was the only study to adjust the risk estimates for colorectal cancer screening in addition to other covariates. One US study[50] has examined the relationship by right and left colon, and found significantly increased risk of cancer in the right colon among former smoking women (OR of 2.4) and non-significantly increased risk of cancer in the left colon and rectum among former smoking men. This study also reported significantly increased risk of colon and rectal cancer associated with pack-years of smoking in the distant and recent past in both sexes[50].

Only more recent epidemiological studies (since 1994) have examined colorectal cancer incidence or mortality in relation to gradients of smoking duration and timing, beyond smoking status[14,15,19,39,43]. Four recent prospective studies have shown increased risk of colorectal cancer incidence and mortality with increased smoking duration in both men and women[14,15,19,39]. The only exception is the Swedish study of men in whom no increased risk was observed with smoking duration[43]. The Health Professionals Follow-up Study[14] reported significantly increased risk among men who had smoked at least 40–44 years (RR of 1.8), and observed a significant trend in the number of pack-years accumulated before age 30. The 16-year follow-up of the Nurses' Health Study[15] reported elevated risk in women who had smoked more than 10 cigarettes for 35–39 years (RR of 1.5), and in women who had accumulated 35 years or more since starting to smoke. The US Veterans Cohort[37] found significantly increasing risk of colorectal cancer death associated with younger age at smoking initiation; this 26-year follow-up of the Veterans Cohort reported that initiating smoking before age 15 years was associated with RR of 1.4 for colon cancer mortality and RR of 1.5 for rectal cancer mortality. Recent studies consistently show increased risk of colorectal cancer associated with long-duration cigarette smoking, after adjustment for multiple covariates.

THE CANCER PREVENTION STUDY II

Study methods and results presented here have been described in detail previously[19]. Briefly, CPS II is a large prospective mortality cohort established by the

American Cancer Society (ACS) in 1982, with 508 351 men and 676 306 women aged 30 years or older recruited by ACS volunteers in 50 states, the District of Columbia, and Puerto Rico. Median age at cohort entry was 57 years for men and 56 years for women.

Deaths due to colon or rectal cancer (ICD-9 codes 153.0–154.9) occurring between enrolment in 1982 and 31 December 1996 were examined; colon and rectal cancer deaths were combined due to the potential for their mutual misclassification on death certificates[53]. Date and cause of death were obtained from death certificates or linkage with the National Death Index. Excluded from this study are individuals who reported a previous cancer (other than non-melanoma skin) at cohort enrollment, and those with missing cigarette smoking status or covariate data. Information on cigar or pipe smoking was collected from men only; those who reported any use were excluded from all analyses on cigarette smoking and were examined separately for cigar/pipe smoking. The final study population included 312 332 men and 469 019 women.

Study participants reported lifetime tobacco use information in a mailed questionnaire that also included questions on diet, alcohol consumption, exercise, occupation, medical history, and family cancer history. Potential confounders were chosen based on their observed associations with colorectal cancer mortality and with cigarette smoking, and on previously reported risk factors associated with colon cancer mortality in CPS II[54–56]. Covariates included in data analyses were age; race; body mass index (kg/m^2) computed from self-reported height and weight at baseline; education; family history of colorectal cancer; exercise; current multivitamin and aspirin use; use of hormone replacement therapy in women; current alcohol consumption; and intake of vegetables, high-fibre grain foods, and meat.

Cox proportional hazards models were used to estimate age- and multivariate-adjusted rate ratios (RR) and 95% confidence intervals (CI) relative to never smokers. We computed the proportion of colorectal cancer deaths attributable to smoking in the general population based on multivariate-adjusted risk estimates and prevalence estimates of current and former smoking in the US adult population in 1997[2,57].

Twenty-eight per cent of men and 21% of women reported current smoking at baseline, and 38% of men and 20% of women reported former smoking at baseline. Men and women who currently smoked had lower body mass index, reported more daily drinks of alcohol, lower intake of vegetables and high-fibre grain foods, and higher intake of fatty meats than never or former smokers. Compared with never and former smokers, male current smokers reported lower educational levels and less physical activity. Former smoking women were more likely to report higher educational levels, current use of multivitamins and oestrogen replacement therapy, regular aspirin use, and lower intake of fatty meats than never or current smoking women.

Current and former smoking men and women in 1982 had significantly higher colorectal cancer mortality rate ratios compared to never smokers, with rate ratios being the highest for current smokers (Table 1). The multivariate-adjusted RR (95% CI) for current smoking status was 1.32 (1.16–1.49) among men and 1.41 (1.26–1.58) among women; RR (95% CI) for former smoking was 1.15 (1.04–1.27) among men and 1.22 (1.09–1.37) among women. Adjusting for

Table 1 Number of colorectal cancer deaths, age- and multivariate-adjusted rate ratio (RR) and 95% confidence interval (CI) by smoking status at cohort enrolment, CPS II men and women, 1982 through 1996

Smoking status	Colorectal cancer deaths	Age-adjusted RR (95% CI)	Multivariate-adjusted RR (95% CI)
Men			
Never	683	1.00 (referent)	1.00 (referent)
Current	558	1.44 (1.28–1.61)	1.32 (1.16–1.49)
Former	915	1.21 (1.10–1.34)	1.15 (1.04–1.27)
Women			
Never	1355	1.00 (referent)	1.00 (referent)
Current	476	1.42 (1.28–1.58)	1.41 (1.26–1.58)
Former	445	1.15 (1.03–1.28)	1.22 (1.09–1.37)

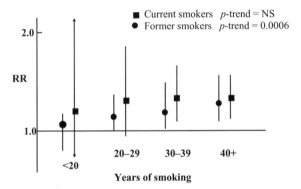

Figure 5 Cigarette smoking duration by current and former smoking status, CPS II men, 1982 through 1996

multiple covariates consistently reduced risk estimates for former and current smoking men, had little impact on estimates for current smoking women, but increased risk estimates for former smoking women (Table 1).

Statistically significant increased risk was observed among current smokers after 30 or more years of smoking in men (Figure 5) and women (Figure 6). In current smoking men the estimated RR (95% CI) was 1.33 (0.96–1.84) for smoking 20–29 years, 1.34 (1.11–1.62) for smoking 30–39 years, and 1.31 (1.13–1.51) for smoking 40+ years. In currently smoking women the estimated RR (95% CI) was 1.33 (1.05–1.69) for smoking 20–29 years, 1.41 (1.19–1.68) for smoking 30–39 years, and 1.51 (1.29–1.76) for smoking 40+ years. Men who were current smokers of exclusively cigars or pipes for 20 years or more were also at increased risk of colorectal cancer mortality compared to never smokers of any tobacco, with multivariate-adjusted RR (95% CI) 1.34 (1.11–1.62).

Risk estimates also increased with cigarettes smoked per day and were statistically significant at nearly all exposure levels in currently smoking men

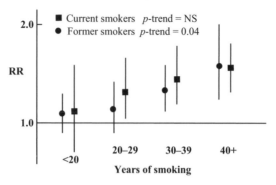

Figure 6 Cigarette smoking duration by current and former smoking status, CPS II women, 1982 through 1996

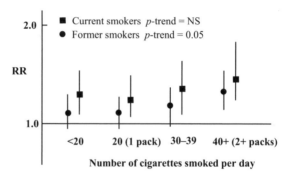

Figure 7 Cigarette smoking amount by current and former smoking status, CPS II men, 1982 through 1996

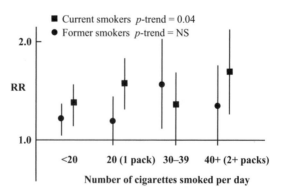

Figure 8 Cigarette smoking amount by current and former smoking status, CPS II women, 1982 through 1996

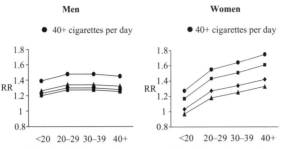

Figure 9 Smoking duration by number of cigarettes smoked per day, CPS II currently smoking men and women, 1982 through 1996

Table 2 Number of colorectal cancer deaths, multivariate-adjusted rate ratio (RR), and 95% confidence interval (CI) by number of years since quit smoking, CPS II men and women, 1982 through 1996

Years since quitting	Men: multivariate-adjusted RR (95% CI)	Women: multivariate-adjusted RR (95% CI)
Current smoker	1.32 (1.16–1.49)	1.41 (1.26–1.58)
≤ 10	1.28 (1.11–1.47)	1.39 (1.18–1.63)
11–19	1.24 (1.08–1.43)	1.10 (0.90–1.33)
20+	0.99 (0.86–1.13)	1.16 (0.98–1.37)
Never	1.00 (referent)	1.00 (referent)
p-trend	0.0009	0.0383

(Figure 7) and women (Figure 8). Among current smokers the multivariate-adjusted RR associated with smoking duration was consistently highest among smokers of 40 or more cigarettes per day in both sexes (Figure 9).

Former smokers of both sexes were also at increased risk after smoking for 30 years, with significant dose–response observed with increasing smoking duration in men (Figure 5) and women (Figure 6). Risk estimates decreased significantly with the number of years since quitting in men and women (Table 2); former smokers who quit 20 or more years ago were not at increased risk compared to never smokers.

Assuming that the associations observed in this study are causal, we estimate the proportion of colorectal cancer deaths in the US population attributable to cigarette smoking to be approximately 12.0% among men and 12.3% among women.

DISCUSSION

Based on the consistently observed association between cigarette smoking and adenomatous polyps and the association between colorectal cancer and long-duration smoking in recent studies, Giovannucci and others have proposed that cigarette smoking plays a role early in colorectal carcinogenesis[14–17]. Two large cohort studies found that smoking for two decades or more was associated with large adenomas, and smoking for less than 20 years was associated with small adenomas[14,15]. Cigarette smoking for at least three decades, or younger age at smoking initiation, has also been associated with increased risk of colorectal cancer incidence and mortality[14,15,19,37,39]. An initiating role of tobacco in the formation of adenomas is further supported by the fact that smokers who quit continue to have an elevated risk of adenoma recurrence after 10 years of smoking cessation[58].

The aggregate epidemiological evidence supports the hypothesis by Giovannucci *et al.* that a long induction-latent period of several decades is necessary for cigarette smoking to affect colorectal cancer incidence or mortality, and that cigarette smoking probably plays an early role in colorectal carcinogenesis[14–17]. Under this hypothesis early studies may have missed an association due to insufficient follow-up time for the necessary tumour growth, particularly among women in whom the smoking epidemic began later than among men in the US[18]. CPS II data on smoking cessation[19] are consistent with both an early and late stage effect of cigarette smoking in colorectal carcinogenesis, and highlight the importance of earlier smoking cessation as well as the avoidance of smoking initiation. These data are consistent with results from the Leisure World cohort, that found men who quit smoking over 20 years ago were at lower risk of colorectal cancer incidence than those that quit within the past 20 years[59].

CPS II is the largest cohort study[19] reporting increased risk of colorectal cancer mortality associated with current smoking status in men and women, and with smoking for 30 or more years. The size of CPS II allowed for detailed examination of gradients in smoking characteristics separately in current and former smokers, and separately in men and women. Other than CPS II, the Nurses' Health Study is the only other prospective study reporting an association in women, with RR of 1.47 (1.07–2.01) after 35–39 years since start of smoking at least 10 cigarettes per day and adjusting for age and body mass index[15]. CPS II data also allowed us to examine the effect of cigarette smoking among men who reported no cigar or pipe smoking, and to examine the effect of long-term cigar or pipe smoking among men who reported no cigarette smoking.

Confounding by unmeasured factors has been proposed as an alternative explanation for the association between cigarette smoking and colorectal cancer, particularly since risk estimates range between 1.1 and 2.0 in most studies[14,15,19,37–39,47,50,51,59]. However, the small but statistically significant increase in risk associated with smoking is remarkably consistent across studies, regardless of the number or type of covariates adjusted for in analysis. Most studies had no information on screening for colorectal cancer; the only study of incidence or mortality that adjusted for screening sigmoidoscopy (as well as other variables) in women[51] reported relative risk estimates similar to CPS II and other results for smoking duration and years since quitting.

In CPS II, adjusting for measured potential confounders for colorectal cancer affected the association with smoking differently by gender and smoking status[19]. Covariate adjustment increased risk estimates among female former smokers, had little impact on risk estimates among female current smokers, and decreased risk estimates in men. The slight decrease in adjusted estimates in men was comparable to that reported by the Health Professionals Follow-up Study[14], which controlled for saturated fat, folate, and dietary fibre, and was one of the few studies that reported age- and multivariate-adjusted risk estimates. Although the possibility of residual confounding cannot be completely excluded, the internal consistency of our findings, and the fact that adjusting for measured potential confounders actually strengthened the association between smoking and colorectal cancer mortality in CPS II female former smokers, a particularly health conscious subgroup, suggest that confounding cannot solely explain the observed associations.

Like all studies of colorectal cancer mortality, CPS II risk estimates potentially reflect an association between cigarette smoking and either survival or incidence. However, in the epidemiological literature, smoking risk estimates have been similar in studies of colorectal cancer incidence and mortality. Another limitation of prospective studies that obtained smoking status only once at cohort enrolment, such as CPS II, is that risk estimates based on longer follow-up may have underestimated the true risk among long-term continuing smokers since some current smokers may have quit smoking during the cohort follow-up period.

Cigarette smoke contains approximately 50 carcinogens including polycyclic aromatic hydrocarbons (PAH), heterocyclic aromatic amines, and N-nitrosamines[60] that can reach the large bowel systemically or by direct ingestion[16,17]. One small study has documented DNA adducts to metabolites of benzo[a]pyrene, a potent PAH, in colonic mucosa more frequently and at higher concentrations in smokers than in non-smokers[61]. This study provides direct evidence that tobacco carcinogens bind to DNA in the human colonic epithelium. DNA adduct levels in the colon epithelium also have been found at higher levels in colonic tissue from patients with colorectal cancer cases than in controls[62].

Several studies suggest that the strength of association between cigarette smoking and colorectal cancer may be larger within subgroups of individuals defined by indices of genetic susceptibility, such as DNA repair or carcinogen metabolism or detoxification gene polymorphisms. One recent study[63] found cigarette smoking to be associated with mismatch repair deficiency in colorectal cancers, reflected by current smoking being associated with a six-fold increased risk of colon tumours with microsatellite instability, in contrast to a two-fold increased risk of colon tumours without microsatellite instability. A large case–control study[64] also reported that, compared to non-smokers, smoking 20 or more cigarettes per day is associated with a 30% increased risk of colon tumours without microsatellite instability but with a two-fold increased risk of colon tumours with microsatellite instability. While these results need to be replicated, they offer a potential explanation for the observed inconsistency in the association between smoking and colorectal cancer, and may help to explain differences in the observed proportion of colon tumours that exhibit microsatellite instability in various study populations[65]. Furthermore, if smoking plays a role early in colon carcinogenesis, then this lifestyle factor may help to determine the genetic or epigenetic pathway by which colonic tumours develop[64].

Colorectal cancer incidence rates increased in the US from 1973 until 1985 and began decreasing steadily in the mid-1980s; mortality rates increased through 1991 and then decreased rapidly through 1997, with patterns different between men and women[66,67]. Cigarette smoking has been proposed as a lifestyle factor that may be partially responsible for the divergent colorectal cancer incidence and mortality trends in men and women between the mid-1940s and early-1980s[67]. Since the smoking epidemic in US women began later in time than in men[18], and is only emerging or maturing in many countries around the world, the impact of long-term cigarette smoking could still be reflected in future colorectal cancer incidence and mortality trends.

If the associations we observed in CPS II between prolonged cigarette smoking and colorectal cancers are causal, then the proportion of colorectal cancer deaths in the general population estimated to be attributable to smoking in 1997 is approximately 12% in men and 12% in women[19]. This approximates estimates obtained from other studies of colorectal cancer incidence and mortality[14,37,51]. The addition of colorectal cancer to the list of smoking-attributable cancers would increase the total number of deaths in the general US population attributable to smoking by over 6800 per year[19].

In summary, the precise risk estimates derived from this and other large prospective studies show a modest but consistently increased risk of colorectal cancer associated with cigarette smoking, especially long-duration smoking. The accumulated evidence supports the hypothesis that cigarette smoking increases the risk of colorectal carcinogenesis, and supports the classification of colorectal cancer as a tobacco-related cancer. Further research is warranted to examine the role of smoking in different genetic and epigenetic pathways of colon and rectal carcinogenesis.

Acknowledgements

The authors gratefully acknowledge the CPS II study participants and colleagues in the Epidemiology and Surveillance Research Department of the American Cancer Society, especially Drs Eugenia E. Calle, Eric Jacobs, Marjorie McCullough, and Carmen Rodriguez. Cancer Prevention Study II is funded by the American Cancer Society. Ann Chao is supported by the American Cancer Society and grant K07-CA75062 from the US National Cancer Institute.

References

1. World Bank. Curbing the epidemic: Governments and the economics of tobacco control. Tobacco Control 1999;8:196–201. http://www.who.int/toh/worldbank/wbr.html.
2. CDC. Cigarette smoking among adults – United States, 1997. Morb Mortal Wkly Rep. 1999;48:993–6.
3. CDC. Tobacco use among high school students – United States, 1997. Morb Mortal Wkly Rep. 1998;47:229–33.
4. Peto R, Lopez AD, Boreham J, Thun M, Heath C. Mortality from tobacco in developed countries: indirect estimation from national vital statistics. Lancet. 1992;339:1268–78.
5. Murray CJL, Lopez AD. Alternative projections of mortality and disability by cause 1990–2020: Global Burden of Disease Study. Lancet. 1997;349:1498–504.
6. The Health Benefits of Smoking Cessation: a report of the Surgeon General. Rockville, MD: US Department of Health and Human Services, Public Health Service, Centers for Disease Control, Center for Chronic Disease Prevention and Health Promotion, Office on Smoking and Health, 1990.
7. Nelson DE, Kirkendall RS, Lawton RL et al. Office on Smoking and Health National Center for Chronic Disease Prevention and Health Promotion. Surveillance for smoking-attributable mortality and years of potential life lost, by State – U.S., 1990. Morb Mortal Wkly Rep. 1994; 43:1–8.

8. Parkin DM, Pisani P, Lopez AD, Masuyer E. At least one in seven cases of cancer is caused by smoking: global estimates for 1985. Int J Cancer. 1994;59:494–504.

9. International Agency for Research on Cancer. IARC monographs on the evaluation of the carcinogenic risk of chemicals to humans: tobacco smoking. Vol. 38. Lyon: International Agency for Research on Cancer, 1986.

10. Jemal A, Thomas A, Murray T, Thun M. Cancer statistics, 2002. CA Cancer J Clin. 2002; 52:23–47.

11. Parkin DM, Pisani P, Ferlay J. Estimates of the worldwide incidence of 25 major cancers in 1990. Int J Cancer. 1999;80:827–41.

12. Pisani P, Parkin DM, Bray F, Ferlay J. Estimates of the worldwide mortality from 25 cancers in 1990. Int J Cancer. 1999;83:18–29.

13. Doll R. Cancers weakly related to smoking. Br Med Bull. 1996;52:35–49.

14. Giovannucci E, Rimm EB, Stampfer MJ et al. A prospective study of cigarette smoking and risk of colorectal adenoma and colorectal cancer in U.S. Men. J Natl Cancer Inst. 1994;86:183–91.

15. Giovannucci E, Colditz GA, Stampfer MJ et al. A prospective study of cigarette smoking and risk of colorectal adenoma and colorectal cancer in U.S. women. J Natl Cancer Inst. 1994;86:192–9.

16. Giovannucci E, Martínez ME. Tobacco, colorectal cancer, and adenomas: a review of the evidence. J Natl Cancer Inst. 1996;88:1717–30.

17. Giovannucci E. An updated review of the epidemiological evidence that cigarette smoking increases risk of colorectal cancer. Cancer Epidemiol Biomarkers Prev. 2001;10:725–31.

18. Pierce JP, Fiore MC, Novotny TE, Hatziandreu EJ, Davis RM. Trends in cigarette smoking in the United States. Projections to the year 2000. J Am Med Assoc. 1989;261:61–5.

19. Chao A, Thun MJ, Jacobs EJ, Henley J, Rodriguez C, Calle EE. Cigarette smoking and colorectal cancer mortality in the Cancer Prevention Study II. J Natl Cancer Inst. 2000;92:1888–96.

20. Breuer-Katschinski B, Nemes K, Ma M et al. and the Colorectal Adenoma Study Group. Alcohol and cigarette smoking and the risk of colorectal adenomas. Dig Dis Sci. 2000;45:487–93.

21. Kato I, Tominaga S, Matsuura A, Yoshii Y, Shirai M, Kobayashi S. A comparative case–control study of colorectal cancer and adenoma. Jpn J Cancer Res. 1990;81:1101–8.

22. Baron JA, Sandler RS, Haile RW, Mandel JS, Mott LA, Greenberg ER. Folate intake, alcohol consumption, cigarette smoking, and risk of colorectal adenomas. J Natl Cancer Inst. 1998;90:57–62.

23. Zahm SH, Cocco P, Blair A. Tobacco smoking as a risk factor for colon polyps. Am J Public Health. 1991;81:846–9.

24. Monnet E, Allemand H, Farina H, Carayon P. Cigarette smoking and the risk of colorectal adenoma in men. Scand J Gastroenterol. 1991;26:758–62.

25. Nagata C, Shimizu H, Kametani M, Takeyama N, Ohnuma T, Matsushita S. Cigarette smoking, alcohol use, and colorectal adenoma in Japanese men and women. Dis Colon Rectum. 1999;42:337–42.

26. Inoue H, Kiyohara C, Marugame T et al. Cigarette smoking, CYP1A1 MspI and GSTM1 genotypes, and colorectal adenomas. Cancer Res. 2000;60:3749–52.

27. Cope GF, Wyatt JI, Pinder IF, Lee PN, Heatley RV, Kelleher J. Alcohol consumption in patients with colorectal adenomatous polyps. Gut. 1991;32:70–2.

28. Olsen J, Kronborg O. Coffee, tobacco and alcohol as risk factors for cancer and adenoma of the large intestine. Int J Epidemiol. 1993;22:398–402.

29. Martínez ME, McPherson RS, Annegers JF, Levin B. Cigarette smoking and alcohol consumption as risk factors for colorectal adenomatous polyps. J Natl Cancer Inst. 1995;87:274–9.

30. Longnecker MP, Chen MJ, Probst-Hensch NM et al. Alcohol and smoking in relation to the prevalence of adenomatous colorectal polyps detected at sigmoidoscopy. Epidemiology. 1996;7:275–80.

31. Potter JD, Bigler J, Fosdick L et al. Colorectal adenomatous and hyperplastic polyps: smoking and N-acetyltransferase 2 polymorphisms. Cancer Epidemiol Biomarkers Prev. 1999;8:69–75.

32. Almendingen K, Hofstad B, Trygg K, Hoff G, Hussain A, Vatn MH. Smoking and colorectal adenomas: a case–control study. Eur J Cancer Prev. 2000;9:193–203.

33. Kikendall JW, Bowen PE, Burgess MB, Magnetti C, Woodward J, Langenberg P. Cigarettes and alcohol as independent risk factors for colonic adenomas. Gastroenterology. 1989;97:660–4.

34. Lee WC, Neugut AI, Garbowski GC et al. Cigarettes, alcohol, coffee, and caffeine as risk factors for colorectal adenomatous polyps. Ann Epidemiol. 1993;3:239–44.

35. Boutron MC, Faivre J, Dop MC, Quipourt V, Senesse P. Tobacco, alcohol, and colorectal tumors: a multistep process. Am J Epidemiol. 1995;141:1038–46.
36. Sandler RS, Lyles CM, McAuliffe C, Woosley JT, Kupper LL. Cigarette smoking, alcohol, and the risk of colorectal adenomas. Gastroenterology. 1993;104:1445–51.
37. Heineman EF, Zahm Sh, McLaughlin JK, Vaught JB. Increased risk of colorectal cancer among smokers: results of a 26-year follow-up of US veterans and a review. Int J Cancer. 1995; 59:728–38.
38. Chyou PH, Nomura A, Stemmermann GN. A prospective study of colon and rectal cancer among Hawaii Japanese men. Ann Epidemiol. 1996;6:276–82.
39. Hsing AW, McLaughlin JK, Chow WH et al. Risk factors for colorectal cancer in a prospective study among U.S. white men. Int J Cancer. 1998;77:549–53.
40. Stürmer T, Glynn RJ, Lee IM, Christen WG, Hennekens CH. Lifetime cigarette smoking and colorectal cancer incidence in the Physicians' Health Study I. J Natl Cancer Inst. 2000; 92:1178–81.
41. Tverdal A, Thelle D, Stensvold I, Leren P, Bjartveit K. Mortality in relation to smoking history: 13 years' follow-up of 68,000 Norwegian men and women 35–49 years. J Clin Epidemiol. 1993;46:475–87.
42. Engeland A, Andersen A, Holdorsen T, Tretli S. Smoking habits and risk of cancers other than lung cancer: 28 years' follow-up of 26,000 Norwegian men and women. Cancer Causes Control. 1996;7:497–506.
43. Nyrén O, Bergström R, Nyström, L et al. Smoking and colorectal cancer: a 20-year follow-up study of Swedish construction workers. J Natl Cancer Inst. 1996;88:1302–7.
44. Doll R, Peto R, Wheatley K, Gray R, Sutherland I. Mortality in relation to smoking: 40 years' observations on male British doctors. Br Med J. 1994;309:901–11.
45. Chute CG, Willett WC, Colditz GA et al. A prospective study of body mass, height, and smoking on the risk of colorectal cancer in women. Cancer Causes Control. 1991;2:117–24.
46. Klatsky AL, Armstrong MA, Friedman GD, Hiatt RA. The relations of alcoholic beverage use to colon and rectal cancer. Am J Epidemiol. 1988;128:1007–15.
47. Knekt P, Hakama M, Järvinen R, Pukkala E, Heliövaara M. Smoking and risk of colorectal cancer. Br J Cancer. 1998;78:136–9.
48. Kune GA, Kune S, Vitetta L, Watson LF. Smoking and colorectal cancer risk: data from the Melbourne Colorectal Cancer Study and brief review of literature. Int J Cancer. 1992;50:369–72.
49. D'Avanzo B, La Vecchia C, Franceschi S, Gallotti L, Talamini R. Cigarette smoking and colorectal cancer: a study of 1,584 cases and 2,879 controls. Prev Med. 1995;24:571–9.
50. Le Marchand L, Wilkens LR, Kolonel LN, Hankin JH, Lyu LC. Associations of sedentary lifestyle, obesity, smoking, alcohol use, and diabetes with the risk of colorectal cancer. Cancer Res. 1997;57:4787–94.
51. Newcomb PA, Storer BE, Marcus PM. Cigarette smoking in relation to risk of large bowel cancer in women. Cancer Res. 1995;55:4906–9.
52. Baron JA, Gerhardsson de Verdier M, Ekbom A. Coffee, tea, tobacco, and cancer of the large bowel. Cancer Epidemiol Biomarkers Prev. 1994;3:565–70.
53. Percy C, Stanek E, Gloeckler L. Accuracy of cancer death certificates and its effect on cancer mortality statistics. Am J Public Health. 1981;71:242–50.
54. Thun MJ, Calle EE, Namboodiri MM et al. Risk factors for fatal colon cancer in a large prospective study. J Natl Cancer Inst. 1992;84:1491–2.
55. Calle EE, Miracle-McMahill HL, Thun MJ, Health CW. Estrogen replacement therapy and risk of fatal colon cancer in a prospective cohort of postmenopausal women. J Natl Cancer Inst. 1995;87:517–23.
56. Murphy TK, Calle EE, Rodriguez C, Kahn HS, Thun MJ. Body mass index and colon cancer mortality in a large prospective study. Am J Epidemiol. 2000;152:847–54.
57. Greenland S. Applications of stratified analysis methods. In: Rothman K, Greenland S, editors. Modern Epidemiology, 2nd edn. Philadelphia: Lippincot-Raven, 1998;281–300.
58. Jacobson JS, Neugut AI, Murray T et al. Cigarette smoking and other behavioral risk factors for recurrence of colorectal adenomatous polyps (New York City, NY, USA). Cancer Causes Control. 1994;5:215–20.
59. Wu AH, Paganini-Hill A, Ross RK, Henderson BE. Alcohol, physical activity and other risk factors for colorectal cancer: a prospective study. Br J Cancer. 1987;55:687–94.

60. Hoffmann D, Hoffmann I. The changing cigarette, 1950–1995. J Toxicol Environ Health. 1997;50:307–64.
61. Alexandrov K, Rojas M, Kadlubar FF, Lang NP, Bartsch H. Evidence of anti-benzo[a]pyrene diolepoxide–DNA adduct formation in human colon mucosa. Carcinogenesis. 1996;17:2081–3.
62. Pfohl-Leszkowicz A, Grosse Y, Carrière V et al. High levels of DNA adducts in human colon are associated with colorectal cancer. Cancer Res. 1999;55:5611–16.
63. Yang P, Cunningham JM, Halling KC et al. Higher risk of mismatch repair-deficient colorectal cancer in α_1-antitrypsin deficiency carriers and cigarette smokers. Mol Genet Metab. 2000;71:639–45.
64. Slattery ML, Curtin K, Anderson K et al. Associations between cigarette smoking, lifestyle factors, and microsatellite instability in colon tumors. J Natl Cancer Inst. 2000;92:1831–6.
65. Chao A, Gilliland F, Willman C et al. Patient and tumor characteristics of colon cancers with microsatellite instability: a population-based study. Cancer Epidemiol Biomarkers Prev. 2000; 9:539–44.
66. Ries LAG, Wingo PA, Miller DS et al. The annual report to the nation on the status of cancer, 1973–1997, with a special section on colorectal cancer. Cancer. 2000;88:2398–424.
67. Chu KC, Tarone RE, Chow WH, Hankey BF, Ries LAG. Temporal patterns in colorectal cancer incidence, survival, and mortality from 1950 through 1990. J Natl Cancer Inst. 1994;86: 997–1006.

20
Bacteria in the pathogenesis of colorectal cancer

J. H. CUMMINGS and G. T. MACFARLANE

INTRODUCTION

It is now over 30 years since Hill and colleagues proposed that colorectal cancer (CRC) was due to 'a metabolite produced *in situ* in the colon by bacterial action on a benign substrate'. In 1969, in order to explain the observed relationship between diet and the worldwide variation in CRC incidence, Aries *et al.*[1] proposed that gut bacteria formed carcinogens from diet or digestive secretions such as bile acids, a process determined largely by the composition of the diet and the flora. They went on to show, in a study of six widely diverse populations, that the faecal flora from high-risk regions had higher counts of *Bacteroides* and lower numbers of aerobes, and that they excreted higher concentrations of steroids that had been chemically modified by the microbiota[2,3].

What progress have we made over the past 30 years in determining the role of bacteria in CRC? Most striking has been the explosion of knowledge of the genetics of the disease. Mutations in more than 12 genes are now thought to contribute, for example, K ras, APC, hMLH1, hMSH2, p53, DCC, etc.[4,5]. Many of these mutations are acquired during life and could be the result of carcinogens present in the large bowel lumen. However, the multiplicity of genetic changes involved clearly indicates that in this form of cancer we are not dealing with a single mutagen, but a variety of different forms; it is therefore likely that diverse bacteria–diet interactions are relevant.

While the principal dietary risk factors for large bowel cancer have not really changed over the years, there has been a move to seeing our food as providing both promoting and protective factors. High intakes of red and processed meats increase risk, vegetables are protective[6,7], whilst fibre, immortalized in Burkitt's seminal 1971 paper[8], has struggled to live up to its role, but has undoubtedly been a most important catalyst in our understanding of protective mechanisms.

Our diets are complex, the genetics of CRC are complex, and so is the large intestinal microbiota. We are therefore unlikely to be looking at a single process, individual bacterium or dietary component to explain large bowel cancer. Moreover, new concepts are emerging that may shape a different future for prevention of this disease. In this context the roles of probiotic bacteria and prebiotic carbohydrates are important.

PROBIOTIC BACTERIA AND COLORECTAL CANCER

Whereas in the 1970s and 1980s much of the work designed to uncover the relationship between CRC and bacteria was focused on bile acid metabolism and mutagen formation (see review by Rowland[9]), by the early 1990s a new and unexpected concept began to emerge. How did the seemingly unlikely strategy of giving bacteria by mouth to prevent CRC develop?

From studies on the metabolism of intestinal microorganisms it became clear that bacterial enzymes, such as β-glucuronidase, nitroreductase, azoreductase and steroid 7α-dehydroxylase, that acted to convert dietary and endogenous secretions to potential carcinogens, could be influenced by diet[10–12]. Moreover, populations at high risk of CRC had higher activities of these enzymes in faeces[10]. At the back of people's minds at this time was the work of Metchnikoff[13], who attributed the longevity of Bulgarian peasants to consumption of a cultured dairy product produced by fermentation with lactobacilli. As a result of this a number of researchers had looked at the potential benefits of feeding *Lactobacillus acidophilus* in diarrhoeal and other diseases[14–17]. A study, coordinated by the International Agency for Research on Cancer Intestinal Microecology Group[18] (which showed that in two Scandinavian populations, Danes and Finns, counts of faecal lactobacilli were significantly higher in the Finns who had only one-quarter of the incidence of CRC) prompted Goldin and Gorbach to conduct what were probably the first studies of probiotics in the prevention of cancer[19–21]. They showed that feeding *Lactobacillus acidophilus* to rats reduced the levels of carcinogen- metabolizing enzymes and tumour incidence. In a study using three small groups of humans these authors demonstrated that daily *Lactobacillus acidophilus* supplements for 1 month reduced β-glucuronidase and nitroreductase activity[22].

Since then a number of studies on the effects of probiotic bacteria in animal models have been published (Table 1) and the topic of cancer prevention by probiotics has been the subject of several recent reviews[23–27]. With the exception of one study there is an unusual consistency in the results of these experiments. Although in the original paper by Goldin and his co-workers[20], tumour numbers were reported to be reduced at 20 weeks but not at 36 weeks, five further studies have shown global reduction in tumour numbers in the colon[28–32] using a variety of carcinogens, probiotic species and one knockout mouse model.

Because of the impossibility of doing similar investigations in humans the search has begun for intermediate markers of cancer risk, of which aberrant crypt foci (ACF) have gained popularity. Table 1 shows that, using these as bio-markers of exposure to carcinogens, there is a consistent reduction with probiotic bacteria. However, in the study of Gallaher et al.[33], protection was seen only when a prebiotic was added with the probiotic (see Table 2), and in Bolognani et al.'s report[34], an effect was found only with a high-fat diet. Overall, when compared with, for example, the conflicting and often-indifferent results

Table 1 Animal studies of probiotics and colorectal cancer

Probiotic	Model	Result	Reference
L. caseii	MNNG rats	Reduced DNA damage in colonic cells	73
L. gasseri, L. confusus, L. delbrueckii, S. thermophilus, B. breve, B. longum	MNNG and DMH rats	All strains anti-genotoxic using Comet assay. Heat-treated species without benefit	74
Lactobacillus sp.	DMH rats	Fewer tumours at 20 weeks, but not at 36 weeks	20
B. longum	IQ rats	Reduced tumours from 0.43 per rat to zero (males)	28
B. longum	AOM rats	ACF formation reduced by 53%, β-glucuronidase decreased	75
Bifidobacterium sp. Bio	DMH rats	Probiotic given in skimmed milk significantly reduced aberrant crypts	76
Bifidobacterium sp., L. acidophilus	DMH rats	No effect on ACF except where combined with FOS (see Table 2)	33
Lactobacillus GG	DMH rats	LGG reduced incidence and numbers of colon tumours if given early and with high-fat diet	29
B. longum	AOM rats	Tumour numbers significantly reduced at 40 weeks. Cell proliferation also reduced	30
B. longum	AOM rats	Total ACF reduced from 187 to 143 (see Table 2) Colonic mucosal GST increased	66
B. longum	AOM rats	Small ACF reduced by 26% (see Table 2)	71
L. acidophilus, L. acidophilus ssp. rhamnosus, B. animalis, S. thermophilus	DMH rats	L. acidophilus gave small but significant reduction in tumours. Others not significant	31
L. casei (Shirota)	AOM rats	Large ACF significantly reduced in both short- and long-term experiments	77
B. longum, L. acidophilus	AOM rats	ACF reduced by 35% and 45% for each species. Combining both probiotics did not increase protective effect. Increased β-glucuronidase and reduced nitroreductase	78, 79
S. bovis	AOM rats	Promoted progression of preneoplastic lesions and ACF, enhanced expression of proliferation markers and production of IL-8. Extracted cell wall material even more potent	36
B. longum, L. casei, L. acidophilus	AOM rats, DMH rats, MNU rats	No consistent changes in ACF, except with high-fat diet	34
L. salivarius	IL-10(−) mice	Probiotic reduced incidence of adenocarcinoma, deaths and mucosal inflammation	32

Table 2 Mechanisms of protection against colorectal cancer by probiotics

---

Binding of mutagens, e.g. heterocyclic amines, to bacterial cell wall
Reduction of procarcinogen activating bacterial enzyme activity, e.g. β-glucuronidase, azoreductase,
  nitrate reductase, nitroreductase, β-glucosidase
Reduction of bile acid 7α-dehydroxylase (reduced synthesis of tumour promoters)
Induction of protective detoxifying enzymes in colonic epithelium (e.g. GST, μ and π)
Butyrate formation from fermentation of carbohydrate
Stimulation of immune responses

---

that were reported for the protective effect of dietary fibre in the 1970s and 1980s[35], probiotic bacteria have a remarkable effect.

One notable exception to all this is the study using *Streptococcus bovis*[36] in azoxymethane (AOM)-treated rats. In marked contrast to the protective role of the various bifidobacteria, lactobacilli and streptococci used in the other studies, *Streptococcus bovis* promoted progression of preneoplastic lesions, ACF and enhanced proliferation markers. *Streptococcus bovis* was one of the early bacterial species thought to be associated with increased risk of CRC[37], although it did not feature in Moore and Moore's more recent population studies[38]. However, trying to relate intestinal carriage of individual bacteria to CRC risk is probably not a worthwhile exercise, since there is considerable metabolic redundancy in the microbiota, with many different species being able to participate in the formation and destruction of genotoxic substances. Studying environmental, physiological and biochemical factors that control bacterial metabolism in the bowel is more likely to increase our understanding of CRC aetiology.

GERMFREE ANIMAL STUDIES

Germfree (GF) animals are useful models for studying the role of intestinal bacteria in disease. They have, for example, provided powerful evidence for the involvement of bacteria in the initiation and perpetuation of inflammation in the large intestine in inflammatory bowel disease[39,40]. When used to study the aetiopathogenesis of CRC, however, they do not present a clear message. GF rats and mice, treated with dimethylhydrazine (DMH), develop adenomas and ACF[41,42]. In the former study, conventional rats had only 42% as many ACF as GF, although 147% as many large ACF. In GF rats associated with a mixture of *Escherichia coli*, *Enterococcus faecium*, *Bacteroides* sp. and *Clostridium* sp. bacteria not thought to be protective against CRC, large increases in preneoplastic lesions were seen, with 168% of animals having ACF and 442% large ACF compared to GF. When these animals were also associated with *Bifidobacterium. breve* fewer large ACF were seen and crypt multiplicity was less. In DMH-treated mice[42], 74% of GF animals had adenomas compared with 58% and 69% of two groups of con-ventionalised animals. When GF were monoassociated with various species, *Bifidobacterium longum* gave no protection (63% with adenoma) whilst *Lactobacillus acidophilus* did (30% with adenoma). Clearly, bacteria are not *a priori* required for the development of CRC. This is understandable if preformed carcinogens are present in the diet. However, some species promote carcinogenesis, possibly due to their abilities to secrete mutagens, or synthesize hydrolytic and reductive enzymes involved in the formation of genotoxic substances, while some bifidobacteria and lactobacilli are protective.

MECHANISMS OF PROTECTION (TABLE 2)

Mutagen binding

In vitro probiotic bacteria bind dietary mutagens in a pH-dependent manner[43–48]. This is thought to be due to interactions with the bacterial cell wall[49]. If this process were to occur *in vivo* then it might be a valuable protective mechanism. However, Rowland's group[46] has shown that *in-vivo* mutagenicity of various heterocyclic amines is not reduced by *Bifidobacterium longum* or *Lactobacillus acidophilus* despite binding *in vitro*. Furthermore, using radiolabelled carcinogen there was no reduction in the amount reaching target organs such as the liver, lungs and heart when the probiotic was given; neither was the amount entering the blood reduced. When similar probiotic species were tested in the mouse for their ability to reduce uptake of ^{14}C-labelled Trp-P-2 that were shown to bind *in vitro*, there was a 29–73% reduction in radioactivity in the lung, thymus, liver and other organs, suggesting some protection[48]. Using the same mutagen[47] and an *in-situ* loop technique in rats, *Lactobacillus acidophilus* ssp. *delbrueckii* reduced absorption from the loop but *Streptococcus thermophilus* did not.

Mutagen binding to Gram-positive bacterial peptidoglycan remains a possible protective mechanism in CRC. However, mutagens and bacteria need to be brought together in an appropriate place in the gut, presumably the gastroduodenal region for pre-existing dietary mutagens such as heterocyclic amines, and in the large bowel for bacterial carcinogens such as N-nitroso compounds. Moreover, the physicochemical environment such as pH and bile acid concentration must be appropriate. Binding would need to be irreversible, otherwise high concentrations of mutagens might be delivered to a lower segment of the gut.

Bacterial enzymes

Modulation of the enzymic/metabolic activities of the indigenous microflora by probiotics is another possible mechanism whereby probiotics may protect against CRC. The early work of Goldin and Gorbach[19–22] showed that cancer risk was associated with lower activities of enzymes such as β-glucuronidase and nitroreductase, and that these activities could be changed by feeding *Lactobacillus acidophilus*[50]. Studies of human intestinal contents have shown that azoreductase and arylsulphatase activities are much higher in the distal than the proximal colon, whilst nitroreductase and β-glucuronidase are higher proximally[51,52]. Most of this activity is bacterial cell-associated in the microbiota. When faecal β-glucuronidase activity was measured in faeces of colon cancer patients and compared with healthy controls, it was found to be 12-fold higher in the cancer patients after sonication of faeces, but only twice as high without sonication[53]. *In-vitro* modelling of fermentation in a three-stage continuous culture using *Bifidobacterium longum* as a model probiotic showed significant reduction in β-glucosidase and β-glucuronidase activities, whilst nitroreductase was stimulated. Addition of the prebiotic carbohydrate oligofructose stimulated enzyme activity in vessels modelling the proximal colon[51], showing the overriding effect of substrate availability on bacterial metabolism.

The wide diversity of toxic and genotoxic compounds produced by intestinal bacteria[9], the importance of substrate availability[51] and the moderating effect of probiotic microorganisms[21,54] may provide an important mechanism whereby bacteria influence the development of CRC, although this is not a simple story.

Bile acids

The role of bile acids in CRC has been much investigated and written about. From putative carcinogen to promoter of cell proliferation, bacterially modified bile acids have been part of the mechanistic hypothesis relating fat to CRC risk. However, there are almost no studies of probiotics and prebiotics on bile acid metabolism. Those that have been published show no effect in humans[55–58] and rarely are they measured in animal studies. This is surprising since the colonic microflora is intimately involved in the deconjugation and dehydroxylation of bile acids, events which a change in the composition and metabolism of the microbiota by probiotics and prebiotics might influence.

Immune function of the gut mucosa

One of the mechanisms of action proposed for probiotic bacteria is strengthening the basic barrier function of the gut, through its effect on the mucosal immune system. The general principle of this effect has recently been reviewed[59]. Observed changes in the mucosal immune system that are thought to be beneficial include increased production of macrophages and activation of phagocytosis; reduced TNFα and increased IFNγ; an increase in mucosal IgA, as well as suppression of lymphocyte proliferation and T cell cytokine production, leading to suppression of inflammation and enhanced antibody response to vaccines and pathogens.

In the context of cancer prevention, studies in Min mice show reduced inflammatory responses, an increase in IgA secretory cells and in CD4(+) T cells when yoghurt is given[60] and increased tumour development in mice that were fed oligofructose, but depleted of CD4(+) and CD8(+) cells[61]. In humans given *Lactobacillus brevis* for 4 weeks a significant dose-dependent increase in virus-induced IFNα production was found with live cells, but not with heat-treated bacteria[62]. However, in a well-designed study that was placebo-controlled in 20 men, *Lactobacillus casei* did not alter any immune parameter, including natural killer cell activity, phagocytosis and cytokine production[63].

Other mechanisms

Of the many other proposed mechanisms whereby probiotics and prebiotics may protect the gut against development of CRC, that of stimulating fermentation with increased production of butyrate is important. Much has been written about butyrate and CRC, and is discussed in detail by Menzel (Chapter 29, this volume). Feeding prebiotic carbohydrate to DMH-treated rats enhances apoptosis[64], which is thought to be a protective mechanism, but whether this is specific to prebiotics, or a general effect of fermented carbohydrate, remains to be seen.

PREBIOTICS

The diet, gut bacteria and cancer story comes full circle with the emergence in recent years of some prebiotic carbohydrates as being protective. Whilst oligofructose (FOS) and inulin are the prebiotics best supported by evidence at the present time, early studies were made with lactulose[65,66] and show clear reduction in DNA damage to colon cells or in ACF in human flora associated DMH rats or azoxymethane-treated conventional rats. Subsequently a number of studies with FOS or inulin[31,34,67–70] have shown either reductions in tumour

Table 3 Animal studies of prebiotics and colorectal cancer

Prebiotics	Animal model	Result	Reference
FOS	Min mouse	Reduced total tumours per animal from 2.01 to 0.7. Increased GALT count from 27 to 32	67
FOS or inulin	AOM rats	Total ACF/colon reduced from 120 to 92 by FOS and to 78 by inulin	68
FOS	Transplanted tumours – mice	Growth of subcutaneous transplanted tumours reduced by both FOS and inulin	80
Lactulose	AOM rats	Total ACF reduced from 187 to 145 (see Table 1)	66
FOS	Min mice	Mice depleted of CD4(+) and CD8(+) T lymphocytes developed more tumours	61
Inulin	AOM rats, ACF	Reduced small ACF by 41% (see Table 1)	71
FOS, soybean, oligosaccharide (SBO), wheat bran, oligosaccharide (WBO)	DMH rats	No effect of FOS on ACF except when combined with probiotic. WBO and SBO – no consistent effect (see Table 1)	33, 69
Lactulose	DMH rats	DNA damage measured by Comet assay was less for lactulose compared with sucrose	65
Inulin	DMH, AOM and MNU rats	No consistent change except when high-fat diet given	34
FOS, inulin	DMH mice	FOS and inulin reduced ACF from 76% (control) to 54% and 53%. Also reduced density of *Candida albicans* and obviated mortality from infection with *Listeria monocytogenes* and *Salmonella typhimurium*	70

numbers[67] or in ACF. Interestingly, where only modest production against tumorigenesis was observed, either with probiotics or prebiotics, combining the two as a symbiotic often produced a much more dramatic effect[33,66,69,71]. This is seen particularly well in Rowland's studies[71] where consumption by AOM-treated rats of either *Bifidobacterium longum* or inulin led to 26% and 41% reductions in small ACF, but no change in large ACF, whereas combined administration reduced small ACF by 80% and large ACF by 59%. Rowland noted a reduction of ammonia levels in caecal contents with the symbiotic, a decrease in β-glucuronidase, and an increase in caecal β-glucosidase.

Prebiotics should by definition selectively increase the number of bifidobacteria or lactobacilli in the gut. Other effects on the flora have also been noted, including reduced numbers of *Clostridium perfringens*[33] and *Candida albicans*, and increased resistance to infection by *Listeria monocytogenes* and *Salmonella typhimurium*[70].

Putative prebiotics and conventional sources of dietary fibre, have also been used in this context. Wheat bran and resistant starch were without consistent benefit[67], an observation made in many previous studies. In another study in which FOS and bifidobacteria reduced ACF numbers, neither soybean oligosaccharides nor wheat bran oligosaccharides were protective[69].

The studies listed in Table 3 were all done using animal models of CRC. Whether the same protective effect of prebiotics will be seen in humans is more difficult to demonstrate. However, Ponz de Leon and Roncucci[72] used lactulose in a study to prevent polyp recurrence in polypectomy patients. After an average of 18 months follow-up in 209 patients there was recurrence in 36% of untreated controls and 15% of those given lactulose. In the same investigation antioxidant vitamins (A, C and E) reduced recurrent rates to 5.7%.

CONCLUSION

The interactions between the multidimensional facets of diet and the complex intestinal microflora, which lead to the various mutations that contribute to the eventual expression or repression of CRC, is not a simple story. The evidence from epidemiology, animal studies and genetics has produced many theories and proposed mechanisms, perhaps too many. There is a need for debate and prioritization of the most fruitful avenues to follow. The scope for more work in humans is especially great, although it brings problems of endpoints and study duration, as well as other interacting factors such as diet, stress and lifestyle events. However, there is a striking consistency in the results of investigations on probiotics and prebiotics that we have not seen before in the many studies using other dietary components, especially wheat bran, pectin and resistant starch.

Does this help us towards a better understanding of the genesis of CRC? The obvious difference between the probiotic and prebiotic data and those of earlier studies is the selective pressures on the colonic microflora that, by definition, occur with probiotics and prebiotics. Changing the composition of the microflora towards one dominated by bifidobacteria and lactobacilli may be crucial. The potential of probiotics and prebiotics to increase intestinal resistance to pathogens and to enhance immune function comprises mechanisms that have not really been studied in the context of CRC. Moreover, there is a complete lack of epidemiological data relating prebiotic carbohydrates and the intestinal microflora to CRC. However, after more than 30 years of research into CRC, an important protective factor and accompanying mechanism may now be emerging.

References

 1. Aries V, Crowther JS, Drasar BS, Hill MJ, Williams REO. Bacteria and the aetiology of cancer of the large bowel. Gut. 1969;10:334–5.
 2. Hill MJ, Crowther JS, Drasar BS, Hawksworth G, Aries V, Williams REO. Bacteria and aetiology of cancer of the large bowel. Lancet. 1971;1:95–100.
 3. Hill MJ, Aries VC. Faecal steroid composition and its relationship to cancer of the large bowel. J Pathol. 1971;104:129–39.
 4. Hardy RG, Meltzer SJ, Jankowski JA. Molecular basis for risk factors. Br Med J. 2000; 321:886–9.
 5. Lengauer C, Kinzler KW, Vogelstein B. Genetic instabilities in human cancers. Nature. 1998; 396:643–9.
 6. World Cancer Research Fund and American Institute for Cancer Research. Food, Nutrition and the Prevention of Cancer: a global perspective. Washington, DC: World Cancer Research Fund in association with American Institute for Cancer Research, 1997.
 7. Department of Health. Nutritional aspects of the development of cancer. Report on Health and Social Subjects. London: Stationery Office, 1998. Report No. 48.
 8. Burkitt DP. Epidemiology of cancer of the colon and rectum. Cancer. 1971;28:3–13.
 9. Rowland IR. Toxicology of the colon: role of the intestinal microflora. In: Gibson GR, Macfarlane GT, editors. Human Colonic Bacteria. Role in nutrition, physiology, and pathology. Boca Raton, FL: CRC Press, 1995:155–74.
10. Reddy BS, Wynder EL. Large-bowel carcinogenesis: fecal constituents of populations with diverse incidence rates of colon cancer. J Natl Cancer Inst. 1973;50:1437–42.
11. Reddy BS, Weisburger JH, Wynder EL. Fecal bacterial beta-glucuronidase: control by diet. Science. 1974;183:416–17.
12. Goldin BR, Gorbach SL. The relationship between diet and rat fecal bacterial enzymes implicated in colon cancer. J Natl Cancer Inst. 1976;57:371–5.
13. Metchnikoff E. The Prolongation of Life. New York: Putnam, 1908.
14. Rettger LF, Levy MN, Weinstein L, Weiss JE. *Lactobacillus acidophilus* and its Therapeutic Applications. New Haven, Conn: Yale University Press, 1935.
15. Beck C, Necheles H. Beneficial effects of administration of *Lactobacillus acidophilus* in diarrheal and other disorders. Am J Gastroenterol. 1961;35:522–30.
16. Paul D, Hoskins LC. Effect of oral lactobacillus feedings on fecal lactobacillus counts. Am J Clin Nutr. 1972;25:763–5.
17. Gilliland SE, Speck ML, Nauyok JR, Geisbrecht FG. Influence of consuming nonfermented milk containing *Lactobacillus acidophilus* on fecal flora of healthy males. J Dairy Sci. 1978;61:1–10.
18. IARC. Dietary fibre, transit time, faecal bacteria, steroids, and colon cancer in two Scandinavian populations. Lancet. 1977;2:207–11.
19. Goldin BR, Gorbach SL. Alterations in fecal microflora enzymes related to diet, age, *Lactobacillus* supplements, and dimethylhydrazine. Cancer. 1977;40:2421–6.
20. Goldin BR, Gorbach SL. Effect of *Lactobacillus acidophilus* dietary supplements on 1,2-dimethylhydrazine dihydro-chloride induced intestinal cancer in rats. J Natl Cancer Inst. 1980;64:263–5.
21. Goldin BR, Gorbach SL. Alterations of the intestinal microflora by diet, oral antibiotics, and *Lactobacillus*: decreased production of free amines from aromatic nitro compounds, azo dyes, and glucuronides. J Natl Cancer Inst. 1984;73:689–95.
22. Goldin BR, Swenson L, Dwyer J, Sexton M, Gorbach SL. Effect of diet and *Lactobacillus acidophilus* supplements on human fecal bacterial enzymes. J Natl Cancer Inst. 1980;64:255–61.
23. Reddy BS. Prevention of colon cancer by pre- and probiotics: evidence from laboratory studies. Br J Nutr. 1998;80:S219–23.
24. Parodi PW. The role of intestinal bacteria in the causation and prevention of cancer: modulation by diet and probiotics. Aust J Dairy Technol. 1999;54:103–21.

25. Hirayama K, Rafter J. The role of lactic acid bacteria in colon cancer prevention: mechanistic considerations. Antonie Van Leeuwenhoek Int J Gen Mol Microbiol. 1999;76:391–4.
26. Brady LJ, Gallaher DD, Busta FF. The role of probiotic cultures in the prevention of colon cancer. J Nutr. 2000;130:410–14S.
27. Wollowski I, Rechkemmer G, Pool-Zobel BL. Protective role of probiotics and prebiotics in colon cancer. Am J Clin Nutr. 2001;73:451–5S.
28. Reddy BS, Rivenson A. Inhibitory effect of *Bifidobacterium longum* on colon, mammary and liver carcinogenesis induced by 2-amino-3-methylimidazo[4,5-f] quinoline, a food mutagen. Cancer Res. 1993;53:3914–18.
29. Goldin BR, Gualtieri LJ, Moore RP. The effect of *Lactobacillus* GG on the initiation and promotion of DMH-induced intestinal tumors in the rat. Nutr Cancer Int J. 1996;25:197–204.
30. Singh J, Rivenson A, Tomita M, Shimamura S, Ishibashi N, Reddy BS. *Bifidobacterium longum*, a lactic acid-producing intestinal bacterium, inhibits colon cancer and modulates the intermediate biomarkers of colon carcinogenesis. Carcinogenesis. 1997;18:833–41.
31. McIntosh GH, Royle PJ, Playne MJ. A probiotic strain of *L. acidophilus* reduces DMH-induced large intestinal tumors in male Sprague-Dawley rats. Nutr Cancer Int J. 1999;35:153–9.
32. O'Mahony L, Feeney M, O'Halloran S *et al*. Probiotic impact on microbial flora, inflammation and tumour development in IL-10 knockout mice. Aliment Pharmacol Ther. 2001;15:1219–25.
33. Gallaher DD, Stallings WH, Blessing LL, Busta FF, Brady LJ. Probiotics, cecal microflora, and aberrant crypts in the rat colon. J Nutr. 1996;126:1362–71.
34. Bolognani F, Rumney CJ, Pool-Zobel BL, Rowland IR. Effect of lactobacilli, bifidobacteria and inulin on the formation of aberrant crypt foci in rats. Eur J Nutr. 2001;40:293–300.
35. Jacobs LR. Enhancement of rat colon carcinogenesis by wheat bran consumption during the stage of 1,2-dimethylhydrazine administration. Cancer Res. 1983;43:4057–61.
36. Ellmerich S, Scholler M, Duranton B *et al*. Promotion of intestinal carcinogenesis by *Streptococcus bovis*. Carcinogenesis. 2000;21:753–6.
37. Klein RS, Recco RA, Catalano MT, Edberg SC, Casey JI, Steigbigel NH. Association of *Streptococcus bovis* with carcinoma of the colon. N Engl J Med. 1977;297:800–2.
38. Moore WEC, Moore LH. Intestinal floras of populations that have a high risk of colon cancer. Appl Environ Microbiol. 1995;61:3202–7.
39. Rath HC, Herfarth HH, Ikeda JS *et al*. Normal luminal bacteria, especially *Bacteroides* sp, mediate chronic colitis, gastritis, and arthritis in HLA-B27/Human β_2 microglobulin transgenic rats. J Clin Invest. 1996;98:945–53.
40. Sellon RK, Tonkonogy S, Schultz M *et al*. Resident enteric bacteria are necessary for development of spontaneous colitis and immune system activation in Interleukin-10-deficient mice. Infect Immun. 1998;66:5224–31.
41. Onoue M, Kado S, Sakaitani Y, Uchida K, Morotomi M. Specific species of intestinal bacteria influence the induction of aberrant crypt foci by 1,2-dimethylhydrazine in rats. Cancer Lett. 1997;113:179–86.
42. Horie H, Kanazawa K, Okada M, Narushima S, Itoh K, Terada A. Effects of intestinal bacteria on the development of colonic neoplasm: an experimental study. Eur J Cancer Prev. 1999; 8:237–45.
43. Morotomi M, Mutai M. *In vivo* binding of potent mutagenic pyrolysates. J Natl Cancer Inst. 1986;77:195–201.
44. Zhang XB, Ohta Y. *In vitro* binding of mutagenic pyrolyzates to lactic acid bacterial cells in human gastric juice. J Dairy Sci. 1991;74:752–7.
45. Orrhage K, Sillerstrom E, Gustaffson J-A, Nord CE, Rafter J. Binding of mutagenic heterocyclic amines by intestinal and lactic acid bacteria. Mutat Res. 1994;311:239–48.
46. Bolognani F, Rumney CJ, Rowland IR. Influence of carcinogen binding by lactic acid-producing bacteria on tissue distribution and *in vivo* mutagenicity of dietary carcinogens. Food Chem Toxicol. 1997;35:535–45.
47. Terahara M, Meguro S, Kaneko T. Effects of lactic acid bacteria on binding and absorption of mutagenic heterocyclic amines. Biosci Biotechol Biochem. 1998;62:197–200.
48. Orrhage KM, Annas A, Nord CE, Brittebo EB, Rafter JJ. Effects of lactic acid bacteria on the uptake and distribution of the food mutagen Tro-P-2 in mice. Scand J Gastroenterol. 2002; 37:215–21.
49. Mital BK, Garg SK. Anticarcinogenic, hypocholesterolemic, and antagonistic ativities of *Lactobacillus acidophilus*. J Med Microbiol. 1995;4:451–9.

50. Goldin BR, Lombardi P, Mayhew J, Gorbach SL. Factors that affect intestinal bacterial activity: implications for colon carcinogenesis. In: Bruce WR, Correa P, Lipkin M, Tannenbaum SR, Wilkins TD, editors. Banbury Report 7: Gastrointestinal Cancer: Endogenous Factors. Cold Spring Harbour: Cold Spring Harbor Press, 1981:1–468.

51. McBain AJ, Macfarlane GT. Investigation of bifidobacterial ecology and oligosaccharide metabolism in a three-stage compound continuous culture system. Scand J Gastroenterol. 1997;32 (Suppl. 222):32–40.

52. McBain AJ, Macfarlane GT. Ecological and physiological studies on large intestinal bacteria in relation to production of hydrolytic and reductive enzymes involved in formation of genotoxic metabolites. J Med Microbiol. 1998;47:407–16.

53. Kim DH, Jin YH. Intestinal bacterial beta-glucuronidase activity of patients with colon cancer. Arch Pharm Res. 2001;24:564–7.

54. Bouhnik Y, Flourie B, Andrieux C, Bisetti N, Briet F, Rambaud J-C. Effects of *Bifidobacterium* sp fermented milk ingested with or without inulin on colonic bifidobacteria and enzymatic activities in healthy humans. Eur J Clin Nutr. 1996;50:269–73.

55. Bartram H-P, Scheppach W, Gerlach S, Ruckdeschel G, Kelber E, Kasper H. Does yogurt enriched with *Bifidobacterium longum* affect colonic microbiology and fecal metabolites in healthy subjects? Am J Clin Nutr. 1994;59:428–32.

56. Bouhnik Y, Flourie B, Riottot M *et al.* Effects of fructo-oligosaccharides ingestion on fecal bifidobacteria and selected metabolic indexes of colon carcinogenesis in healthy humans. Nutr Cancer. 1996;26:21–9.

57. Ellegard L, Andersson H, Bosaeus I. Inulin and oligofructose do not influence the absorption of cholesterol, or the excretion of cholesterol, Ca, Mg, Zn, Fe, or bile acids but increase energy excretion in ileostomy subjects. Eur J Clin Nutr. 1997;51:1–5.

58. Alles MS, Hartemink R, Meyboom S *et al.* Effect of transgalactooligosaccharides on the composition of the human intestinal microflora and on putative risk markers for colon cancer. Am J Clin Nutr. 1999;69:980–91.

59. Isolauri E, Sutas Y, Kankaanpaa P, Arvilommi H, Salminen S. Probiotics: effects on immunity. Am J Clin Nutr. 2001;73:444–50S.

60. Shortt C. Living it up for dinner. Chem Ind. 1998;8:300–3.

61. Pierre F, Perrin P, Bassonga E, Bornet F, Meflah K, Menanteau J. T cell status influences colon tumor occurrence in *Min* mice fed short chain fructo-oligosaccharides as a diet supplement. Carcinogenesis. 1999;20:1953–6.

62. Kishi A, Uno K, Matsubara Y, Okuda C, Kishida T. Effect of the oral administration of *Lactobacillus brevis* subsp *coagulans* on interferon-alpha producing capacity in humans. J Am Coll Nutr. 1996;15:408–12.

63. Spanhaak S, Havenaar R, Schaafsma G. The effect of consumption of milk fermented by *Lactobacillus casei* strain *Shirota* (*L. casei Shirota*) on the composition and metabolic activities of the intestinal microflora, and immune parameters in humans. Eur J Clin Nutr. 1998;52: 899–907.

64. Hughes R, Rowland IR. Stimulation of apoptosis by two prebiotic chicory fructans in the rat colon. Carcinogenesis. 2001;22:43–7.

65. Rowland IR, Bearne CA, Fischer R, Pool-Zobel BL. The effect of lactulose on DNA damage induced by DMH in the colon of human flora-associated rats. Nutr Cancer. 1996;26:37–47.

66. Challa A, Ramkishan R, Chawan CB, Shackelford L. *Bifidobacterium longum* and lactulose suppress azoxymethane-induced colonic aberrant crypt foci in rats. Carcinogenesis. 1997;18:517–21.

67. Pierre F, Perrin P, Champ M, Bornet F, Meflah K, Menanteau J. Short-chain fructo-oligosaccharides reduce the occurrence of colon tumors and develop gut-associated lymphoid tissue in *Min* mice. Cancer Res. 1997;57:225–8.

68. Reddy BS, Hamid R, Rao CV. Effect of dietary oligofructose and inulin on colonic preneoplastic. Carcinogenesis. 1997;18:1371–4.

69. Gallaher DD, Khil J. The effect of symbiotics on colon carcinogenesis in rats. J Nutr. 1999; 127:1483–7S.

70. Buddington KK, Donahook JB, Buddington RK. Dietary oligofructose and inulin protect mice from enteric and systemic pathogens and tumor inducers. J Nutr. 2002;132:472–7.

71. Rowland IR, Rumney CJ, Coutts JT, Lievense LC. Effect of *Bifidobacterium longum* and insulin on gut bacterial metabolism and carcinogen-induced aberrant crypt foci in rats. Carcinogenesis. 1998;19:281–5.

72. Ponz de Leon M, Roncucci L. Chemoprevention of colorectal tumors: role of lactulose and of other agents. Scand J Gastroenterol. 1997;32:72–5.
73. Pool-Zobel BL, Bertram B, Knoll M *et al*. Antigenotoxic properties of lactic-acid bacteria *in vivo* in the gastrointestinal tract of rats. Nutr Cancer J. 1993;20:271–81.
74. Pool-Zobel BL, Neudecker C, Domizlaff *et al*. *Lactobacillus*- and *Bifidobacterium*-mediated antigenotoxicity of the colon of rats. Nutr Cancer Int J. 1996;26:365–80.
75. Kulkarni N, Reddy BS. Inhibitory effect of *Bifidobacterium-longum* cultures on the azoxymethane-induced aberrant crypt foci formation and fecal bacterial beta-glucuronidase. Proc Soc Exp Biol Med. 1994;207:278–83.
76. Abdelali H, Cassand P, Soussotte V, Daubeze M, Bouley C, Narbonne JF. Effect of dairy products on initiation of precursor lesions of colon cancer in rats. Nutr Cancer Int J. 1995;24:121–32.
77. Yamazaki K, Tsunoda A, Sibusawa M *et al*. The effect of an oral administration of *Lactobacillus casei* strain *Shirota* on azoxymethane-induced colonic aberrant crypt foci and colon cancer in the rat. Oncol Rep. 2000;7:977–82.
78. Lee SM, Lee WK. Inhibitory effects of lactic acid bacteria (LAB) on the azoxymethane-induced colonic preneoplastic lesions. J Microbiol. 2000;38:169–75.
79. Lee SM, Lee WK. Effects of lactic acid bacteria on intestinal microbial enzyme activity and composition in rats treated with azoxymethane. J Microbiol. 2001;39:154–61.
80. Taper HS, Lemort C, Roberfroid MB. Inhibition effect of dietary inulin and oligofructose on the growth of transplantable mouse tumor. Anticancer Res. 1998;18:4123–6.

Section VI
Carcinogens and co-carcinogens

21
The role of nitric oxide and oxygen radicals in colon carcinogenesis

S. R. TANNENBAUM and D. SCHAUER

INTRODUCTION

The role of oxidative stress in carcinogenesis is confusing, complex and poorly understood. This is because the effects of oxygen and nitrogen reactive species may play a protective role at low concentrations and a destructive role at high concentrations. Sorting this out is a difficult problem in simple cellular systems, but orders of magnitude more complex in whole organisms. In this paper we will cover the essential chemistry of DNA damage, an analysis of the role of oxidative stress in colon cancer as seen from susceptible strains of genetically engineered mice, and some observations in humans. At the end, we will summarize the additional literature pertinent to the role of NO in colon cancer.

OXIDATIVE STRESS AND DNA

Oxidative stress is an undesirable yet unavoidable consequence of aerobic existence, and chronic inflammatory diseases are major additional sources of oxidative stress *in vivo*. Such conditions liberate reactive nitrogen and oxygen species that have been implicated in inflicting damage to cellular proteins, lipids and DNA. We are particularly interested in understanding the chemical nature of the lesions produced in DNA and other biological molecules as a result of oxidative stress since these modifications can potentially be toxic or mutagenic, thereby contributing to the tissue damage and increased cancer risk observed in some chronic inflammatory diseases. We believe that knowing the chemical identity of oxidative DNA lesions along with how they are processed by cellular repair and replication machinery will be essential in elucidating the biological consequences of oxidative stress[1-3].

Oxidative stress was classically believed to arise predominantly from superoxide generation, but the complexity of the problem increased dramatically with the discovery of nitric oxide. Other contributors to the problem are singlet oxygen and, in the case of inflammation, lipid peroxidation. In the absence of NO, superoxide causes DNA damage through metal-catalyzed decomposition of hydrogen peroxide to yield hydroxyl radical. Nitric oxide also reacts to form additional reactive species that can participate in other types of chemistry. One major fate of nitric oxide is reaction with superoxide, to yield peroxynitrite, $ONOO^-$. This is an extremely fast reaction due to the fact that both species are radicals. The rate of the nitric oxide/superoxide reaction is near the diffusion limit with a rate constant of 6.7×10^9 mol/L^{-1}s^{-1}. This rate constant is approximately 3.5 times larger than that for the superoxide dismutase (SOD)-catalysed decomposition of superoxide, indicating that the nitric oxide/superoxide reaction may predominate over the superoxide/SOD reaction. The formation of both nitric oxide and superoxide does indeed occur simultaneously in cells such as macrophages, neutrophils, Kupffer cells, and endothelial cells. In the vicinity of these cells, peroxynitrite may be present at high concentrations, although the mechanism and extent of $ONOO^-$ formation are strongly influenced by the relative fluxes of superoxide and NO, and the ubiquitous presence of CO_2. A second fate of the NO· produced by these cells is to autoxidize to yield N_2O_3, a powerful electrophilic nitrosating agent.

In the old paradigm of oxidative damage, the focus was predominantly on hydroxyl radical induced damage of all of the DNA bases and induction of strand breaks by attack on the deoxyribose backbone. In the new paradigm, we seek to account for the specificity of DNA damage resulting from inflammation. The new chemistry results from the attack of N_2O_3 and peroxynitrite on DNA bases and deoxyribose and the formation of reactive secondary oxidation products from deoxyribose and unsaturated lipids. The major reactions of N_2O_3 have been dealt with elsewhere[4]. Briefly, the chemistry revolves around diazotization of exocyclic amino groups on the DNA bases, leading to deamination, and crosslinks. In the case of peroxynitrite, dG is the most reactive base, but 8-oxodG is even more reactive, requiring a 1000-fold excess of dGuo to provide 50% protection against the reaction with 8-oxodGuo. This result is thermodynamically predictable from the oxidation potentials of the DNA bases. G is the most oxidizable base, and 8-oxodG has an oxidation potential about 0.5 V lower than G. We have also confirmed this result in synthetic oligonucleotides. Therefore, it seems reasonable that 8-oxodGuo is a potentially important target in DNA, and that the structures of the reaction products with $ONOO^-$ should be characterized. Using 3′,5′-di-O-acetyl-8-oxodGuo and 2′,3′,5′-tri-O-acetyl-8-oxoGuo as model compounds, the reaction products with $ONOO^-$ have been isolated and identified under simulated physiological reaction conditions[5]. The major reaction product is unstable and undergoes base-mediated hydrolysis to 2,5-diaminoimidazol-4-one. Other important products include oxaluric acid (major), cyanuric acid (major), and parabanic acid (minor)[6]. The primary products formed from dG include 8-oxodG, 8-nitrodG, and a 5-guanido-4-nitroimidazole[7]. We have also shown that 8-nitrodG is susceptible to further attack by peroxynitrite to give 8-oxodG and its breakdown products[8]. To confirm that the above reactions occurred in DNA, synthetic oligonucleotides containing 8-oxoguanine were treated with $ONOO^-$ and the reaction products were analysed by liquid chromatography/electrospray ionization mass spectrometry[9]. All of these oligos were found to readily react with peroxynitrite via the same transformations as those observed for free 8-oxodG. The exact location of a modified base within a DNA sequence was determined using exonuclease digestion of oligonucleotide products followed by LC–MS analysis of the fragments. For all 8-oxo-G-containing oligomers, independent of the sequence, the reactions with ONOO⁻ took place at the 8-oxo-G residues. These results suggest that 8-oxo-G, if present in DNA, is rapidly oxidized by peroxynitrite and that oxaluric acid is a likely secondary oxidation product of 8-oxo-G under physiological conditions.

The recognition of the oxidative lesions by formamidopyrimidine glycosylase (Fpg enzyme) was examined in double-stranded versions of the synthetic oligodeoxynucleotides[10]. Fpg efficiently excised 8-oxo-G and oxaluric acid and, to some extent, oxazolone, but not cyanuric acid. These data suggest that some DNA lesions formed via ONOO⁻ exposures (cyanuric acid) are not repaired by Fpg and are not uncovered by assays based on piperidine cleavage at the site of lesion. Our results indicate that cryptic secondary and tertiary oxidation products arising from 8-oxo-G may contribute to the overall mutational spectra arising from oxidative stress. To obtain more detailed information on ONOO⁻-induced DNA damage, a restriction fragment from the pSP189 plasmid containing the supF gene (135 bp) was ³²P-end-labelled and treated with ONOO⁻. PAGE analysis of the products revealed sequence-specific lesions at guanine nucleobases, including the sites of mutational 'hotspots'. These lesions were repaired by Fpg glycosylase and cleaved by hot piperidine treatment, but they were resistant to depurination at 90 °C. Since 8-nitro-G is subject to spontaneous depurination, and 8-oxo-guanine is not efficiently cleaved by piperidine, then results suggest that alternative DNA lesions (e.g. oxaluric acid) contribute to mutations induced by ONOO⁻. Further research demonstrated that the damage spectrum was highly correlated with the mutational spectrum when the gene was expressed in either *E. coli* or in human kidney cells[11].

Finally, the results of all of the experiments carried out by exposure of DNA or plasmids *in vitro* must be judged against the results in which either cells in culture or intact animals are exposed to NO or peroxynitrite. Here we have worked with several different systems: *S. typhimurium* exposed to NO; TK-6 cells exposed to NO; RAW 264 macrophages stimulated to produce NO and superoxide; and the SJL mouse with a B-cell lymphoma.

S. typhimurium[12]

Six tester strains, each containing one of the six possible point mutations in the target codon of a gene in the histidine biosynthetic pathway, were similarly treated with NO and induction of mutation was detected by reversion to histidine auxotrophy. Significant increases were observed in frequencies of each of the six possible base mutations, with the highest occurring in G : C → A : T transitions.

TK-6 cells[12]

Exposure of TK6 cells continuously for 60 min decreased viability by 88%, and survivors exhibited a six-fold increase in mutant fraction in the hprt gene. Independent mutants were isolated and mutations characterized by RT-PCR and DNA sequencing. Base substitutions were present in 18 mutants, 12 occurring at

A: T base pairs. Seven mutants contained deletions of 1–27 bp and one a 13-bp insertion; the 15 remaining RT-PCR products contained whole-exon deletions, 14 involving single exons. The patterns of NO-induced hprt mutations in TK6 cells are similar to the spectrum of spontaneous mutants, suggesting that reactive species derived from NO may contribute to spontaneous mutagenesis of the endogenous hprt gene in human cells.

RAW 264 cells[13]

Controlled exposure to low doses of LPS and IFN-γ allows continuous exponential growth and NO production. Mutant fractions in the hprt gene of NO-producing cells were elevated above 10-fold compared with untreated cells. Addition of an NO synthase inhibitor, N-monomethyl-L-arginine, to the culture medium decreased NO production and MF by 90% and 85%, respectively. Reverse transcription-PCR and DNA sequencing revealed that mutation spectra in NO-associated hprt mutants did not differ significantly from those arising spontaneously, with the exception that certain small deletions/insertions and multiple exon deletions were observed only in the former.

SJL mouse

We recently reported development of an experimental model for the study of nitric oxide (NO) toxicology *in vivo*. SJL mice were injected with superantigen-bearing RcsX (pre-B-cell lymphoma) cells, which migrated to the spleen and lymph nodes, where their rapid growth induced activation of macrophages to produce large amounts of NO over a period of several weeks. In order to investigate specific DNA damage caused by nitric oxide (NO)-induced lipid peroxidation, levels of promutagenic etheno adducts were measured in spleen DNA[14]. εdA and εdC levels were quantified by an ultrasensitive immunoaffinity-^{32}P-post-labelling method. In RcsX cell-injected mice, levels of these adducts were elevated ~6-fold compared with controls. Mice injected with RcsX cells and also treated with NG-methyl-L-arginine (NMA), an inhibitor of inducible nitric oxide synthase, had significantly reduced levels of both εdA and εdC. These findings constitute the first available evidence of formation of etheno adducts associated with NO overproduction *in vivo*. The adducts were presumably formed from lipid peroxidation products such as trans-4-hydroxy-2-nonenal (HNE), generated via oxidation of lipids by peroxynitrite, or alternatively from small reactive molecules generated from deoxyribose oxidation. The results suggest that etheno-DNA adducts, among other types of damage, may contribute to the aetiology of cancers associated with chronic infection/inflammation in which NO is over-produced. This model was also used to investigate mutagenesis in splenocytes exposed to NO during RcsX cell growth[15]. Transgenic mice were produced by crossbreeding animals of the pUR288 transgenic C56BL/6 and SJL strains. RcsX cells were injected into F1 mice and NO production was confirmed by quantification of urinary nitrate, the ultimate metabolite of NO. Mutant frequency in the lacZ gene of the pUR288 plasmid was determined in DNA isolated from spleen (target) and kidney (non-target) tissues. A significant elevation in mutant frequency was found in the spleen, but not in the kidney, of tumour-bearing mice. Furthermore, increases in mutant frequency in the spleen as well as NO production were abrogated by administration of N-methylarginine, a NO inhibitor, to mice following injection of RcsX cells. These results indicate that NO had mutagenic activity in RcsX tumour-bearing mice and thus support a possible role for its involvement in the carcinogenic process. However, in contrast to *in-vitro* experiments which demonstrate oxidation damage, deamination, and strand breaks, the *in-vivo* experiments show that there is increased complexity in DNA modification *in vivo*.

OXIDATIVE STRESS AND COLON CANCER

Over a decade ago, Fearon and Vogelstein proposed a multistep genetic model for the development of human colorectal cancer[16]. Inactivation of the *Apc* tumour suppressor gene and DNA hypomethylation are early events that result in epithelial hyperproliferation and the development of early adenomas. Subsequent oncogene activation and/or inactivation of other tumour suppressor genes are associated with progressive adenoma growth and dysplasia. Inactivation of the *p53* tumour suppressor gene is a late event that results in the development of carcinoma from late adenoma. Additional changes are then associated with metastasis. Although the distinct stages of this model (hyperproliferation, early, intermediate, and late adenoma, carcinoma, and metastasis) can only approximate what is a complex continuum, they serve to emphasize two key points. First, multiple genetic changes are required for the development of a malignant cancer, and, second, although genetic changes often occur in a favoured sequence, it is the accumulation of changes and not the order in which they arise that determines the behaviour of a neoplasm.

The probability that mutations leading to colorectal cancer will accumulate in an individual in the general population is relatively low, but approximately half of all individuals in Western populations develop adenomas (benign polyps) by the age of 70. A fraction of these adenomas progress to cancer, and the lifetime risk of sporadic colorectal cancer is approximately 5%. On the other hand, individuals with inherited mutations in *Apc* develop hundreds to thousands of adenomas in the colon, and the lifetime risk of colorectal cancer in these familial adenomatous polyposis (FAP) patients approaches 100%. Loss of *Apc* function results in the cellular accumulation of β-catenin, which in turn inappropriately activates genes responsive to TCF/LEF family transcription factors, including cyclin D and *c-myc*[17]. Tumour suppressor genes, such as *Apc*, that keep cell growth in check have been designated 'gatekeepers' because, in their absence, cells become neoplastic and exhibit runaway growth.

Laboratory mice carrying a germline mutation in *Apc* have been used as a model to study human colorectal cancer. One such model is the multiple intestinal neoplasia (Min) mouse, which is heterozygous for a nonsense mutation (*Apc^Min*) that encodes an inactive truncated gene product[18]. Homozygosity for an *Apc* mutation results in embryonic lethality. Min mice on a C57BL/6 background develop numerous adenomas in the small intestine and fewer in the large intestine. The large number of adenomas in these animals results in bleeding in the gastrointestinal tract and anaemia. It is rare for C57BL/6 Min mice to live beyond 6 months of age. On other genetic backgrounds, Min mice develop fewer adenomas, live longer, and some of the adenomas become locally invasive carcinomas[19]. Metastasis is not seen in these animals. The main factor influencing tumour development in different inbred strains of mice is secretory phospholipase A_2 ($sPla_2$)[20]. C57BL/6 Min mice are homozygous for a mutation in $sPla_2$, while AKR/J and BALB/c mice are wild type for $sPla_2$. The mechanism by which $sPla_2$ confers a delayed onset and a reduced number of adenomas remains to be determined. Targeted *Apc* mutant mice, or knockout (KO) mice, have also been described[21,22].

It has been known for some time that prolonged use of aspirin and other NSAIDs is associated with reduced relative risk of colorectal cancer. COX-2 expression is induced in adenomas in both FAP patients and in Min and *Apc* KO mice. Furthermore, NSAIDs reduce the number and the size of adenomas in FAP patients and in Min and *Apc* KO mice[23]. Sulindac in particular has received considerable attention. Sulindac is a pro-drug that is metabolized to the pharmacologically active sulindac sulphide, which inhibits COX-1 and COX-2. However, sulindac sulphone, a second derivative, also appears to have anti-neoplastic activity although it does not inhibit prostaglandin synthesis. Thus, the mechanism by which sulindac exerts its antineoplastic effect remains unclear. In addition, because it is not a selective COX-2 inhibitor, sulindac can cause serious adverse reactions, including gastric ulceration and bleeding. More recently, selective COX-2 inhibitors, including celecoxib (Celebrex; Searle) and rofecoxib (Vioxx, Merck), have been shown to inhibit adenoma development in Min and *Apc* KO mice[24,25]. For this reason, selective COX-2 inhibitors are now approved for use in reducing adenomas in FAP patients. Finally, COX-2 *Apc* double KO mice have a reduced number of adenomas that are also smaller in size compared with those in *Apc* KO mice with functional COX-2[26].

While it is clear that COX-2 plays a role in the development of colorectal cancer, some controversy remains about the relative contribution of COX-2 expression by tumour cells and by stromal cells in carcinogenesis. Indeed, different investigators have detected COX-2 activity in different cell populations in adenomas in Min and *Apc* KO mice[26–28]. It appears that COX-2 both inhibits apoptosis when expressed in neoplastic cells and stimulates angiogenesis when expressed by macrophages and myofibroblasts in tumours and cancers. COX-2 expression is also induced during inflammation. Chronic inflammation is known to be a risk factor for cancer. One example is idiopathic inflammatory bowel disease (IBD), including ulcerative colitis and Crohn's disease. IBD patients have an increased risk of developing colorectal cancer. Several KO mouse models have been used to study the pathogenesis of IBD, but only a limited number of reports have investigated the relationship between IBD and tumour development. One such model is the IL-10 KO mouse. When infected with microbial pathogens, IL-10 KO mice develop large bowel inflammation that resembles IBD[29]. Some affected IL-10 KO mice develop highly dysplastic lesions in the large intestine[30]. Unlike the adenomas in Min and *Apc* KO mice on a C57BL/6 background, these areas of dysplasia remain flat and can invade locally, leading investigators to characterize them as carcinomas. The neoplastic lesions in IL-10 KO mice morphologically resemble those that develop in IBD patients, but the ability of these areas of dysplasia to progress to frank carcinoma has not been established. It has been suggested that IBD-associated colorectal cancer follows a different favoured sequence of genetic alterations than sporadic colorectal cancer or FAP. In IBD-associated colorectal cancer, *p53* mutations and microsatellite instability appear to be early common events, while *Apc* mutations occur at a low frequency. Additional studies are needed to definitively characterize the pathway to colorectal cancer in IBD and to determine the mechanism by which chronic inflammation increases cancer risk.

The generation of NO by iNOS is a key feature of chronic inflammation, including chronic inflammation in the gastrointestinal tract. Two recent reports describe adenoma development in Min mice lacking iNOS activity. Scott *et al.* generated iNOS KO Min mice on a C57BL/6 background[31]. There was no significant difference in the number of adenomas in the large intestine or in the proximal two thirds of the small intestine of iNOS KO and iNOS +/+ Min mice. There was a small, but significant, increase in the number of adenomas in the distal third of the small intestine in iNOS KO Min mice compared with iNOS +/+ Min mice, suggesting that iNOS protects against tumorigenesis. On the other hand, Ahn and Oshima found that iNOS contributes to adenoma development in Min mice[32]. These investigators reported that iNOS KO and iNOS +/− Min mice had significantly fewer adenomas than iNOS +/+ Min mice in the small intestine. The number of adenomas in the large intestine was not significantly different. Both studies used Min mice on a C57BL/6 background, and both studies evaluated adenoma number at approximately 4 months of age. However, the number of adenomas in the iNOS +/+ Min mice in the first study was considerably less, with approximately 50 adenomas per animal in the small intestine compared with over 125 adenomas per animal in the second study. One possibility is that environmental factors, including microbial pathogens, enhanced adenoma development in the study by Ahn and Oshima. Thus, the ability of iNOS to contribute to adenoma development would become more apparent with increasing degrees of intestinal inflammation. No information on the degree of mucosal inflammation or the presence of microbial pathogens was provided in these reports, and this hypothesis remains to be tested. In addition, iNOS may play multiple roles in tumorigenesis. NO as an endogenous mutagen, an angiogenesis factor, and an inhibitor of apoptosis would all favour adenoma development. NO as a cytotoxic product directed against transformed cells would inhibit tumorigenesis. Perhaps under conditions of little to no mucosal inflammation, this latter activity is predominant.

We have recently reported that infection with a microbial pathogen enhances adenoma development in the colon of Min mice[33]. The microbial pathogen *Citrobacter rodentium* causes severe but self-limiting epithelial hyperproliferation in the colon of mice[34]. The resulting epithelial hyperplasia has been shown to promote the development of carcinogen-initiated adenomas[35]. We observed an approximately four-fold increase in the number of colon adenomas in infected Min mice compared with uninfected Min mice. As expected, no increase in the number of adenomas in the small intestine was observed, consistent with the fact that *C. rodentium* infection is limited to the colon[34]. The increase in colon adenomas occurred in the absence of significant mucosal inflammation, and indeed COX-2 expression was observed in adenomas but not in hyperplastic colonic mucosa. Thus, infection with microbial pathogens can contribute to tumorigenesis in mouse models of colorectal cancer. The presence of adventitious microbial pathogens should not be overlooked when using these model systems. In humans, chronic inflammation and its attendant hyperproliferation in IBD are risk factors for colorectal cancer. Although its aetiology is unknown, there are considerable similarities between colon cancer risk with IBD and gastric cancer risk with *Helicobacter pylori* infection, which is a Group 1 carcinogen. Indeed, the search for an infectious cause of IBD is currently underway. Additional studies are needed to determine if infection contributes to human colorectal cancer. We are currently characterizing the mechanisms by which microbial infection leading to hyperproliferation and/or chronic inflammation increase cancer risk, particularly with regard to the role of NO.

ROLE OF NO IN COLON CANCER

The process of carcinogenesis is currently viewed as a series of steps involving the inactivation of tumour suppressor genes and the activation of oncogenes. Both types of genetic change involve damage to DNA in the form of either mutations or deletions. In addition, the sequence of steps for transformation of a somatic cell requires alternation of DNA damage and cell division, resulting in expansion of the new target cell population.

The overall hypothesis presented in this paper is that DNA damage, mutation and cytotoxicity will arise as a result of nitrosative deamination, NO· radical reactions, and oxygen radical damage when target cells are exposed to generator cells that produce NO·. Depending upon the dose rate, total dose, types of cells, and other circumstances, NO· may drive cells into apoptosis through multiple pathways, or inhibit apoptosis and enhance mutation through damage to bases, strand breaks and cross-links.

There appear to be significant differences between the effects of NO generated by cells *in vitro* vs. *in vivo*, as will be amplified below. We have already described the major role that microbial pathogens play in activating the inflammatory process, and a major source of free radicals will be from the leukocytes that invade tissue in response to an infection. Thus, NO may first appear as a result of inflammation but, as will be explained below, colon cancer cells also acquire a constitutive NO synthase gene somewhere along the path to cancer, and this NO synthase has different effects *in vitro* and *in vivo*.

The first part of this paper focused on the chemistry of NO and its contribution to DNA damage through multiple pathways. A comprehensive analysis of the NO literature, however, would reveal a much more complex mechanistic relationship to the process of carcinogenesis. NO activates GMP cyclase leading to the formation of cGMP and profound effects on a cell's phenotype. NO also has either a promoting or an inhibitory effect on apoptosis, depending upon the cell type. NO has a cytostatic effect due either to inhibition of ribonucleotide reductase or to damage to the electron-transfer system in the mitochondrion. NO also has been shown to upregulate VEGF, which is critical for blood supply to a solid tumour.

The picture of what COX inhibitors are doing is equally complex[36,37]. 'At the cellular level, COX inhibitors have been shown to inhibit proliferation, induce apoptosis, inhibit angiogenesis, reduce carcinogen activation, and stimulate the immune system.' The overlap between NO and COX effect is so large that it is impossible to separate the two in terms of their mechanistic impact on colon cancer. The biochemical connection between NO and COX lies in peroxynitrite, which has been shown to be essential for activation of the peroxidase function of COX *in vivo*[38]. Loss of COX activity may lead to compensation through an increase in arachidonic acid metabolism via the lipoxygenase pathway. Shureiqi *et al.*[39] have shown that inhibition of COX-2 leads to upregulation of 15-LOX-1, and the products of this enzyme can induce apoptosis in colon cancer cells.

The work of Moncada and co-workers is also instructive on the role of NO both in cancer cell phenotype and in tumour growth[40]. Transfection of iNOS into colon tumour cells causes them to divide more slowly *in vitro* than their wild-type parental cells but, when nude mice were infected with the iNOS tumour cells, the tumours grew faster, were more vascularized, more invasive, and gave higher tumour volume. The discovery that colon cancer cell lines have low NO synthase activity poses the question of the function of NO in these cells[41,42]. Confounding the picture, there also appears to be both constitutive and inducible iNOS in the intestinal tract of mice[43], with the constitutive response confined to the ileum, and the inducible (by LPS) to caecum and colon. In both cases, the enzyme was located in villus epithelium.

Curt Harris laboratory has demonstrated that a significant relationship exists between iNOS and p53 that might help to explain why the low level of NO produced in colon cancer cell lines is important. Ambs and co-workers[44] demonstrated that NO synthase activity is capable of inducing mutations in p53 in human colorectal cancer. They also demonstrated that p53 KO mice had upregulated iNOS[45]. Finally, cancer cell lines expressing iNOS that had wild-type p53 had reduced tumour growth in nude mice, whereas those with mutated p53 had accelerated tumour growth associated with increased VEGF and neovascularization[46]. Thus, data from the Harris laboratory and the Moncada laboratory are consistent with the differing effects of NO *in vivo* vs. *in vitro*, and the difference may be the physiological role of VEGF. The associated finding of increased p53 mutation load in non-cancerous colon tissue from ulcerative colitis patients suggests a significant role for NO in causing these mutations in human subjects[47].

Acknowledgements

This research was supported by NIH grant number DK52413 and grant number P01-CA26731-23 from the National Cancer Institute. Its contents are solely the responsibility of the authors and do not necessarily represent the official views of the National Cancer Institute.

References

1. Davies KJA. The broad spectrum of responses to oxidants in proliferating cells: a new paradigm for oxidative stress. IUBMB Life. 1999;48:41–7.
2. Joshi MS, Ponthier JL, Lancaster Jr JR. Cellular antioxidant and pro-oxidant actions of nitric oxide. Free Radical Biol Med. 1999;27:1357–66.
3. Surh YJ, Chun KS, Cha HH et al. Molecular mechanisms underlying chemopreventive activities of anti-inflammatory phytochemicals: Down-regulation of COX-2 and iNOS through suppression of NF-κB activation. Mutat Res. 2001;480–1:243–68.

4. Caulfield JL, Wishnok JS, Tannenbaum SR. Nitric oxide-induced deamination of cytosine and guanine in deoxynucleosides and oligonucleotides. J Biol Chem. 1998;273:12689–95.

5. Niles JC, Barney S, Singh SP, Wishnok JS, Tannenbaum SR. Peroxynitrite reaction products of 3',5'-di-O-acetyl-8-oxo-7,8-dihydro-2'-deoxyguanosine. Proc Natl Acad Sci USA. 1999;96: 11729–34.

6. Burney S, Caulfield JL, Niles JC, Wishnok JS, Tannenbaum SR. The chemistry of DNA damage from nitric oxide and peroxynitrite. Mutat Res. 1999;424:37–49.

7. Niles JC, Wishnok JS, Tannenbaum SR. A novel nitroimidazole compound formed during the reaction of peroxynitrite wioth 2',3'5'-tri-O-acetyl-guanosine. J Am Chem Soc. 2001;123: 12147–51.

8. Lee JM, Niles JC, Wishnok JS, Tannenbaum SR. Peroxynitrite reacts with 8-nitropurines to yield 8-oxopurines. Chem Res Toxicol. 2002;15:7–14.

9. Tretyakova NY, Niles JC, Burney S, Wishnok JS, Tannenbaum SR. Peroxynitrite-induced reactions of synthetic oligonucleotides containing 8-oxoguanine. Chem Res Toxicol. 1999;12:459–66.

10. Tretyakova NY, Wishnok JS, Tannenbaum SR. Peroxynitrite-induced secondary oxidative lesions at guanine nucleobases: Chemical stability and recognition by the Fpg DNA repair enzyme. Chem Res Toxicol. 2000;13:658–64.

11. Tretyakova NY, Burney S, Pamir B et al. Peroxynitrite-induced DNA damage in the supF gene: Correlation with mutational spectrum. Mutat Res. 2000;447:287–303.

12. Zhuang JC, Wright TL, deRojas-Walker T, Tannenbaum SR, Wogan GN. Nitric oxide-induced mutations in the HPRT gene of human lymphoblastoid TK6 cells and in Salmonella typhimurium. Env Molec Mutag. 2000;35:39–47.

13. Zhuang JC, Lin D, Lin C, Wogan GN. Mutagenesis associated with nitric oxide production in macrophages. Proc Natl Acad Sci USA. 1998;95:8286–91.

14. Nair J, Gal A, Tamir S, Tannenbaum SR, Wogan GN, Bartsch H. Etheno adducts in spleen DNA of SJL mice stimulated to overproduce nitric oxide. Carcinogenesis. 1998;19:2081–4.

15. Gal A, Wogan GN. Mutagenesis associated with nitric oxide production in transgenic SJL mice. Proc Natl Acad Sci USA. 1996;93:15102–7.

16. Fearon ER, Vogelstein BA. Genetic model for colorectal tumorigenesis. Cell. 1990;61:759–67.

17. Wong NA, Pignatelli M. Beta-catenin – a linchpin in colorectal carcinogenesis? Am J Pathol. 2002;160:389–401.

18. Moser AR, Pitot HC, Dove WF. A dominant mutation that predisposes to multiple intestinal neoplasia in the mouse. Science. 1990;247:322–4.

19. Shoemaker AR, Moser AR, Midgley CA, Clipson L, Newton MA, Dove WF. A resistant genetic background leading to incomplete penetrance of intestinal neoplasia and reduced loss of heterozygosity in ApcMin/+ mice. Proc Natl Acad Sci USA. 1998;95:10826–31.

20. Cormier RT, Hong KH, Halberg RB et al. Secretory phospholipase Pla2g2a confers resistance to intestinal tumorigenesis. Natl Genet. 1997;17:88–91.

21. Oshima M, Oshima H, Kitagawa K, Kobayashi M, Itakura C, Taketo M. Loss of Apc heterozygosity and abnormal tissue building in nascent intestinal polyps in mice carrying a truncated Apc gene. Proc Natl Acad Sci USA. 1995;92:4482–6.

22. Smits R, van der Houven van Oordt W, Luz A. Apc1638N: a mouse model for familial adenomatous polyposis-associated desmoid tumors and cutaneous cysts. Gastroenterology. 1998;114: 275–83.

23. Taketo MM. Cyclooxygenase-2 inhibitors in tumorigenesis (Part II). J Natl Cancer Inst. 1998;90:1609–20.

24. Jacoby RF, Seibert K, Cole C, Kelloff G, Lubet RA. The cyclooxygenase-2 inhibitor celecoxib is a potent preventive and therapeutic agent in the min mouse model of adenomatous polyposis. Cancer Res. 2000;60:5040–4.

25. Oshima M, Murai N, Kargman S et al. Chemoprevention of intestinal polyposis in the Apcdelta716 mouse by rofecoxib, a specific cyclooxygenase-2 inhibitor. Cancer Res. 2001;61:1733–40.

26. Oshima M, Dinchuk JE, Kargman SL et al. Suppression of intestinal polyposis in Apc delta716 knockout mice by inhibition of cyclooxygenase 2 (COX-2). Cell. 1996;87:803–9.

27. Hull MA, Booth JK, Tisbury A et al. Cyclooxygenase 2 is up-regulated and localized to macrophages in the intestine of Min mice. Br J Cancer. 1999;79:1399–405.

28. Shattuck-Brandt RL, Varilek GW, Radhika A, Yang F, Washington MK, DuBois RN. Cyclooxygenase 2 expression is increased in the stroma of colon carcinomas from IL-10($-/-$) mice. Gastroenterology. 2000;118:337–45.

29. Rennick DM, Fort MM. Lessons from genetically engineered animal models. XII. IL-10-deficient IL-10(−/−) mice and intestinal inflammation. Am J Physiol Gastrointest Liver Physiol. 2000;278:G829–33.
30. Berg DJ, Davidson N, Kuhn R et al. Enterocolitis and colon cancer in interleukin-10-deficient mice are associated with aberrant cytokine production and CD4(+) TH1-like responses. J Clin Invest. 1996;98:1010–20.
31. Scott DJ, Hull MA, Cartwright EJ et al. Lack of inducible nitric oxide synthase promotes intestinal tumorigenesis in the Apc(Min/+) mouse. Gastroenterology. 2001;121:889–99.
32. Ahn B, Oshima H. Suppression of intestinal polyposis in Apc(Min/+) mice by inhibiting nitric oxide production. Cancer Res. 2001;61:8357–60.
33. Newman JV, Kosaka T, Sheppard BJ, Fox JG, Schauer DB. Bacterial infection promotes colon tumorigenesis in Apc(Min/+) mice. J Infect Dis. 2001;184:227–30.
34. Luperchio SA, Schauer DB. Molecular pathogenesis of *Citrobacter rodentium* and transmissible murine colonic hyperplasia. Microbes Infect. 2001;3:333–40.
35. Barthold SW, Beck D. Modification of early dimethylhydrazine carcinogenesis by colonic mucosal hyperplasia. Cancer Res. 1980;40:4451–5.
36. Hawk ET, Viner JL, Dannenberg A, DuBois RN. COX-2 in cancer – a player that's defining the rules. J Natl Cancer Inst. 2002;94:545–91.
37. Song X, Lin HP, Johnson AJ et al. Cyclooxygenase-2, player or spectator in cyclooxygenase-2 inhibitor-induced apoptosis in prostate cancer cells. J Natl Cancer Inst. 2002;94:585–91.
38. Marnett LJ, Wright TL, Crews BC, Tannenbaum SR, Morrow JD. Regulation of prostaglandin biosynthesis by nitric oxide is revealed by targeted deletion of inducible nitric-oxide synthase. J Biol Chem. 2000;275:13427–30.
39. Shureiqi I, Chen D, Lotan R et al. 15-Lipoxygenase-1 mediates nonsteroidal anti-inflammatory drug-induced apoptosis independently of cyclooxygenase-2 in colon cancer cells. Cancer Res. 2000;60:6846–50.
40. Jenkins DC, Charles IG, Thomsen LL et al. Roles of nitric oxide in tumor growth. Med Sci. 1995;92:4392–6.
41. Jenkins DC, Charles IG, Baylis SA, Lelchuk R, Radomski MW, Moncada S. Human colon cancer cell lines show a diverse pattern of nitric oxide synthease gene expression and nitric oxide generation. Br J Cancer. 1994;70:847–9.
42. Radomski MW, Jenkins DC, Holmes L, Moncada S. Human colorectal adenocarcinoma cells: differential nitric oxide synthesis determines their ability to aggregate platelets. Cancer Res. 1991;51:6073–8.
43. Hoffman RA, Zhang G, Nussler NC et al. Constitutive expression of inducible nitric oxide synthase in the mouse ileal mucosa. Am J Physiol. 1997;272:G383–92.
44. Ambs S, Bennett WP, Merriam WG et al. Relationship between p53 mutations and inducible nitric oxide synthase expression in human colorectal cancer. J Natl Cancer Inst. 1999;91:86–8.
45. Ambs S, Ogunfusika MO, Merriam WG, Bennett WP, Billiar TR, Harris CC. Up-regulation of inducible nitric oxide synthase expression in cancer-prone p53 knockout mice. Proc Natl Acad Sci USA. 1998;95:8823–8.
46. Ambs S, Merriam WG, Ogunfusika MO et al. P53 and vascular endothelian growth factor regulate tumor growth of NOS2-expressing human carcinoma cells. Nature Med. 1990;4:1371–6.
47. Hussain SP, Amstad P, Raja K et al. Increased p53 mutation load in noncancerous colon tissue from ulcerative colitis: A cancer-prone chronic inflammatory disease. Cancer Res. 2000;60:3333–7.

22
The role of *N*-nitrosation in colon carcinogenesis: some recent insights

D. E. G. SHUKER

INTRODUCTION

Cancer of the colon and rectum is one of the four major cancers in the UK[1]. Unlike lung cancer, for which tobacco smoking is clearly the major underlying cause, there is no single clear major risk factor for colorectal cancer. Apart from the small percentage of hereditary cancers, which have well-defined gene defects, the vast majority of colorectal cancers arise in a so-called 'spontaneous' manner. A number of hypotheses which link various aspects of diet to colorectal cancer risk have been proposed on the basis of a large number of epidemiological studies[2]. The earliest of these suggested that increasing levels of saturated fat were associated with increased risk but much of this was based on comparisons of population groups. More recently, case–control studies have revealed a consistent association between consumption of red meat, particularly when it is well-cooked, and colorectal cancer. This has led to much interest in the possibility that pyrolysis of amino acid/carbohydrate mixtures leading to formation heterocyclic amines may be important. However, the level of exposure to heterocyclic amines is actually rather low (of the order of <10 μg/kg body weight per day) and these products are only formed to a significant extent if meat is heated to a very high temperature.

Some years ago, Shephard and Lutz[3] suggested that dietary amino acids were the major substrate for another kind of chemical transformation which could not only lead to the formation of carcinogens but would also proceed under very mild conditions, such as those found in the stomach and lower gastrointestinal tract, namely, *N*-nitrosation.

N-NITROSATION

N-Nitrosation is a relatively simple organic chemical transformation but the biological consequences are dramatic (Figure 1). Most dietary nitrogen-containing

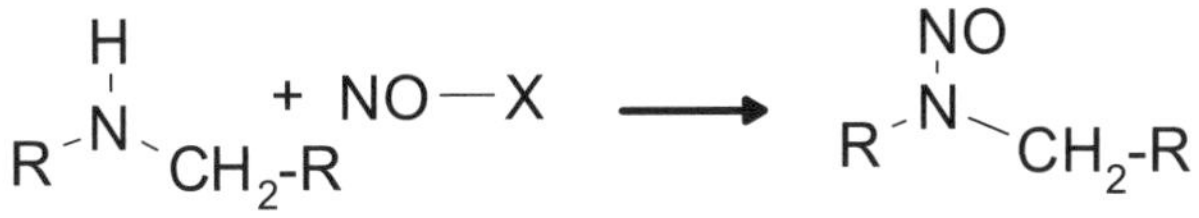

$$H \qquad\qquad\qquad NO$$
$$R^{-N}{}^{\backslash}CH_2\text{-}R \quad + \; NO-X \quad \longrightarrow \quad R^{-N}{}^{\backslash}CH_2\text{-}R$$

Amine + **Nitrosating agent** ➜ *N*-nitrosocompound
or amide

Non-toxic   *Non-toxic (?)*   *Toxic*

Figure 1   A general reaction scheme for the formation of *N*-nitrosocompounds from nitrogenous precursors and nitrosating agents

compounds are non-toxic but replacement of one of the hydrogens by a nitroso group results in the production of derivatives which are almost invariably toxic and usually mutagenic and carcinogenic. As a consequence, there has been a large research effort directed towards identifying environmental and dietary *N*-nitrosocompounds (NOC) and, not surprisingly, many such compounds have been detected[4]. However, the role of *N*-nitrosocompounds in human cancer has been difficult to elucidate. It would appear that the relationship between *N*-nitrosation, *N*-nitrosocompounds and human cancer is perhaps more subtle than was imagined and involves more than just low-level exposure to some obvious candidate carcinogens. One factor which has emerged is the role of endogenous nitrosation as a major route of human exposure to *N*-nitrosocompounds.

ENDOGENOUS NITROSATION

The discovery of endogenous synthesis of NOC, firstly by Sander and Bürkle in 1969[5] and then by Ohshima and Bartsch in 1981[6], opened up a whole new area of research which has irrevocably changed our view of human exposure to NOC and their role in cancer[7]. The *N*-nitrosoproline (NPRO) test was devised by Ohshima and Bartsch to measure endogenous nitrosation in humans. NPRO is an unusual nitrosamine in that it is resistant to metabolic activation and is excreted unchanged in urine. Furthermore, the precursor L-proline (PRO), a natural amino acid, is capable of being efficiently nitrosated under mildly acidic conditions whereas the more basic dialkylamines are protonated and are thus much less reactive.

N-NITROSATION AND COLON CANCER

In 1998, the Committee on Medical Aspects of Food and Nutrition Policy found moderate evidence of a relationship between red and processed meat and colorectal cancer. It stated that the nature and mechanisms of the observed association between meat consumption and the risk of cancers should be the subject of research[2]. Nitrogenous residues from meat and other protein-containing foods enter the large bowel where they are substrates for fermentation by proteolytic

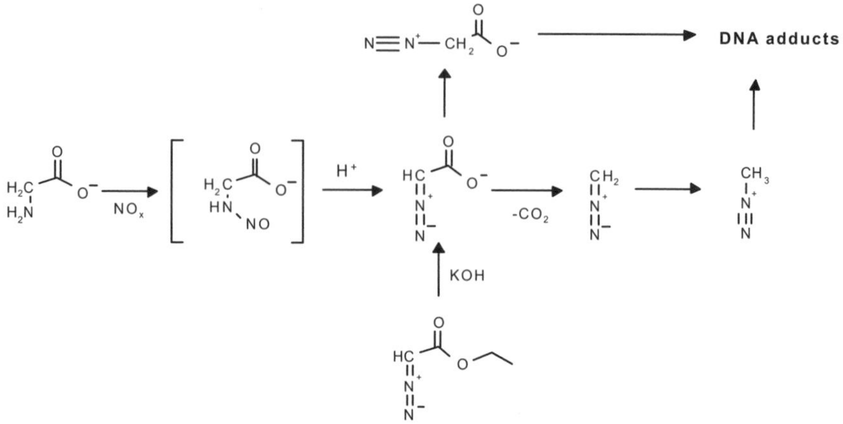

Figure 2 A summary of the transformations which occur on nitrosation of glycine. The key intermediate, diazoacetate, can also be prepared by alkaline hydrolysis of commercially available ethyldiazoacetate

bacteria leading to increased ammonia, amines and amides[8]. These residues are available for N-nitrosation mediated by colonic bacteria which generate nitrosating agents via nitrite and nitrate reductases[9–11]. The amount of nitrogenous residues entering the colon are known to increase with increasing protein intake[12] and Bingham and colleagues have shown that increased intake of red meat increases faecal NOC levels in human volunteers in a dose-responsive manner[13–15].

Glycine is the simplest α-amino acid and is among the most abundant amino acids in dietary proteins. Free glycine occurs in biological fluids at millimolar concentrations[16]. Nitrosation of glycine esters to give stable diazoacetic esters was first reported in 1904[17] and salts of diazoacetic acid itself were reported in 1908[18] (Figure 2). Remarkably, apart from kinetic studies on decomposition[19], there has been no examination of the potential toxicity or carcinogenicity of this simple compound. However, there has been a recent resurgence of interest in the chemistry and biology of diazo- and N-nitrosopeptides and this was reviewed by Challis[20]. Diazo- and N-nitrosopeptides are consistently mutagenic in many test systems and several are potent carcinogens in animal models[21].

NITROSATION OF GLYCINE

We have recently shown that nitrosation of glycine proceeds under mild conditions that model those likely to be found in the upper gastrointestinal tract and that the resulting products are stable enough to alkylate DNA (Cupid *et al.*, manuscript in preparation). Solutions of glycine (10 μmol/L–50 mM) were exposed to nitric oxide. An HPLC assay was developed to measure the resulting nitrosated glycine derivative, diazoacetate (DA). The amount of nitrosating agent present in the reaction, determined by colorimetric measurement of nitrite, was typically 200–600 μmol/L. DA formation was found to be linear with glycine and nitrite concentration.

DNA ALKYLATION BY NITROSATED GLYCINE

A previous observation[22] that an N-nitroso-N-carboxymethyl derivative reacts with DNA to give both O^6-carboxymethyl-2'-deoxyguanosine (O^6-CMdG) and O^6-methyl-2'-deoxyguanosine (O^6-MedG) has been confirmed using a range of nitrosated glycine derivatives (N-acetyl-N'-nitroso-N'-prolylglycine (APNG), azaserine (AS), and potassium diazoacetate (KDA))[23,24]. O^6-CMdG and O^6-MedG were assessed in enzymatic hydrolysates of treated calf thymus DNA using a combined immunoaffinity/HPLC/fluorescence procedure. The ratio of O^6-CMdG to O^6-MedG varied somewhat between the different compounds with APNG giving the most methylation (O^6-CM : O^6-Me ratio of 10) and AS the least (ratio = 39), with KDA giving intermediate amounts (ratio = 16). The formation of O^6-MedG by the four compounds probably arises through decarboxylation at various stages in the decomposition pathways, but the exact mechanisms remain to be clarified. The formation of O^6-MedG from reactions of nitrosated glycine derivatives with DNA *in vitro* may explain the frequent detection of this adduct in human gastrointestinal DNA, as nitrosation of dietary glycine may occur.

QUANTITATION OF O^6-CMdG IN GASTROINTESTINAL TISSUES

The levels of O^6-CMdG in the *in-vitro* experiments described above could be readily detected using immunoaffinity clean-up followed by HPLC-fluorescence. However, for analysis of the adduct in human DNA we have developed a sensitive immunoslotblot (ISB) assay using a polyclonal antiserum[23]. The principles of the ISB assay have been described in detail elsewhere[25,26]. Briefly, samples of DNA are adsorbed onto nitrocellulose filters and exposed to the antiserum. After several washing steps, a horseradish peroxidase conjugated second antibody is then used to complete the 'sandwich'. Addition of a chemiluminescent reagent system results in the production of light that is proportional to the level of adduct present. Variations in the amounts of DNA which become bound to the filter can be corrected using the DNA-binding flourescent dye, propidium iodide. Recent results indicate that O^6-CMdG can be detected in human gastric DNA at levels ranging from undetectable to 7 adducts per 10^7 normal bases[27], although earlier preliminary results from our laboratory indicated that somewhat higher levels could also be present[28]. A systematic study of the factors affecting levels of O^6-CMdG in DNA is currently under way.

SIGNIFICANCE OF O^6-CMdG

O^6-CMdG was found to be resistant to repair by O^6-alkylguanine alkyl transferase[22] and it was therefore of interest to determine if this adduct resulted in a different mutagenic profile from that of O^6-MeG. Using a functional p53 mutation assay in yeast[29], we have observed that potassium diazoacetate (KDA) gives a significantly different spectrum of mutations from that of methylnitrosourea (MNU). With MNU, the majority of mutations are GC > AT transitions (83%) whereas, with KDA, these mutations account for only 59% of the total (Figure 3)[30].

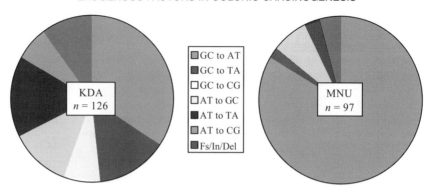

Figure 3 Comparison between the proportions of different types of mutations induced by MNU (2 mmol/L) and KDA (6–10 mmol/L) in the yeast p53 functional mutation assay

It would appear that the O^6-CMdG adduct results in a different mutagenic outcome compared with O^6-MedG. This aspect is curently being addressed through the synthesis of oligonucleotides containing O^6-CMdG which will be used to explore the mispairing and promutagenic properties of this novel adduct.

ANOTHER FACE OF AMINO ACID NITROSATION

Thus far, we have been concerned exclusively with N-nitrosation of the N-terminal of amino acids. Clearly, in many cases, nitrosation of side chains is likely to be a significant pathway. One likely target is the indole nucleus of tryptophan, and, some years ago, Bonnett and colleagues characterized the N-nitroso derivatives of tryptophan and obtained evidence that they are mutagenic[31]. For N-nitrosoindoles, unlike many of the N-nitrosodialkylamines, the N-nitroso group is somewhat labile and we have recently shown that the mutagenic plant derivative 1-nitrosoindole-3-acetonitrile (NIAN) interacts with individual DNA bases exclusively by nitroso group transfer, leading to depurination, deamination and base rearrangement (Figure 4)[32]. To determine the likely biological relevance of these modification pathways, the reactivity of NIAN, a model 3-substituted N-nitrosoindole, with oligonucleotides and calf thymus DNA, was examined at physiological pH and temperature[33]. Reaction of NIAN with single-stranded oligonucleotides containing various guanine motifs resulted in the production of single-strand break products at guanine sites due to the formation of alkali-labile lesions. The number of lesions increased with NIAN concentration and incubation time. Modification of calf thymus DNA by NIAN resulted in: depurination, which gave the corresponding purine bases; deamination coupled with depurination, which gave xanthine; and, the formation of oxanine. The former pathway was clearly the most important, and all reaction products exhibited a dose–response relationship. Cytosine and thymine residues were inactive toward NIAN. Further studies revealed an additional product in NIAN-treated duplex DNA containing a CCGG motif that was characterized as an interstrand cross-link, the yield of which increased with increasing NIAN concentration. These

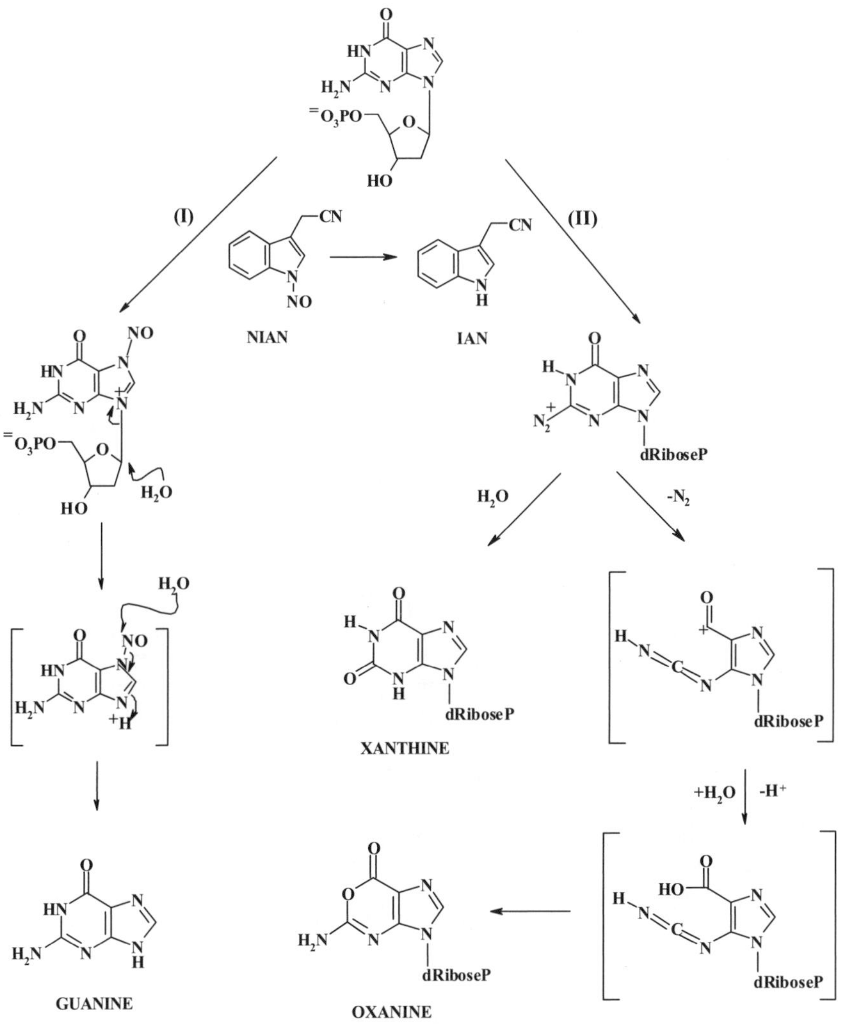

Figure 4 Scheme of NIAN-induced depurination, deamination and formation of oxanine via transnitrosation from 2'-deoxyguanosine-5'-monophosphate. (I) Transnitrosation to the N-7 atom of guanine followed by cleavage of the N-glycosidic bond and hydrolysis of the N-nitrosopurine affords depurination products. (II) Transnitrosation to the exocyclic amino group of guanine results in the formation of purine diazonium ion. Subsequent reactions give rise to deamination products and the formation of oxanine

results indicated that the transnitrosating ability of NIAN to modify purine residues is preserved at the macromolecular level, with guanine residues appearing to be a primary site of reaction. All of these modification processes are potentially mutagenic events if they occur *in vivo*. In fact, we found that intragastric instillation of NIAN in experimental animals results in increased levels of base depurination in gastric DNA[34]. Unfortunately, base depurination occurs at relatively high levels as a result of inherent DNA instability so the search for a characteristic marker of DNA base nitrosation is being focussed on oxanine.

DISCUSSION

The role of N-nitrosation and N-nitrosocompounds in colorectal cancer remains to be elucidated. Various pieces of evidence are consistent with such a role – the association between increased meat protein intake and cancer risk is indicative that nitrogenous food constituents may be involved, there are a number of sources of nitrosating agents within the gastrointestinal tract (NO from inflammation or from bacterial reduction of nitrate) and the detection of alkylation damage in DNA extracted from colorectal tissue. Despite many years of searching for a particular N-nitrosocompound or a group of such compounds, there is little evidence that such isolable or stable species are involved in the aetiology. In contrast, there is accumulating evidence that transient and highly reactive chemical species which are generated as a result of N-nitrosation may be responsible for relevant DNA damage. We have shown that nitrosation of the most common amino acid glycine gives rise to diazoacetic acid which, although unstable at physiological pH, is stable enough to travel across the cell membrane and attack DNA. The adducts which are formed, in this case O^6-CMdG and O^6-MedG, provide the evidence of the pathway and give us the tools to investigate the matter further. Not only do these adducts give us usable biomarkers but they themselves possess interesting promutagenic properties which suggest that they may have a direct role in the development of colorectal cancer.

More subtly, the transfer of the nitroso group from nitrosated indoles results in base changes, such as the rearrangement of guanine to give oxanine, which are likely to be mutagenic.

The most satisfactory outcome of this investigation will be the development of tools which allow us to more clearly pose questions about the relationship between N-nitrosation and colorectal cancer. Without such approaches, we will continue to get only tantalizing glimpses of possibilities rather than the ability to ask very direct questions. There is an additional prospect available to us once the kind of molecular biomarkers that have been discussed in this paper have been validated (i.e. found to be informative about underlying causative factors in colorectal cancer) and that is that these markers can be used as short-term indicators of the efficacy of interventions. Thus, rather than waiting for many years in a prospective investigation to discover if a change in dietary habits is actually beneficial (or not), we could use short-term markers of DNA damage to evaluate whether the expected change has in fact occurred.

Acknowledgements

Much hard work carried out by a number of postdoctoral fellows, research students and project officers is gratefully acknowledged and their names appear on the cited papers. Generous support for this work from the Food Standards Agency, World Cancer Research Fund and the Open University is gratefully acknowledged.

References

1. Statbase. http://www.statistics.gov.uk/statbase/ (accessed 12 July, 2002). UK National Statistics. 2002.
2. UK Department of Health. Nutritional aspects of the development of cancer. Report of the Working Group on Diet and Cancer of the Committee on Medical Aspects of Food and Nutrition Policy. Rep Health Soc Subj (London) 1998; 48.
3. Shephard SE, Lutz, WK. Nitrosation of dietary precursors. Cancer Surveys. 1989;8:401–21.
4. Hotchkiss JH. Preformed N-nitroso compounds in foods and beverages. Cancer Surveys. 1989;8:295–321.
5. Sander J, Bürkle G. Induktion maligner Tumoren bei Ratten durch gleichzeitige Verfuttung von Nitrit und sekundaren Aminen. Zeit Krebsforsch. 1969;76:93–6.
6. Ohshima H, Bartsch H. Quantitative estimation of endogenous nitrosation in humans by monitoring N-nitrosoproline excreted in the urine. Cancer Res. 1981;41:3658–62.
7. Bartsch H, Ohshima H, Shuker DEG, Pignatelli B, Calmels S. Exposure of humans to endogenous N-nitroso compounds – implications in cancer etiology. Mutation Res. 1990;238:255–67.
8. Macfarlane G, Cummings JH. The colonic flora, fermentation, and large bowel digestive function. In: Phillips S, Pemberton JH, Shorter RG, editors. The Large Intestine: Physiology, Pathophysiology and Disease. New York: Raven Press, 1991:51–92.
9. Calmels S, Ohshima H, Vincent P, Gounot AM, Bartsch H. Screening of microorganisms for nitrosation catalysis at pH 7 and kinetic studies on nitrosamine formation from secondary amines by E. coli strains. Carcinogenesis. 1985;6:911–15.
10. Calmel S, Ohshima H, Bartsch, H. Nitrosamine formation by denitrifying and non-denitrifying bacteria: implication of nitrite reductase and nitrate reductase in nitrosation catalysis. J of Gen Microbiol. 1988;134:221–6.
11. Calmels S, Ohshima H, Henry Y, Bartsch H. Characterisation of bacterial cytochrome cd1-nitrite reductase as one enzyme responsible for catalysis of secondary amines. Carcinogenesis. 1996;17:533–6.
12. Silvester KR, Cummings JH. Does digestibility of meat protein help to explain large bowel cancer risk? Nutrition Cancer. 1995;24:279–88.
13. Bingham SA, Pignatelli B, Pollock JRA et al. Does increased endogenous formation of N-nitroso compounds in the human colon explain the association between red meat and colon cancer? Carcinogenesis. 1996;17:515–23.
14. Silvester KR, Bingham SA, Pollock JRA, Cummings JH, O'Neill IK. Effect of meat and resistant starch on fecal excretion of apparent total N-nitroso compounds and ammonia from the human large bowel. Nutrition Cancer. 1997;29:13–15.
15. Hughes R, Cross, AJ, Pollock JRA, Bingham SA. Dose-dependent effect of dietary red meat on endogenous colonic N-nitrosation. Carcinogenesis. 2001;22:199–202.
16. Komorowska M, Szafran H, Popiela T, Szafran Z. Free amino acids of human gastric juice. Acta Physiol Pol. 1981;32:559–67.
17. Curtius T. Uber die freiwillige Zerzetzung des glycollesters. Chem Ber. 1904;37:1285–300.
18. Müller E. Uber pseudo diazoessigsaüre. Chem Ber. 1908;41:3116–39.
19. Kreevoy MM, Konasewich DE. The mechanism of hydrolysis of diazoacetate ion. J Phys Chem. 1970;74:4464–72.
20. Challis BC. Chemistry and biology of nitrosated peptides. Cancer Surveys. 1989;8:363–4.
21. Anderson D, Blowers SD. Limited cancer bioassay to test a potential food chemical. Lancet. 1994;344:343–4.
22. Shuker DEG, Margison GP. Nitrosated glycine derivatives as a potential source of O-6-methylguanine in DNA. Cancer Res. 1997;57:366–9.
23. Harrison KL, Fairhurst N, Challis BC, Shuker DEG. Synthesis, characterization, and immunochemical detection of O-6-(carboxymethyl)-2'-deoxyguanosine: a DNA adduct formed by nitrosated glycine derivatives. Chem Res Toxicol. 1997;10:652–9.
24. Harrison KL, Jukes R, Cooper DP, Shuker DEG. Detection of concomitant formation of O-6-carboxymethyl- and O-6-methyl-2'-deoxyguanosine in DNA exposed to nitrosated glycine derivatives using a combined immunoaffinity/HPLC method. Chem Res Toxicol. 1999;12:106–11.
25. Nehls P, Adamkiewicz J, Rajewsky MF. Immuno-slot-blot: A highly sensitive immunoassay for the quantitation of carcinogen-modified nucleosides in DNA. J Cancer Res Clin Oncol. 1984;108:23–9.

26. Leuratti C, Singh R, Lagneau C *et al*. Determination of malondialdehyde-induced DNA damage in human tissues using an immunoslot blot assay. Carcinogenesis. 1998;19:1919–24.
27. Singh R, Leuratti C, Griech E *et al*. The role of *Helicobacter pylori* infection on the modulation of O^6carboxymethylguanine DNA adducts in gastric tissue arising from the nitrosation of amino acids and peptides. Proc Am Assoc Cancer Res. 2000;41:422.
28. Shuker DEG. The role of nitrosation: Exogenous vs. endogenous exposure to N-nitroso compounds In: Eisenbrand G, editor, Carcinogenic/Anticarcinogenic Factors in Foods: Novel Concepts. DFG-SKLM Symposium Series, Wiley-VCH, 2000:205–16.
29. Fronza G, Inga A, Monti P *et al*. The yeast p53 functional assay: a new tool for molecular epidemiology. Hopes and realities. Mutat Res. 2000;462:293–301.
30. Gottschalg E. Detection, stability and factors influencing the formation of promutagenic endogenous DNA damage. PhD thesis. Leicester (UK): University of Leicester, 2002.
31. Bonnett R, Holleyhead R, Johnson BL, Randall EW. Reaction of acidified nitrite solutions with peptide derivatives: Evidence for nitrosamine and thionitrite formation from 15 N N.M.R. studies. J Chem Soc. Perkin Trans. 1975;1:2261–4.
32. Lucas LT, Gatehouse D, Shuker DEG. Efficient nitroso group transfer from *N*-nitrosoindoles to nucleotides and 2′-deoxyguanosine at physiological pH. J Biol Chem. 1999;274:18319–26.
33. Lucas LT, Gatehouse D, Jones GDD, Shuker DEG. Characterization of DNA damage at purine residues in oligonucleotides and calf thymus DNA induced by the mutagen 1-nitrosoindole-3-acetonitrile. Chem Res Toxicol. 2001;14:158–64.
34. Lucas LT. Detection of DNA damage caused by nitrosoindoles. PhD thesis. Leicester (UK): University of Leicester, 2001.

23
Heterocyclic aromatic amines

I. C. ROBERTS-THOMSON

INTRODUCTION

Heterocyclic aromatic amines, or heterocyclic amines (HCA), are a group of mutagenic and carcinogenic substances that are formed when meat is cooked. They were first described in 1977 when smoke condensates and extracts from the surface of grilled fish and meat were found to show mutagenic activity in strains of *Salmonella typhimurium*[1]. Subsequently, the structure of a series of mutagenic compounds was determined[2] and chemically synthesized compounds were shown to be carcinogenic in animal models[3]. In recent years several studies have addressed HCA intake in human populations and the potential contribution of HCA to the burden of human cancer[4,5]. These studies have not established a clear link between HCA intake and cancer and, because of this, HCA have been categorized as a possible risk for human carcinogenesis (category 2 in the classification of the IARC). This chapter will summarize data on the formation and metabolism of HCA and the possible relationship between HCA intake and risk for colorectal cancer.

STRUCTURE, FORMATION AND METABOLISM

Structure of HCA

Chemically, HCA have been divided into two classes: those that resemble 2-amino-3-methylimidazo [4,5-f] quinoline (IQ-type HCA) and non-IQ-type HCA[3]. The structure of IQ is shown in Figure 1. The IQ-type HCA appear to be more important carcinogens and include IQ, MeIQ, MeIQx, DiMeIQx and PhIP. They consist of an aminoimidazo moiety which appears to arise from the cyclization of creatine, and quinoline, quinoxaline and phenylpyridine moieties that are Maillard reaction products of amino acids and sugars. The 2-aminoimidazo component is common to all IQ compounds and is largely responsible for mutagenicity. The Maillard reaction produces hundreds of reaction products that are important for the development of flavours, texture and brown pigments during the cooking process. Non-IQ-type HCA are produced by the pyrolysis of amino acids and proteins and generally require higher temperatures than IQ-type HCA.

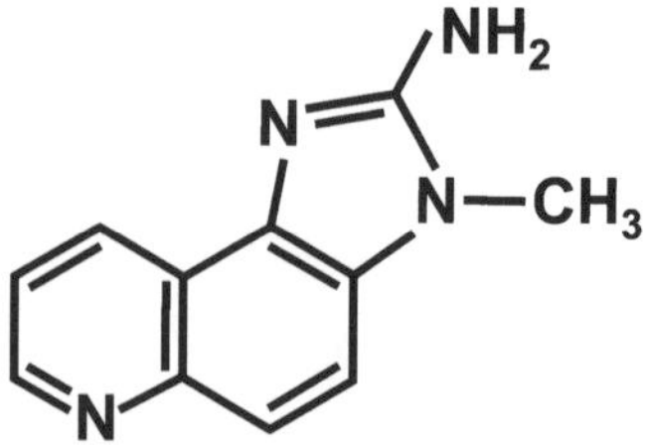

Figure 1   Chemical structure of 2-amino-3-methylimidazo [4,5-f] quinoline (IQ)

Formation of HCA in model systems

The formation of HCA has been studied in various model systems[6]. These have included creatine or creatinine, various amino acids and hexoses such as glucose and fructose. There is minimal formation of HCA below 100 °C. At higher temperatures various HCA have been detected, largely depending on the presence of particular amino acids. For example, IQ formation is favoured by mixtures containing glycine, serine and proline, while PhIP formation is favoured by mixtures containing phenylalanine and leucine. IQ can also be formed by dry-heating creatine or creatinine and various amino acids, but yields are higher in the presence of glucose. Heating sugar–amino acid mixtures can also result in the production of weak mutagens but these are not categorized as HCA.

Some data are available on factors which influence HCA formation in model systems. In general, HCA formation increases with increasing temperature and duration of heating. Different amino acids not only influence the concentrations of individual heterocyclic amines but have also been shown to enhance or inhibit HCA formation when added in different concentrations. Concentrations of individual monosaccharides and disaccharides have also been shown to influence mutagenicity and, for individual monosaccharides, HCA formation appears to be impaired at both low and high concentrations.

Metabolism of HCA

The HCA, particularly those of the IQ-type, require metabolic activation for DNA adduct formation[7–9]. The first step is N-hydroxylation that is largely mediated by the phase I enzyme, CYP1A2. These N-hydroxylamine derivatives react relatively poorly with nucleic acids and normally require a second metabolic activation step to facilitate adduct formation. This second step is mediated by phase II cytosolic enzymes such as N-acetyltransferase (NAT), sulphotransferase, prolyl tRNA synthetase and phosphorylase, and results in the formation of highly reactive esters. These ester moieties then give rise to arylnitrenium ions which are thought to be the ultimate carcinogenic form of IQ-type HCA.

In relation to the site of HCA metabolism, it seems likely that N-hydroxylation largely occurs in the liver. Phase II esterification activity can occur in the liver but may also occur in peripheral tissues including the gastrointestinal tract. For NAT2, however, higher concentrations have been demonstrated in the liver than in the colon. The metabolic pathways described above have led to the hypothesis that risks for colonic adenoma and cancer after exposure to HCA could increase in rapid hydroxylators (CYP1A2) and rapid acetylators (NAT1, NAT2). While this may be the case, detoxification pathways also need to be considered and some, at least, show substantial individual variation.

Formation of HCA in cooked meat

HCA can be produced in all forms of cooked meat. In developed countries the most common meats are beef, lamb, chicken, fish, sausage, pork and bacon. Common cooking methods include frying, grilling (broiling), barbecuing, roasting and stewing. Unfortunately there is some variation in HCA formation for one meat type with one cooking method, perhaps largely because of variation in temperature and duration of cooking. There is also variation across meat types for the same cooking method and across cooking methods for the same meat type[10]. Yet another issue is preference for particular meats and particular cooking methods in different countries.

At least one marker of HCA formation in meat is the degree of browning; i.e. 'rare', 'medium' or 'well done'. This correlates with the maximum internal temperature during cooking and with concentrations of at least some HCA such as PhIP. Weight loss of meat preparations during cooking also correlates with higher internal temperatures[11].

Concentrations of HCA in cooked meats have been assessed in studies from the USA[4,11-13], Sweden[14] and New Zealand[10,15]. The highest concentrations of HCA have been found in barbecued chicken. High concentrations have also been found in chicken, fish and beef which is pan-fried, grilled or broiled. Roasting results in lower concentrations of HCA while HCA formation is minimal with cooking methods such as stewing, casseroling and microwaving. HCA formation from pork and lamb appears to be lower than for other meats but the cause remains unclear. Processed meats such as hamburgers and sausages also have lower HCA levels with 'risky' cooking conditions, perhaps because of containment of meat juices or the effects of additives such as salt, soy protein and starch. Reduced levels of HCA may also be achieved by marination prior to grilling, microwaving prior to pan-frying and insulating meat with coatings such as breadcrumbs. Other sources of HCA include the formation of gravies from pan residues and the reuse of fat for roasting.

Total intake of HCA

Exposure to HCA can be estimated by assessing the intake of particular meats, the frequency of use of various cooking methods and the degree of surface browning. The latter can be assisted by use of colour photographs. Estimates of HCA exposure in adults in the USA, Sweden and New Zealand are shown in Table 1. In general, more recent estimates of intake have been lower than earlier estimates in the mid-1990s. Variation between countries may reflect true differences or may be due to different assignments of HCA concentrations to cooked meats, differences in estimated meat consumption and differences in assumed cooking practices. In Sweden[16], intakes of HCA vary widely from very low levels to intakes of more than 5000 ng/person per day (a 60-fold increase over mean values).

Table 1 Approximate daily intake of heterocyclic amines (ng) in adults in different countries

	Amount (ng)	Reference
USA	1800	Layton et al.[4]
	440	Byrne et al.[13]
	440	Keating and Bogen[11]
Sweden	160	Augustsson et al.[14]
	77	Augustsson et al.[16]
New Zealand	1000	Thomson[10]
	146	Norrish et al.[15]

Intake of individual HCA

In Western countries the major dietary HCA is PhIP. This accounts for approximately half to two-thirds of the total intake. Other HCA such as AαC, MeIQx, DiMeQx and IQ accounted for 20%, 10%, 3% and 1% of the total intake, respectively, in the USA[4] but there was a higher percentage of MeIQx in Sweden[14]. In the USA most of the PhIP comes from beef and fish, whereas in New Zealand the most important source of PhIP is chicken.

MUTAGENICITY AND CARCINOGENICITY IN ANIMALS AND HUMANS

Carcinogenicity in animal models

The potential for HCA to cause cancer in humans is supported by studies in laboratory animals[3,8]. In rodents liver cancer is relatively common. However, cancer has also been described in a number of other tissues including the intestine, bladder, blood vessels, Zymbal gland, clitoral gland and lymphoid tissue. In some rat strains challenged with PhIP liver cancer is uncommon, but cancers have been described in the large intestine, prostate and mammary gland. One of the HCA, IQ, has also been shown to cause liver cancer in monkeys.

Mutagenicity *in vitro*

The mutagenicity of HCA has been evaluated in bacterial assays and in cultured mammalian cells[8]. In the Ames assay, using *Salmonella* strains, HCA are relatively potent mutagens in the order of MeIQ > IQ > DiMeIQx > MeIQx > PhIP. More potent mutagens show greater binding to bacterial DNA with a preference for adduct formation at guanine. In cultured mammalian cells genotoxicity has been assessed by several methods including mutagenesis, chromosomal aberrations, sister-chromatid exchange, DNA repair synthesis and DNA strand breaks.

The issue of DNA changes induced by HCA adducts will be addressed in Chapter 26. It is of interest, however, that colon cancer in rats induced by PhIP showed a 'signature' mutation of G deletion from the GGGA sequence in the *Apc* gene. This type of mutation can also be found in the TP53 gene of human cancers[17].

Relative carcinogenicity of HCA

The cancer potency for various HCA have been estimated by Bogen[12], largely on the basis of rodent studies. The most potent carcinogen is IQ. The relative potencies of other carcinogens are DiMeIQx > MeIQx > PhIP > AαC. These cancer potencies are almost in the reverse order to the relative frequencies of various HCA in the diet (see above).

Potential carcinogenesis in humans

On the basis of dietary data and data on HCA formation from various cooking methods, Bogen[12] and Layton et al.[4] have attempted to estimate the risk of cancer from HCA exposure in humans. Although there are several potential sources of error they calculated that, at most, the ingestion of HCA would be responsible for only 0.25% of all colorectal cancers. However, as colorectal cancer is a common disease (cumulative lifetime risk of 4–4.5%), the risk is not negligible from a public health viewpoint.

The incremental cancer risk from individual HCA can be calculated from the amount of HCA ingested and the potency of the carcinogen. Estimates in the USA[4] indicate that PhIP accounts for 46% of the total risk followed by MeIQx (27%), DiMeIQx (15%), IQ (7%) and AαC (6%). However, data from Sweden and New Zealand suggest a somewhat higher contribution from MeIQx[14,15].

Epidemiological studies in humans

The ideal cancer study in humans would quantitate intake of HCA for individual participants, would include data on metabolic genotypes influencing carcinogenicity and would include markers of exposure to HCA such as DNA adducts or metabolites of HCA in urine. Furthermore, the study would be prospective and would monitor intakes of HCA over a period of at least 10 years. No such study exists, although prospective studies which include at least some of the above components are currently in progress.

The first case–control study to examine the relationship between meat intake, meat browning, metabolic phenotypes and risk for colorectal cancer was reported by Lang et al.[7] from Little Rock, Arkansas. The participants were 41 patients with adenomas, 34 with cancer and 205 community controls. Diet was assessed by a modified Block questionnaire that was supplemented with more detailed information on cooking practices. The activities of HCA-metabolizing enzymes (CYP1A2 and NAT2) were determined by ratios of urinary metabolites of caffeine.

The results showed that rapid phenotypes for CYP1A2 and NAT2 were slightly more prevalent in patients than in controls. These differences reached statistical significance only for the rapid CYP1A2-rapid NAT2 phenotype (odds ratio (OR) = 2.79; 95% CI 1.69–4.47). Univariate analysis indicated that age, rapid–rapid phenotype and consumption of well-done red meat were associated with an increased risk of colorectal neoplasia. Data were also analysed for combinations of phenotype and cooked meat preference. The OR ranged from 1.0 for rare–medium meat with the slow–slow phenotype to 6.45 for well-done meat with the rapid–rapid phenotype. These figures were not influenced by other dietary components such as vegetables and cooking oils.

The second case–control study was performed in white subjects in Adelaide, Australia[18]. The participants included 110 patients with colorectal cancer, 89 with adenomatous polyps and 110 control subjects who had a normal colonoscopy or barium enema X-ray within the preceding 12 months. Diet was assessed by a self-administered dietary questionnaire (CSIRO) and converted to nutrient consumption with the programme FREQUAN. The questionnaire did not include data on cooking methods or degree of browning. Acetylator status (NAT2) was determined by the rate of acetylation of sulphamethazine given orally, and was confirmed by genotyping in a subset of individuals.

The OR for the rapid acetylator phenotype in patients with adenoma and cancer were 1.1 (0.6–2.1) and 1.8 (1.0–3.3), respectively. Estimates of risk in rapid versus slow acetylators were highest in the youngest tertile of subjects (< 64 years) but were not influenced by gender or tumour characteristics. Furthermore, when risks for adenoma and cancer were analysed across tertiles of dietary items, there was no significant association with consumption of fat, protein, fibre, carbohydrate or meat. However, when the analysis was stratified by NAT2 phenotype, rapid acetylators with adenoma or with cancer or in the combined group showed increasing levels of risk with increasing intakes of meat. Differences were statistically significant for the combined group of patients. In contrast, there was no pattern of increasing risk with increasing intake of meat in slow acetylators.

The third case–control study was reported by Welfare et al.[19] from Newcastle, UK. The study included 201 patients with colorectal cancer and 174 randomly selected community controls. Diet was assessed by a food-frequency question-naire which focused on foods known to have a high content of HCA. Acetylator status was determined by genotyping while data were dichotomized and propor-tions between cases and controls compared by McNemar's test. The results showed that risks for proximal colon cancer were higher with higher intakes of roast meat and gravy. In addition, there was a higher-than-expected risk in rapid acetylators who ate fried meat at least twice per week (OR 6.0; 95% CI 1.34–55).

The fourth case–control study was performed by Sinha et al.[20] from Maryland, USA. The study included 146 patients with colorectal adenomas and 228 controls who did not have adenomas at sigmoidoscopy. Diet was assessed by a food-frequency questionnaire and included detailed questions on meat consumption and cooking practices. Cases and controls were well matched for age and ethnic origin but the cases included fewer women and a lower use of non-steroidal anti-inflammatory drugs.

There was a non-significant increase in risk for adenomas of 4% per 10 g/day increase in total meat intake. This increase in risk was associated with red meat (in comparison to white meat). When red meats were partitioned by 'doneness' level, the risk increased by 29% per 10 g/day (OR 1.29; CI 1.08–1.54) for red meat cooked well-done/very well-done in contrast to 10% per 10 g/day (OR 1.10; CI 0.96–1.26) for red meat cooked rare–medium. Higher risks were also observed when the well-done/very well-done category was subdivided into very well-done (OR 2.11; CI 0.90–4.93) and well-done groups (OR 1.21; CI 0.99–1.48). Risks were also higher with cooking methods which generate high temperatures on the surface of meat; i.e. grilling > frying > baking > oven broiling > microwaving.

The final case–control study was reported by Augustsson et al.[16] from Sweden. The study included patients with colon cancer (352), rectal cancer (249), bladder cancer (273) and kidney cancer (138). Controls were randomly selected from a population register and were matched for age and gender. Diet was assessed by an extensive food-frequency questionnaire (including cooking methods) and was related to eating habits 5 years previously. Extensive preliminary studies on HCA formation from cooked meat permitted an assessment of daily intakes of HCA. Data on metabolic genotypes–phenotypes were not included.

For colon and rectal cancer there was no evidence of an increased risk with increasing intakes of HCA. Indeed, there was a trend for patients with the highest intakes of HCA to have lower risks for cancer (OR = 0.6 and 0.7 for colon and rectal cancer, respectively). Furthermore, these risks did not appear to be affected by potential confounding factors such as smoking, physical activity or dietary components such as fibre, vegetables and fruits. When risks were determined for individual HCA there was a trend towards higher risks for colon cancer with the highest intakes of IQ (OR 1.1; 95% CI 0.7–1.6) and MeIQ (OR 1.3; 95% CI 0.9–1.8). In this study the highest recorded intake of HCA in controls was 1816 ng/day. Of seven cancer patients with higher intakes, four had colon cancer.

One prospective study on red meat intake, NAT genotype and risk for colorectal cancer has been reported from the USA[21]. The study involved 22 071 physicians, largely white men, who completed a food questionnaire and donated a blood sample in the early 1980s. The food questionnaire included data on intakes of red meat, chicken and fish but did not include details of cooking methods. Genotyping was performed for NAT1 and NAT2.

After 13 years of follow-up, blood samples were available from 212 physicians who developed colon cancer and these were matched for age and smoking with 221 controls. Genotype for NAT1, NAT2 or the combined NAT1/NAT2 did not influence risk for cancer. However, there was a trend towards higher risks for cancer with higher intakes of meat in rapid acetylators for NAT1, NAT2 and the rapid–rapid (NAT1/NAT2) genotype. Risks for those with the rapid–rapid genotype were statistically significant in subjects over 60 years who ate red meat at least once per day (OR 5.82; 95% CI 1.11–30.6).

OVERVIEW

Although environmental factors are important for colorectal carcinogenesis the relevant factors have been difficult to define. This is likely to reflect the complex nature of carcinogenesis which involves multiple facilitating and inhibitory factors that not only relate to diet but also include factors such as alcohol, smoking, exercise and perhaps psychological influences such as depression. In addition, there are potential errors in dietary surveys, changes in diet over time and uncertainty about the time interval between adduct-driven mutations and the evolution of adenomas and cancer.

Despite the clear demonstration of carcinogenicity in rodents, the evidence for colorectal carcinogenesis in humans is not compelling. In particular, the study by Augustsson et al.[16] failed to show increasing risks for cancer with increasing intakes of HCA. However, the issue was not completely settled, as the highest intakes of HCA were found in patients with cancer. In the study by Sinha et al.[20] there were higher risks for adenoma in individuals who cooked red meat to a well-done or very well-done state or who used high-temperature cooking techniques such as grilling and frying. Furthermore, at least three case–control studies and one prospective study have shown that rapid acetylators (NAT1, NAT2 or both) had higher risks for cancer with increasing intakes of meat or with use of 'risky' cooking methods. Thus far, this association has been explained only by enhanced metabolism of HCA to more potent carcinogens. It must be remembered, however, that the formation of more potent carcinogens is dependent not only on CYP1A2, NAT1 and NAT2 activity but also on the activity of a variety of detoxifying enzymes including glucuronosyltransferases.

In relation to future research, it seems unlikely that the issue of carcinogenicity of HCA will be resolved by additional case–control studies. Prospective studies which include multiple assessments of diet may be of help, and some are already in progress. Another avenue is to determine whether human cancers contain mutations which are sensitive and specific for HCA exposure. In the meantime it would seem wise for the health-conscious individual to use cooking methods that minimize exposure to HCA, perhaps without being over-zealous.

References

1. Nagao M, Honda M, Seino Y, Kawachi T, Sugimura T. Mutagenicities of smoke condensates and the charred surface of fish and meat. Cancer Lett. 1977;2:221–6.
2. Wakabayashi K, Nagao M, Esumi H, Sugimura T. Food-derived mutagens and carcinogens. Cancer Res. 1992;52:2092–8s.
3. Sugimura T. Nutrition and dietary carcinogens. Carcinogenesis. 2000;21:387–95.
4. Layton DW, Bogen KT, Knize MG, Hatch FT, Johnson VM, Felton JS. Cancer risk of heterocyclic amines in cooked foods: an analysis and implications for research. Carcinogenesis. 1995;16:39–52.
5. Forman D. Meat and cancer: a relation in search of a mechanism. Lancet. 1999;353:686–7.
6. Jägerstad M, Skog K, Grivas S, Olsson K. Formation of heterocyclic amines using model systems. Mutat Res. 1991;259:219–33.
7. Lang NP, Butler MA, Massengill J et al. Rapid metabolic phenotypes for acetyltransferase and cytochrome P4501A2 and putative exposure to food-borne heterocyclic amines increase the risk for colorectal cancer or polyps. Cancer Epidemiol Biomarkers Prev. 1994;3:675–82.
8. Schut HAJ, Snyderwine EG. DNA adducts of heterocyclic amine food mutagens: implications for mutagenesis and carcinogenesis. Carcinogenesis. 1999;20:353–68.
9. Synderwine EG, Wirth PJ, Roller PP, Adamson RH, Sato S, Thorgeirsson SS. Mutagenicity and in vitro covalent DNA binding of 2-hydroxyamino-3-methylimidazo [4,5-f] quinoline. Carcinogenesis. 1988;9:411–18.
10. Thomson B. Heterocyclic amine levels in cooked meat and the implication for New Zealanders. Eur J Cancer Prev. 1999;8:201–6.
11. Keating GA, Bogen KT. Methods for estimating heterocyclic amine concentrations in cooked meats in the US diet. Food Chem Toxicol. 2001;39:29–43.
12. Bogen KT. Cancer potencies of heterocyclic amines found in cooked foods. Food Chem Toxicol. 1994;32:505–15.
13. Byrne C, Sinha R, Platz EA et al. Predictors of dietary heterocyclic amine intake in three prospective cohorts. Cancer Epidemiol Biomarkers Prev. 1998;7:523–9.
14. Augustsson K, Skog K, Jägerstad M, Steineck G. Assessment of the human exposure to heterocyclic amines. Carcinogenesis. 1997;18:1931–5.
15. Norrish AE, Ferguson LR, Knize MG, Felton JS, Sharpe SJ, Jackson RT. Heterocyclic amine content of cooked meat and risk of prostate cancer. J Natl Cancer Inst. 1999;91:2038–44.

16. Augustsson K, Skog K, Jägerstad M, Dickman PW, Steineck G. Dietary heterocyclic amines and cancer of the colon, rectum, bladder and kidney: a population-based study. Lancet. 1999; 353:703–7.
17. Nagao M. A new approach to risk estimation of food-borne carcinogens – heterocyclic amines – based on molecular information. Mutat Res. 1999;431:3–12.
18. Roberts-Thomson IC, Ryan P, Khoo KK, Hart WJ, McMichael AJ, Butler RN. Diet, acetylator phenotype, and risk of colorectal neoplasia. Lancet. 1996;347:1372–4.
19. Welfare MR, Cooper J, Bassendine MF, Daly AK. Relationship between acetylator status, smoking, diet and colorectal cancer risk in the north-east of England. Carcinogenesis. 1997;18: 1351–4.
20. Sinha R, Chow WH, Kulldorff M et al. Well-done, grilled red meat increases the risk of colorectal adenomas. Cancer Res. 1999;59:4320–4.
21. Chen J, Stampfer MJ, Hough HL, Garcia-Closas M et al. A prospective study of N-acetyltransferase genotype, red meat intake and risk of colorectal cancer. Cancer Res. 1998;58:3307–11.

24
Secondary bile acids

F. M. NAGENGAST

Colonic carcinogenesis is a multistep process and involves interaction between luminal and mucosal factors. Genetic predisposition (familial polyposis coli and HNPCC) can lead to cancer at an early age and occurs in about 5–10% of cases. In the adenoma–carcinoma sequence genetic events in the colonic mucosa lead to an accumulation of mutations in specific genes and an imbalance in cell proliferation, differentiation and apoptosis. Dietary and lifestyle factors influence the colonic micro-environment and indirectly probably these mucosal events. Intermediate compounds in the large bowel lumen with genotoxic and cytotoxic potential are long chain fatty acids and bile acids. They can influence signal transduction pathways in colonic epithelial cells resulting in altered cell kinetics. The interaction is assumed to take place through the medium of the water phase of the colonic contents. Circumstantial epidemiological evidence and animal experiments show a promoting role for soluble secondary bile acids in colon carcinogenesis. These amphiphilic molecules are formed after enzymatic deconjugation and dehydroxylation of primary bile acids in the large bowel by anaerobic bacteria. The process is pH-dependent and inhibited in an acidic environment. Secondary bile acids can be co-mutagenic and can cause strand breaks in DNA. Moreover they are cytotoxic and can disrupt the integrity of the cell membrane of colonic mucosal cells. The increased cell loss will stimulate a compensatory cell renewal by increased cellular proliferation. There is also evidence of a direct stimulatory effect on proliferation mediated by protein kinase C (PKC) activation in the colonic cells. In many cell systems this activation of PKC can lead to induction of proteins that form the transcription factor AP-1. Bile acids and lipid components of faecal water can activate AP-1, whose activation has been associated with promotion of neoplastic transformation. Apoptosis is the physiological removal of cells in the human gut. Inhibition of apoptosis by deregulation of a number of oncogenes results in clonal expansion. One of the secondary bile acids, deoxycholic acid (DCA), was an effective inducer of apoptosis. The enhanced apoptosis by bile acids might be the result of their DNA-damaging properties, which possibly makes it a carcinogenic event. A recent interesting observation was the induction of COX-2 promotor activity in a colon cancer cell line by the dihydroxy bile salts chenodeoxycholic acid and deoxycholic acid.

Inhibition of secondary bile acid formation might be an interesting tool to inhibit colonic carcinogenesis. Lowering the intraluminal colonic pH is one way of achieving this goal. Dietary factors such as resistant starch and/or oligosaccharides (prebiotics) are fermented in the large bowel and have been shown to inhibit secondary bile acid formation and in some experiments colonic cell proliferation as well. Formation of short chain fatty acids such as butyrate might also be chemopreventive by other effects in human carcinogenesis. In summary, soluble bile acids are fascinating molecules, which probably play an intermediate role in colon cancer development, though their exact mode of action has not completely been revealed. More insight in the process of the interaction of luminal and genetic events in the large bowel could provide us with chemopreventive tools to decrease the mortality of this tumour in the future.

25
Carcinogens and co-carcinogens: polyamines

V. MILOVIC and J. STEIN

INTRODUCTION

Polyamines were discovered by van Leeuwenhoek in 1678, who described crystallization of spermine on microscopical inspection of human seminal fluid[1]. In spite of their early discovery, the exact physiological roles of polyamines were not fully recognised until as late as the 1960s. The evidence about enhanced polyamine synthesis in rapidly growing normal and neoplastic tissues raised universal attention; it was realized that polyamines are necessary for growth of both normal and neoplastic cells, and they have even been called growth factors[2,3]. Over 15 years of extensive research, polyamine metabolism in mammalian cells was almost completely elucidated[4-7]. Additional attention has been paid also to the understanding of an 'alternative route' of cellular polyamine supply – their uptake from the extracellular space. It was recognized early that, in addition to fine regulatory mechanisms of polyamine synthesis, the polyamine uptake system does contribute significantly to intracellular polyamine pools. Studies on polyamine uptake were triggered after it was realized that, in spite of selective blockade of polyamine-synthesizing enzymes, the neoplastic cells keep on proliferating because they readily absorb polyamines from the extracellular space – the intestinal and colonic lumen being the major source of exogenous polyamines for the body.

CELLULAR FUNCTIONS OF POLYAMINES

In terms of chemical structure, the polyamines, putrescine, spermidine and spermine, are aliphatic cations with two, three and four charges in their molecules, respectively (Figure 1).

At physiological pH, polyamines are fully protonated. Their positive charges are not point charges of inorganic ions (such as Ca^{2+} or Mg^{2+}), but are distributed along the hydrocarbon chain. Due to their unique structure, polyamines can

POLYAMINES

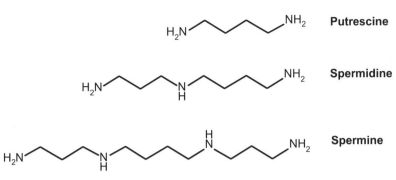

Putrescine

Spermidine

Spermine

Figure 1 Structure of polyamines

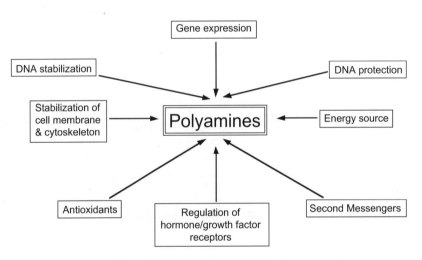

Figure 2 Cellular functions of polyamines

form bridges between distant negative charges. They rapidly bind to all negatively charged molecules in the cell, including DNA, proteins and phospholipids, and, as a result, exert various specific actions in the cell (Figure 2).

Spermidine and spermine bind to phosphate groups of the DNA double helix. Studies utilizing computer-aided molecular modelling showed that, in cell-free systems, spermidine and spermine but not putrescine cause DNA to condense and aggregate, by inducing B–Z and B–A transitions, occupying the small grove and stabilizing the double helix by binding its two strands together[8–12].

Natural spermine specifically prevents oxidative damage of isolated DNA[13–15]. It has been recently shown that similar structural effects of spermidine and spermine occur also in the cell culture systems, and that the major biological function of the polyamines is therefore related to polyamine-induced structural changes in DNA[16,17].

227

Polyamines protect membranes against lipid peroxidation by binding to the polar head groups of the membrane[18] and, in general, stabilize cellular membranes due to their interaction with the cytoskeleton[19-21]. This is a highly specific action, effective only from the cytoplasmic side of the membrane. As a result, polyamines regulate membrane-bound enzymes, calcium homeostasis, polyphosphoinositide metabolism, protein kinase C activity, development of the cytoskeleton, and transport of ions and metabolites[22].

Polyamines regulate the expression of growth-related genes, such as c-myc, c-fos and c-jun[23-30], therefore being directly involved in the regulation of cellular growth. An increase in ODC and in the expression c-myc occur concomitantly with enhanced growth. In polyamine-depleted cells, the expression of the *c-myc* protooncogene is reduced by >90%. The decrease appears to occur at the transcriptional level, since, in isolated nuclei from control cells, addition of spermidine increased thymidine incorporation 3–4-fold and increased *c-myc* and *c-fos* transcription 4–8-fold[31]. Furthermore, it has been recently shown that polyamines can trigger neoplastic transformation of immortalized cultured cells, exerting their effect, at least in part, by stimulating proto-oncogene expression[32-34].

Polyamines act at a second messenger level, and therefore regulate cell growth also indirectly by interfering with the expression and activity of various growth factor- and hormone receptors[35-40]. There is recent evidence that an increase in polyamine content may occur after physical stimuli, and subsequently enhance hormonal actions in target tissues[41].

Polyamines are involved in programmed cell death, but their exact mode of action is at present still unclear. In contrast to earlier reports that polyamines *per se* can inhibit apoptosis in cell culture systems by influencing endonuclease activity and p53 expression[42,43], recent evidence rather suggests that the sequence of events leading to apoptosis does require polyamines, although in much smaller amounts than those necessary for growth[44-47], and that polyamine hyperaccumulation, rather than depletion, triggers apoptosis[48].

BIOCHEMISTRY OF POLYAMINES

The polyamine metabolic pathway in mammalian cells is well understood (Figure 3). L-ornithine, a product of the arginase activity in the urea cycle, is the substrate for the first regulatory enzyme of the polyamine metabolic pathway, ornithine decarboxylase (ODC). ODC decarboxylates L-ornithine forming putrescine. Putrescine is converted to spermidine and spermine by the successive actions of spermidine and spermine synthases. The action of the two synthases is limited by the bioavailability of the aminopropyl donor, decarboxylated S-adenosylmethionine (SAMDC, AdoMet-DC).

Spermine is catabolized to putrescine by the activity of the two-step catabolic pathway, which is rate-limited by the first enzymatic step, spermine/spermidine-N'-acetyltransferase (SSAT). SSAT transfers the acetyl group from acetyl coenzyme A to the N' position of spermidine and spermine. The acetylated spermidine and spermine are catabolized by polyamine oxidase (PAO) to spermidine and putrescine, respectively. This highly regulated and responsive pathway allows the fine regulation of intracellular polyamine concentrations.

POLYAMINES

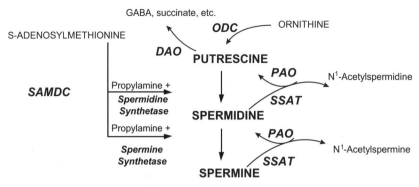

Figure 3 Polyamine metabolic pathway. ODC, ornithine decarboxylase; SAMDC, S-adenosylmethionine decarboxylase; SSAT, spermidine/spermine-N^1-acetyltransferase; PAO, polyamine oxidase; DAO, diamine oxidase

On another pole of the polyamine metabolic cascade, diamine oxidase (DAO), the enzyme present in large amounts in the gut and in endothelial cells, is responsible for degradation of putrescine to succinate and γ-aminobutyric acid (GABA). DAO seems to play a peculiar role in regulating polyamine homeostasis in the body, and all its actions have not yet been elucidated. However, intestinal mucosal DAO activity is reduced in patients with inflammatory bowel disease, coeliac disease, and in those receiving total parenteral nutrition[49–51]. DAO secretion is also stimulated by growth stimuli such as EGF[52]. This all may point to some still unexplained growth-related and polyamine catabolism-related roles of this enzyme in the gut.

SMALL INTESTINAL AND COLONIC LUMINAL POLYAMINES

'Exogenous' polyamines, originating from food, intestinal microflora and from sloughed epithelial cells play an essential role in normal, adaptive and neoplastic epithelial cell growth in the gut[53–56]. Gastrointestinal and colonic luminal polyamines were initially understood only as local factors involved in the processes related to cellular growth and differentiation in the gut. Polyamine hyperaccumulation in the intestinal epithelial cells was found to be increased, by enhanced synthesis, during intestinal adaptive growth after resection[57–61], but the same was also observed when putrescine was administered intraluminally into the adapting gut[62]. Luminal polyamines were found to be necessary not only for growth in the gut, but also for intestinal maturation in rodents[63], and for differentiation of an enterocyte-like cell line in culture[64]. Luminal putrescine *per se* stimulated DNA synthesis and thereby enhanced mucosal proliferation[65].

The evidence that luminal polyamines may stimulate growth of tumours of non-intestinal origin[66], that polyamine content in erythrocytes is markedly increased after a polyamine-rich meal[67–70], and that radioactivity originating from luminal polyamines was detected in all growing tissues and organs, including tumour tissue and skeletal muscle stimulated to grow by clenbuterol[71], has pointed out that luminal polyamines are not utilized only in the gut, but also rapidly absorbed and utilized for growth processes throughout the body.

In 1993, after a detailed analysis of more than 40 food items, Bardocz *et al.* reported that a typical human diet contributes hundreds of micromoles of polyamines per day to the gut lumen[72]. Apart from meat and meat products (rich in spermidine and spermine), all other types of food contain putrescine in amounts far exceeding those of spermidine and spermine, being as high as 400–500 μmol/L. Bardocz was also the first to show that, in the rat, luminal polyamines are readily taken up by the small intestinal mucosa if the gut is stimulated to grow, and that this uptake, unexpectedly, occurs predominantly via the basolateral side of the small intestinal epithelium[73–75].

Studies of Sawada *et al.*[76,77] showed that food is the dominant source of exogenous polyamines in the duodenum and upper jejunum. The contribution of biliopancreatic secretions was negligible in comparison with the amounts of polyamines obtained from food. Using the intubation technique in healthy volunteers, he showed that putrescine, when given perorally in concentrations comparable to those normally present in the duodenal lumen after a meal, disappears from both duodenal and jejunal lumen rapidly, its concentration reaching baseline values as early as 120 min after the 'test meal'. Subsequent studies[78,79] showed that polyamines cross the intestinal barrier by simple diffusion, and that the absorbed amounts are not influenced to a larger extent if intestinal epithelial cells are stimulated to grow. Furthermore, in humans, there is a mild but significant increase in spermidine and spermine concentration in blood after oral administration of putrescine.

Colonic lumen is also rich in polyamines. In the only studies published to date in humans, the putrescine concentration in the colonic lumen of healthy children can reach several millimoles; in comparison with this, spermidine and spermine concentrations in the colonic luminal contents are negligible[80,81]. Luminal polyamines in the colon apparently do not originate from any other source but from bacteria. Several recent studies[82–86] show that a number of bacterial species, normally present in the human colon, are able to synthesize large amounts of polyamines. As a rather indirect proof that colonic luminal polyamines involved in neoplastic cell growth are indeed of bacterial origin, several studies show that decontamination of the rat colon by broad-spectrum antibiotics does impair polyamine pools of the body and does contribute to impaired growth of cancers of non-intestinal origin[87–92].

POLYAMINES AS A TARGET FOR CANCER TREATMENT AND CHEMOPREVENTION

The role of polyamines in neoplastic cell growth has been thoroughly studied, and also reviewed in detail[93–97]. ODC activity, as well as total polyamine concentration, is increased in a wide range of tumours, including colorectal cancer[98–103]. Increased activity of ODC and increased production of polyamines have been suggested to lead to, and not only to support, malignant growth, and polyamines have been even attributed as markers of neoplastic cell proliferation[104].

The importance of enhanced ODC activity and increased polyamine synthesis in relation to carcinogenesis has been investigated in detail. In fibroblasts transfected with ODC and then injected into mice, the intensity of ODC expression (governed by the strength of the associated promoter) resulted in an increased number of tumours[32-34]. As another proof of the mutual interrelationship between ODC expression/polyamine production and occurrence of tumours, in Min mouse expressing an abnormal genotype for the APC tumour suppressor gene (like humans with familial adenomatous polyposis), ODC blockade suppressed the intestinal polyamine content and tumour number[105]. This study indicates that intestinal tissue polyamine content, elevated in Min mice by a mechanism involving APC-dependent changes in ODC mRNA, is necessary for intestinal tumourigenesis.

Because of the essential role of polyamines in maintaining high cell proliferation rates, polyamine depletion has long been a desired goal in antitumour therapy and cancer chemoprevention. To date, several strategies for modulating polyamine metabolism have been proposed: (1) direct inhibition of ODC activity; (2) combination strategies using ODC inhibition as a 'priming' step for other drugs; and (3) depletion of polyamine content through other mechanisms including inhibition of enzymes in the biosynthetic pathway, such as SAMDC, or the catabolic enzymes, polyamine oxidase (PAO) and spermidine/spermine-N^1-acetyltransferase (SSAT).

Initial interest in the area of polyamine deprivation in the treatment of cancer was focused on the inhibition of polyamine biosynthesis, i.e. the inhibition of ODC and SAMDC. Two agents of early promise in chemotherapy have arisen in recent decades; DFMO (alpha-difluoromethylornithine) and MGBG (methylglyoxal bis(guanylhydrazone)). Initial attempts to inhibit polyamine biosynthesis by blocking ODC activity with its suicide inhibitor, DFMO, failed to demonstrate convincing antitumour effects in man, because increased uptake of exogenous polyamines overcome the inhibitory effects of ODC blockade[106]. On the other hand, MGBG appeared to be of a limited clinical applicability, due to its general toxicity and side-effects (low specificity, antimitochondrial activity, general toxicity)[107]. Recently designed SAMDC inhibitors, MGBG analogues by chemical structure, were less toxic but still had side-effects similar to those of MGBG or, in vitro, exerted one part of their antiproliferative actions independently of SAMDC blockade and polyamine depletion[108,109].

Novel polyamine analogues, products of elegant design of R. Bergeron, A. R. Khomutov and P. Woster[110-117], are a new class of compounds specifically designed to perturb polyamine homeostasis within cells. These polyamine analogues show sufficient structural similarity to the parent polyamines to be taken up by the cell via the polyamine transport system; once within the cell, these compounds are sufficiently dissimilar to the parent polyamines to prevent their functional substitution. Most of the growth-inhibitory effects of these compounds are due to intracellular accumulation of these drugs, leading to the displacement of the natural polyamines from their binding sites within the cell. The uptake of the analogues via the putative polyamine transporter has also been implicated, since the decrease in intracellular polyamines, by the analogues, leads to an up-regulation in the transporter, thereby facilitating increased accumulation of the analogues in the cell. The analogues may interfere with polyamine biosynthesis via inhibition of ODC and SAMDC (known to be negatively regulated by intracellular polyamine pools) or by stimulating SSAT activity and therefore enhancing polyamine acetylation and efflux from the cell.

Cytotoxicity of polyamine analogues tends to correlate with their ability to disrupt cell-cycle progression. The effect on cell-cycle progression is accompanied by chromatin condensation around the nuclear envelope, and a change in the interactions between the natural polyamines and DNA. It appeared that the distance between the positively charged amino groups of the analogue is important in determining the extent of chromatin condensation and naked DNA. This has the effect of altering the susceptibility of DNA to endonuclease attack and fragmentation[118]. Also, certain polyamine analogues interfere with protein synthesis, particularly the synthesis of proteins involved in ATP production in the mitochondria[119,120]. ATP production subsequently decreases and this is accompanied by swelling of the mitochondria and deletion of the mitochondrial DNA.

Another effect of the analogues is the superinduction of the polyamine catabolic enzyme SSAT. The induction of this enzyme leads to a large decrease in intracellular polyamine pools, since the acetylated derivatives of spermine and spermidine have a decreased affinity for DNA and are more readily excreted from the cell[121]. Therefore, superinduction of SSAT, combined with the depletion of the intracellular polyamines, could facilitate the acetylation of substrates with much higher K_m values than the natural substrates, resulting in oxidative radical production and subsequent damage of neoplastic cells.

CLINICAL TRIALS

Recent clinical cancer chemoprevention trials, using dose de-escalation designs, indicate that DFMO can be given over long periods of time at low doses that suppress polyamine contents in gastrointestinal and other epithelial tissues but cause no detectable side-effects[122]. Current clinical chemoprevention trials are investigating the efficacy of DFMO to suppress surrogate end-point biomarkers (e.g. colon polyp recurrence) in patient populations at elevated risk for the development of specific epithelial cancers, mainly those of gastrointestinal origin, such as colon, oesophagus and stomach[123]. Polyamine levels in rectal mucosa were continuously suppressed by daily oral doses of 0.20 g/m^2 DFMO that had few or no side-effects[124]. Another possibility, to combine DFMO with non-steroidal anti-inflammatory drugs (agents of proven benefit in colon cancer chemoprevention), is at present undergoing clinical testing; preliminary results showed little or no side-effects when the dosage recommended in humans was used[125].

SAMDC inhibitors, such as SAM486A, have been recently evaluated as chemotherapeutic agents in patients with solid tumours of various origin[126,127]. Analysis of tumour biopsy specimens taken before and after SAM486A treatment revealed a decrease in SAMDC activity, increased ODC activity, increased levels of putrescine, and depleted levels of decarboxylated SAM and spermine, all of which are consistent with the proposed mode of action of SAM486A[127]. However, there are no ongoing studies evaluating this highly promising drug in colon cancer chemoprevention.

A novel polyamine analogue, N^1–N^{11}-diethylnorspermine, has been shown to induce SSAT and potently deplete cells in culture from their polyamines. This drug has been evaluated in patients with solid tumours, and at a dosage of

$25-118$ mg/m^2/day appeared to be toxic[128]. A subsequent study, evaluating N^1–N^{11}-diethylnorspermine in patients with lung cancer, found N^1–N^{11}-diethylnorspermine to be a suitable agent for chemotherapy in combination with agents possessing different spectrums of toxicities[129]. N^1–N^{11}-diethylnorspermine is taken up via the polyamine transporter, and therefore its use as a possible chemopreventive agent in patients with high risk to develop colorectal cancer would be a next logical step.

Studies evaluating DFMO and non-steroidal anti-inflammatory drugs, such as celecoxib and sulindac, as chemopreventive agents in patients with sporadic colonic polyps and Barret's oesophagus are being carried out at present in different centres[130]. The results of these trials are eagerly awaited, and will be most helpful in estimating a true value of the concept that depletion of gastrointestinal and colonic mucosal polyamines can be preventive in the development of gastrointestinal cancers.

Acknowledgements

The authors are indebted to Gerard M. Murphy (Department of Medicine, King's College London), Alex R. Khomutov (Engelhardt Institute of Molecular Biology, Russian Academy of Science) and Heather M. Wallace (Department of Medicine and Pharmaceutics, University of Aberdeen) for inspiring discussions and sharing their knowledge and ideas during the time. Our own studies, summarized in this chapter, were performed with the generous support of Special Trustees of Guy's Hospital, Arthur & Margarete Ebert Foundation and Else Kröner-Fresenius Foundation.

References

1. Leeuwenhoeck A. Observationes D. Anthonii Leeuwenhoeck, de natis et semini genitali animaliculis. Philos Trans R Soc London. 1678;12:1040–3.
2. Russell DH. Polyamines in growth – normal and neoplastic. In: Russell DH, editor, Polyamines in Normal and Neoplastic Growth. New York: Raven Press, 1973:1–13.
3. Tabor CW, Tabor H. Polyamines. Annu Rev Biochem. 1976;45:285–306.
4. Pegg AE, McCann PP. Polyamine metabolism and function. Am J Physiol. 1982;243:C212–21.
5. Grillo MA. Metabolism and function of polyamines. Int J Biochem. 1985;17:943–8.
6. Pegg AE. Recent advances in the biochemistry of polyamines in eukaryotes. Biochem J. 1986;234:240–62.
7. Seiler N. Polyamine metabolism. Digestion. 1990;46(suppl.2):319–30.
8. Marquet R, Houssier C. Different binding modes of spermine to A–T and G–C base pairs modulate the bending and stiffening of the DNA double helix. Biochem Pharmacol. 1988;37:1857–8.
9. Feuerstein BG, Williams LD, Basu HS, Marton LJ. Implications and concepts of polyamine–nucleic acid interactions. J Cell Biochem. 1991;46:37–47.
10. Basu HS, Feuerstein BG, Marton LJ. Polyamine–DNA interactions and their biological significance. In: Dowling RH, Fölsch UR, editors, Polyamines in the Gastrointestinal Tract. Dordrecht/Boston/London: Kluwer Academic Publishers, 1992:35–47.
11. Basu HS, Wright WD, Deen DF, Roti-Roti J, Marton LJ. Treatment with a polyamine analog alters DNA–matrix association in HeLa cell nuclei: a nucleoid halo assay. Biochemistry. 1993;32:4073–6.
12. Basu HS, Smirnov IV, Peng HF, Tiffany K, Jackson V. Effects of spermine and its cytotoxic analogs on nucleosome formation on topologically stressed DNA *in vitro*. Eur J Biochem. 1997;243:247–58.
13. McLean MJ, Well RD. The role of sequence in the stabilization of left-handed DNA helices *in vitro* and *in vivo*. Biochim Biophys Acta. 1988;950:243–54.

14. Ha HC, Yager JD, Woster PA, Casero RA Jr. Structural specificity of polyamines and polyamine analogues in the protection of DNA from strand breaks induced by reactive oxygen species. Biochem Biophys Res Commun. 1998;244:298–303.
15. Ha HC, Sirisoma NS, Kuppusamy P, Zweier JL, Woster PM, Casero RA Jr. The natural polyamine spermine functions directly as a free radical scavenger. Proc Natl Acad Sci USA. 1998;95:11140–5.
16. Muscari C, Guarnieri C, Stefanelli C, Giaccari A, Caldarera CM. Protective effect of spermine on DNA exposed to oxidative stress. Mol Cell Biochem. 1995;144:125–9.
17. Ha HC, Woster PM, Yager JD, Casero RA Jr. The role of polyamine catabolism in polyamine analogue-induced programmed cell death. Proc Natl Acad Sci USA. 1997;94:11557–62.
18. Tadolini B, Cabrini L, Landi L, Varani E, Pasquall P. Inhibition of lipid peroxidation by spermine bound to phospholipid vesicles. Biogenic Amines. 1985;3:97–106.
19. Schuber F. Influence of polyamines on membrane functions. Biochem J. 1989;260:1–10.
20. McCormack SA, Wang JY, Johnson LR. Polyamine deficiency causes reorganization of F-actin and tropomyosin in IEC-6 cells. Am J Physiol. 1994;267:C715–22.
21. McCormack SA, Ray RM, Blanner PM, Johnson LR. Polyamine depletion alters the relationship of F-actin, G-actin, and thymosin beta-4 in migrating IEC-6 cells. Am J Physiol. 1999;276:C459–68.
22. Johnson LR, Brockway PD, Madsen K, Hardin JA, Gall DG. Polyamines alter intestinal glucose transport. Am J Physiol. 1995;268:G416–23.
23. Celano P, Baylin SB, Giardiello FM, Nelkin BD, Casero RA Jr. Effect of polyamine depletion on c-myc expression in human colon carcinoma cells. J Biol Chem. 1988;263:5491–4.
24. Celano P, Baylin SB, Casero RA Jr. Polyamines differentially modulate the transcription of growth-associated genes in human colon carcinoma cells. J Biol Chem. 1989;264:8922–7.
25. Celano P, Berchtold CM, Giardiello FM, Casero RA Jr. Modulation of growth gene expression by selective alteration of polyamines in human colon carcinoma cells. Biochem Biophys Res Commun. 1989;165:384–90.
26. Wang JY, McCormack SA, Viar MJ et al. Decreased expression of protooncogenes c-fos, c-myc and c-jun following polyamine depletion in IEC-6 cells. Am J Physiol. 1993;265:G331–8.
27. Tabib A, Bachrach U. Activation of the proto-oncogene c-myc and c-fos by c-ras: involvement of polyamines. Biochem Biophys Res Commun. 1994;202:720–7.
28. Wang JY, Wang H, Johnson LR. Gastrin stimulates expression of protooncogene c-myc through a process involving polyamines in IEC-6 cells. Am J Physiol. 1995;269:C1474–81.
29. Patel AR, Wang JY. Polyamines modulate transcription but not posttranscription of c-myc and c-jun in IEC-6 cells. Am J Physiol. 1997;273:C1020–9.
30. Patel AR, Wang JY. Polyamine depletion is associated with an increase in JunD/AP-1 activity in small intestinal crypt cells. Am J Physiol. 1999;276:G441–50.
31. Berchtold CM, Tamez P, Kensler TW, Casero RA Jr. Inhibition of cell growth in Caco-2 cells by the polyamine analogue N1,N12-bis(ethyl)spermine is preceded by a reduction in MYC oncoprotein levels. J Cell Physiol. 1998;174:380–6.
32. Auvinen M, Paasinen A, Andersson LC, Höltta E. Ornithine decarboxylase activity is critical for cell transformation. Nature. 1992;360:355–8.
33. Auvinen M, Paasinen-Sohns A, Hirai H, Andersson LC, Höltta E. Ornithine decarboxylase- and ras-induced cell transformations: reversal by protein tyrosine kinase inhibitors and role of pp130CAS. Mol Cell Biol. 1995;15:6513–25.
34. Auvinen M, Laine A, Paasinen-Sohns A et al. Human ornithine decarboxylase-overproducing NIH3T3 cells induce rapidly growing, highly vascularized tumors in nude mice. Cancer Res. 1997;57:3016–25.
35. Buts JP, De Keyser N, Romain N, Dandrifosse G, Sokal E, Nsengiyumva T. Response of rat immature enterocytes to insulin: regulation by receptor binding and endoluminal polyamine uptake. Gastroenterology. 1994;106:49–59.
36. Paasinen-Sohns A, Höltta E. Cells transformed by ODC, c-Ha-ras and v-src exhibit MAP kinase/Erk-independent constitutive phosphorylation of Sos, Raf and c-Jun activation domain, and reduced PDGF receptor expression. Oncogene. 1997;15:1953–66.
37. McCormack SA, Blanner PM, Zimmerman BJ et al. Polyamine deficiency alters EGF receptor distribution and signaling effectiveness in IEC-6 cells. Am J Physiol. 1998;274:C192–205.
38. Manni A, Wechter R, Verderame MF, Mauger D. Cooperativity between the polyamine pathway and HER-2neu in transformation of human mammary epithelial cells in culture: role of the MAPK pathway. Int J Cancer. 1998;76:563–70.

39. Bauske R, Milovic V, Turchanowa L, Stein J. EGF-stimulated polyamine accumulation in the colon carcinoma cell line, Caco-2. Digestion. 2000;61:230–6.
40. Flamigni F, Facchini A, Capanni C, Stefanelli C, Tantini B, Caldarera CM. p44/42 mitogen-activated protein kinase is involved in the expression of ornithine decarboxylase in leukaemia L1210 cells. Biochem J. 1999;341:363–9.
41. Turchanowa L, Rogozkin VA, Milovic V, Feldkoren BI, Caspary WF, Stein J. Physical loading and testosterone are potent inducers of polyamine-synthesizing enzymes in the rat skeletal muscle. Eur J Clin Invest. 2000;30:72–8.
42. Brüne B, Hartzell P, Nicotera P, Orrhenius S. Spermine prevents endonuclease activation and apoptosis in thymocytes. Exp Cell Res. 1991;195:323–9.
43. Packham G, Cleveland JL. Ornithine decarboxylase is a mediator of c-myc induced apoptosis. Mol Cell Biol. 1994;14:5741–7.
44. Kramer DL, Vujcic S, Diegelman P, White C, Black JD, Porter CW. Polyamine analogue-mediated cell cycle responses in human melanoma cells involves the p53, p21, Rb regulatory pathway. Biochem Soc Trans. 1998;26:609–14.
45. Stefanelli C, Bonavita F, Stanic I et al. Spermine triggers the activation of caspase-3 in a cell-free model of apoptosis. FEBS Lett. 1999;451:95–8.
46. Stefanelli C, Bonavita F, Stanic I et al. Spermine causes caspase activation in leukaemia cells. FEBS Lett. 1998;437:233–6.
47. Li L, Li J, Rao JN, Li M, Bass BL, Wang JY. Inhibition of polyamine synthesis induces p53 gene expression but not apoptosis. Am J Physiol. 1999;276:C946–54.
48. Xie X, Tome ME, Gerner EW. Loss of intracellular putrescine pool-size regulation induces apoptosis. Exp Cell Res. 1997;230:386–92.
49. D'Agostino L, Pignata S, Daniele B et al. Ornithine decarboxylase and diamine oxidase in human colon carcinoma cell line Caco-2 in culture. Gastroenterology. 1989;97:888–94.
50. D'Agostino L, Daniele B, Pignata S, Barone MV, D'Argenio G, Mazzacca G. Modifications in ornithine decarboxylase and diamine oxidase in small bowel mucosa of starved and refed rats. Gut. 1987;28(Suppl):135–8.
51. Rokkas T, Vaja S, Murphy GM, Dowling RH. Postheparin plasma diamine oxidase in health and intestinal disease. Gastroenterology. 1990;98:1493–501.
52. Daniele B, Quaroni A. Effects of epidermal growth factor on diamine oxidase expression and cell growth in Caco-2 cells. Am J Physiol. 1991;261:G669–76.
53. Dowling RH, Hosomi M, Stace NH et al. Hormones and polyamines in intestinal and pancreatic adaptation. Scand J Gastroenterol. 1985;112:84–95.
54. Dowling RH. Update on intestinal adaptation. Triangle. 1989;27:149–64.
55. Dowling RH. Polyamines in intestinal adaptation and disease. Digestion. 1990;46(Suppl 2):331–44.
56. Milovic V. Polyamines in the gut lumen: bioavailability and biodistribution. Eur J Gastroenterol Hepatol. 2001;13:1021–5.
57. Osborne DL, Seidel ER. Gastrointestinal luminal polyamines: cellular accumulation and entero-hepatic circulation. Am J Physiol. 1990;258:G576–84.
58. Luk GD, Baylin SB. Inhibition of intestinal epithelial DNA synthesis and adaptive hyperplasia after jejunectomy in the rat by suppression of polyamine biosynthesis. J Clin Invest. 1984;74:698–704.
59. Luk GD, Baylin SB. Ornithine decarboxylase as a biologic marker in familial colonic polyposis. N Engl J Med. 1984;311:80–3.
60. Luk GD, Yang P. Polyamines in intestinal and pancreatic adaptation. Gut. 1987;28:95–101.
61. Hosomi M, Stace NH, Lirussi F, Smith SM, Murphy GM, Dowling RH. Role of polyamines in intestinal adaptation in the rat. Eur J Clin Invest. 1987;17:375–85.
62. Seidel ER, Haddox MK, Johnson LR. Ileal mucosal growth during infusion of ethylamine or putrescine. Am J Physiol. 1985;249:G234–8.
63. Dufour C, Dandrifosse G, Forget P, Vermesse F, Romain N, Lepoint P. Spermine and spermidine induce intestinal maturation in the rat. Gastroenterology. 1988;95:112–16.
64. Herold G, Besemer F, Rogler D, Rogler G, Stange EF. Polyamine deficiency impairs prolifera-tion and differentiation of cultured enterocytes (Caco-2). Z Gastroenterol. 1993;31:120–8.
65. Ginty DD, Osborne DL, Seidel ER. Putrescine stimulates DNA synthesis in intestinal epithelial cells. Am J Physiol. 1989;257:G145–50.
66. Sarhan S, Knödgen B, Seiler N. The gastrointestinal tract as polyamine source for tumour growth. Anticancer Res. 1989;9:215–24.

67. Moulinoux JP, Quemener V, Khan NA. Biological significance of circulating polyamines in oncology. Cell Mol Biol. 1991;37:773–83.
68. Moulinoux JP, Quemener V, Havouis R, Guille F, Martin C, Seiler N. Accumulation of polyamine analogs in red blood cells: a potential index of tumor proliferation rate. Anticancer Res. 1991;11:2143–6.
69. Quemener V, Bansard JY, Delamaire M et al. Red blood cell polyamines, anaemia and tumour growth in the rat. Eur J Cancer. 1996;32:316–21.
70. Catros-Quemener V, Leray G, Moulinoux JP, Havouis R, de Certaines JD, Chapman J. Tumour growth modifies intravascular polyamine transport by plasma lipoproteins in the mouse. Biochim Biophys Acta. 1997;1346:30–7.
71. Bardocz S, Brown DS, Grant G, Pusztai A, Stewart JC, Palmer RM. Effect of the beta-adrenoceptor agonist clenbuterol and phytohaemagglutinin on growth, protein synthesis and polyamine metabolism of tissues of the rat. Br J Pharmacol. 1992;106:476–82.
72. Bardocz S, Grant G, Brown DS, Ralph A, Pusztai A. Polyamines in food – implications for growth and health. J Nutr Biochem. 1993;4:66–71.
73. Bardocz S, Brown DS, Grant G, Pusztai A. Luminal and basolateral polyamine uptake by rat small intestine stimulated to grow by *Phaseolus vulgaris* lectin phytohaemagglutinin *in vivo*. Biochim Biophys Acta. 1990;1034:46–52.
74. Bardocz S, Grant G, Brown DS, Ewen SW, Nevison I, Pusztai A. Polyamine metabolism and uptake during *Phaseolus vulgaris* lectin, PHA-induced growth of rat small intestine. Digestion. 1990;46(Suppl 2):360–6.
75. Bardocz S, Grant G, Brown DS, Ewen SW, Stewart JC, Pusztai A. Effect of fasting and refeeding on basolateral polyamine uptake and metabolism by the rat small bowel. Digestion. 1991;50:28–35.
76. Sawada Y, Pereira SP, Murphy GM, Dowling RH. Polyamine content in different foods. Gut. 1994;35:S20.
77. Sawada Y, Pereira SP, Murphy GM, Dowling RH. Polyamines in duodenal lumen and biliopancreatic secretions. Biochem Soc Trans. 1994;75:122.
78. Milovic V, Odera G, Murphy GM, Dowling RH. Jejunal putrescine absorption and the 'pharmacokinetics'/biotransformation of ingested putrescine in humans. Gut. 1997;41:A62.
79. Milovic V, Faust D, Turchanowa L, Stein J, Caspary WF. Permeability characteristics of polyamines across intestinal epithelium using the Caco-2 monolayer system: comparison between transepithelial flux and mitogen-stimulated uptake into epithelial cells. Nutrition. 2001;17:462–6.
80. Forget P, Sinaasappel M, Bouquet J, Deutz NE, Smeets C. Fecal polyamine concentration in children with and without nutrient malabsorption. J Pediatr Gastroenterol Nutr. 1997;24:285–8.
81. Forget P, Degraeuwe PL, Smeets C, Deutz NE. Fasting gastric fluid and fecal polyamine concentrations in premature infants. J Pediatr Gastroenterol Nutr. 1997;24:389–92.
82. Bover-Cid S, Holzapfel WH. Improved screening procedure for biogenic amine production by lactic acid bacteria. Int J Food Microbiol. 1999;53:33–41.
83. Olaya J, Neopikhanov V, Uribe A. Lipopolysaccharide of *Escherichia coli*, polyamines, and acetic acid stimulate cell proliferation in intestinal epithelial cells. In Vitro Cell Dev Biol Anim. 1999;35:43–8.
84. Bover-Cid S, Holzapfel WH. Biogenic amine production by bacteria. In: Biologically Active Amines in Food, Vol. IV. Bardocz S, Morgan DML, White A, Sanchez-Jimenez F, editors, COST 917. European Commission, 2000:20–9.
85. Noack J, Dongowski G, Hartmann L, Blaut M. The human gut bacteria *Bacteroides thetaiotaomicron* and *Fusobacterium varium* produce putrescine and spermidine in cecum of pectin-fed gnotobiotic rats. J Nutr. 2000;130:1225–31.
86. Ellmerich S, Scholler M, Duranton B et al. Promotion of intestinal carcinogenesis by *Streptococcus bovis*. Carcinogenesis. 2000;21:753–6.
87. Seiler N, Sarhan S, Grauffel C, Jones R, Knodgen B, Moulinoux JP. Endogenous and exogenous polyamines in support of tumour growth. Cancer Res. 1990;50:5077–83.
88. Sarhan S, Knödgen B, Seiler N. Polyamine deprivation, malnutrition and tumour growth. Anticancer Res. 1992;12:457–66.
89. Quemener V, Moulinoux JP, Havouis R, Seiler N. Polyamine deprivation enhances antitumoral efficacy of chemotherapy. Anticancer Res. 1992;12:1447–53.
90. Quemener V, Blanchard Y, Chamaillard L, Havouis R, Cipolla B, Moulinoux JP. Polyamine deprivation: a new tool in cancer treatment. Anticancer Res. 1994;14:443–8.

91. Quemener V, Chamaillard L, Brachet P, Havouis R, Moulinoux JP. The involvement of polyamines in the malignant proliferative process. The anticancer effect of polyamine deprivation. Ann Gastroenterol Hepatol. 1995;31:181–8.

92. Chamaillard L, Catros-Quemener V, Delcros JG et al. Polyamine deprivation prevents the development of tumour-induced immune suppression. Br J Cancer. 1997;76:365–70.

93. Jänne J, Alhonen L, Leinonen P. Polyamines: from molecular biology to clinical application. Ann Med. 1991;23:241–59.

94. McCann PP, Pegg AE. Ornithine decarboxylase as an enzyme target for therapy. Pharmacol Ther. 1992;54:195–215.

95. Marton LJ, Pegg AE. Polyamines as targets for therapeutic intervention. Annu Rev Pharmacol Toxicol. 1995;35:55–91.

96. Medina MA, Quesada AR, Nunez de Castro I, Sanchez-Jimenez F. Histamine, polyamines, and cancer. Biochem Pharmacol. 1999;57:1341–4.

97. Wallace HM, Caslake R. Polyamines and colon cancer. Eur J Gastroenterol Hepatol. 2001;13:1033–9.

98. Saydjari R, Townsend CM, Barranco SC, Thompson JC. Polyamines in gastrointestinal cancer. Dig Dis Sci. 1989;34:1629–36.

99. Löser C, Fölsch UR, Paprotny C, Creutzfeldt W. Polyamines in colorectal cancer: evaluation of polyamine concentrations in the colon tissue, serum, and urine of 50 patients with colorectal cancer. Cancer. 1990;65:958–66.

100. Löser C, Fölsch UR, Paprotny C, Creutzfeldt W. Polyamines in human gastrointestinal malignancies. Digestion. 1990;46(Suppl 2):430–8.

101. Elitsur Y, Moshier JA, Murthy R, Barbish A, Luk GD. Polyamine levels, ornithine decarboxylase (ODC) activity, and ODC-mRNA expression in normal and cancerous human colonocytes. Life Sci. 1992;50:1417–24.

102. Wang W, Liu LQ, Higuchi CM. Mucosal polyamine measurements and colorectal cancer risk. J Cell Biochem. 1996;63:252–7.

103. Giardiello FM, Hamilton SR, Hylind LM, Yang VW, Tamez P, Casero RA. Ornithine decarboxylase and polyamines in familial adenomatous polyposis. Cancer Res. 1997;57:199–201.

104. Higuchi CM, Wang W. Comodulation of cellular polyamines and proliferation: biomarker application to colorectal mucosa. J Cell Biochem. 1995;57:256–61.

105. Erdman SH, Ignatenko NA, Powell MB et al. APC-dependent changes in expression of genes influencing polyamine metabolism, and consequences for gastrointestinal carcinogenesis, in the Min mouse. Carcinogenesis. 1999;20:1709–13.

106. Alhonen-Hongisto L, Seppanen P, Jänne J. Intracellular putrescine and spermidine deprivation induces increased uptake of the natural polyamines and methylglyoxal bis(guanylhydrazone). Biochem J. 1980;192:941–5.

107. Stanek J, Caravatti G, Capraro HG et al. S-Adenosylmethionine decarboxylase inhibitors: new aryl and heteroaryl analogues of Bis(guanylhydrazone). J Med Chem. 1993;36:46–54.

108. Regenass U, Mett H, Stanek J, Mueller M, Kramer D, Porter CW. CGP 48664, a new S-adenosylmethionine decarboxylase inhibitor with broad spectrum antiproliferative and antitumor activity. Cancer Res. 1994;54:3210–17.

109. Dorhout B, Odink MF, De Hoog E, Kingma AW, Van der Veer E, Muskiet FA. 4-Aminoindan-1-one 2'-amidinohydrazone (CGP 48664A) exerts *in vitro* growth inhibitory effects that are not only related to S-adenosylmethionine decarboxylase inhibition. Biochem Biophys Acta. 1997;1335:144–52.

110. Fukuchi J, Kashiwagi K, Kusama-Eguchi K, Terao K, Shirahata A, Igarashi K. Mechanism of the inhibition of cell growth by N1,N2-bis(ethyl)spermine. Eur J Biochem. 1992;209:689–96.

111. Basu HS, Marton LJ, Pellarin M et al. Design and testing of novel cytotoxic polyamine analogues. Cancer Res. 1994;54:6210–14.

112. Khomutov AR, Shvetsov AS, Vepsalainen JJ et al. Aminooxy analogues of polyamines. Bioorg Khim. 1996;22:557–9.

113. Fogel-Petrovic M, Vujcic S, Brown PJ, Haddox MK, Porter CW. Effects of polyamines, polyamine analogs, and inhibitors of protein synthesis on spermidine-spermine N^1-acetyltransferase gene expression. Biochemistry. 1996;35:14436–44.

114. Fogel-Petrovic M, Kramer DL, Vujcic S et al. Structural basis for differential induction of spermidine/spermine N^1-acetyltransferase activity by novel spermine analogs. Mol Pharmacol. 1997;52:69–74.

115. Antony T, Thomas T, Shirahata A, Thomas TJ. Selectivity of polyamines on the stability of RNA-DNA hybrids containing phosphodiester and phosphorothioate oligodeoxyribonucleotides. Biochemistry. 1999;38:10775–84.

116. Milovic V, Turchanowa L, Khomutov AR, Khomutov RM, Caspary WF, Stein J. Hydroxylamine-containing inhibitors of polyamine biosynthesis and impairment of colon cancer cell growth. Biochem Pharmacol. 2001;61:199–206.

117. Turchanowa L, Shvetsov AS, Demin AV et al. Insufficiently charged isosteric analogue of spermine: interaction with polyamine uptake, and effect on Caco-2 cell growth. Biochem Pharmacol. 2002;64:649–55.

118. Kramer DL, Vujcic S, Diegelman P et al. Polyamine analogue induction of the p53-p21WAF1/CIP1-Rb pathway and G1 arrest in human melanoma cells. Cancer Res. 1999;59:1278–86.

119. Toninello A, Dalla Via L, Siliprandi D, Garlid KD. Evidence that spermine, spermidine, and putrescine are transported electrophoretically in mitochondria by a specific polyamine uniporter. J Biol Chem. 1992;267:18393–7.

120. Tome ME, Fiser SM, Payne CM, Gerner EW. Excess putrescine accumulation inhibits the formation of modified eukaryotic initiation factor 5A (eIF-5A) and induces apoptosis. Biochem J. 1997;328:847–54.

121. Chopra S, Wallace HM. Induction of spermidine/spermine N1-acetyltransferase in human cancer cells in response to increased production of reactive oxygen species. Biochem Pharmacol. 1998;55:1119–23.

122. Meyskens FL Jr, Emerson SS, Pelot D et al. Dose de-escalation chemoprevention trial of alpha-difluoromethylornithine in patients with colon polyps. J Natl Cancer Inst. 1994;86:1122–30.

123. Meyskens FL, Gerner EW. Development of difluoro-methylornithine (DFMO) as a chemoprevention agent. Clin Cancer Res. 1999;5:945–51.

124. Meyskens FL Jr, Gerner EW, Emerson S et al. Effect of alpha-difluoromethylornithine on rectal mucosal levels of polyamines in a randomized, double-blinded trial for colon cancer prevention. J Natl Cancer Inst. 1998;90:1212–18.

125. Carbone PP, Douglas JA, Larson PO et al. Phase I chemoprevention study of piroxicam and alpha-difluoromethylornithine. Cancer Epidemiol Biomarkers Prev. 1998;7:907–12.

126. Paridaens R, Uges DR, Barbet N et al. A phase I study of a new polyamine biosynthesis inhibitor, SAM486A, in cancer patients with solid tumours. Br J Cancer. 2000;83:594–601.

127. Siu LL, Rowinsky EK, Hammond LA et al. A phase I and pharmacokinetic study of SAM486A, a novel polyamine biosynthesis inhibitor, administered on a daily-times-five every-three-week schedule in patients with advanced solid malignancies. Clin Cancer Res. 2002;8:2157–66.

128. Streiff RR, Bender JF. Phase 1 study of N^1–N^{11}-diethylnorspermine (DENSPM) administered TID for 6 days in patients with advanced malignancies. Invest New Drugs. 2001;19:29–39.

129. Hahm HA, Ettinger DS, Bowling K et al. Phase I study of $N^{(1)}$,$N^{(11)}$-diethylnorspermine in patients with non-small cell lung cancer. Clin Cancer Res. 2002;8:684–90.

130. Gwyn K, Sinicrope FA. Chemoprevention of colorectal cancer. Am J Gastroenterol. 2002;97:13–21.

26
Exocyclic DNA adducts derived from lipid peroxidation as oxidative stress markers in human colon carcinogenesis

H. BARTSCH and J. NAIR

INTRODUCTION

Although in the pathways to colorectal cancer multiple genetic changes via inherited and/or acquired mutations and disregulated DNA methylation in cancer-relevant genes[1] have been defined, the total number of genetic alterations, i.e. the extent of genomic instability in sporadic colorectal cancer progression, has been unknown. Recently Stoler et al.[2] analysed colorectal premalignant polyps and carcinoma samples by inter (simple sequence repeat)-PCR. The mean number of genomic alterations in carcinoma and premalignant colonic polyps were found to be approximately 11 000 per cell, suggesting a similar number of events to occur early in tumour progression. These results indicated that genomic destabilization is an early step in sporadic tumour development, and genomic instability is a cause rather than an effect of malignancy, facilitating vastly accelerated somatic cell evolution and colon cancer progressions.

The concept of genetic instability implies that, while cancer initiation is generally assumed to be caused by environmental or genotoxic agents, the additional genetic alterations required for neoplastic progression may be derived from endogenously generated genotoxins produced by oxidative stress and lipid peroxidation (LPO). However, the nature of endogenous processes and agents, causing such vast accumulation of DNA damage/genetic alterations that probably acts as a driving force in colon cancer development, are not well understood. This increased oxidative stress could occur as a consequence of up-regulation of 'emergency enzymes' such as nitric oxide synthase (iNOS), lipoxygenase (LOX) or cyclo-oxygenase (COX)-2 that has been detected in many organs in early and late stages of tumour development. For the former two enzymes we have shown in experimental mouse models a direct correlation between overexpression and extent of LPO-derived DNA damage[3,4]. Colon cancer development is frequently a pathological consequence of persistent oxidative stress, whereby oxidative DNA damage and mutations in cancer-related genes are caused that lead to a cycle of cell death and regeneration. This is supported by an increasing body of evidence. Hereby cellular overproduction of reactive oxygen and nitrogen species (ROS and RNS) are implicated. These are produced at low levels by physiological processes, but in excess amounts during various pathophysiological conditions. For example, as a part of the host antibacterial/antiviral defence system a burst of ROS/RNS, often accompanied by NO overproduction, is produced during chronic infections and inflammatory processes, many of which are recognized as important risk factors for human cancers[5,6]. A previous investigation of primary human colon tumours established a statistically significant positive correlation between iNOS activity in tumours and the frequency of G:C to A:T transitions at CpG sites in the p53 tumour-suppressor gene[7]. The multiple types of DNA damage caused by NO overproduction include, *inter alia*, deamination of cytosine and the formation of oxidized DNA bases from HO$^•$ and peroxynitrite, the latter being generated by reaction of NO and superoxide anion, when formed concomitantly[8]. In addition LPO of polyunsaturated fatty acids (PUFA) by ROS and RNS results in DNA-reactive products such as *trans*-4-hydroxy-2-nonenal (HNE), malonaldehyde and crotonaldehyde, which are increasingly implicated in the carcinogenesis process[9]. These intermediates can react with DNA bases to form exocyclic DNA adducts of which several have been characterized as propano- and etheno (ε)-DNA-base adducts[10,11]. Of the latter, 1,N^6-ethenodeoxyadenosine (εdA), 3, N^4-ethenodeoxycytidine (εdC) and N^2,3-ethenodeoxyguanosine have been detected *in vivo*. These promutagenic, chemically stable secondary oxidation markers appear to be useful for assessing oxidative stress-derived DNA damage. They are also formed from the carcinogens vinyl chloride and urethane[12] via their reactive oxirane intermediates, where they are considered as the major initiating carcinogenic DNA lesions. That NO overproduction can produce LPO-derived DNA modifications such as etheno (ε)-DNA adducts, was previously demonstrated in an SJL mouse model whereby NO overproduction after injection of pre-B lymphoma cells *in vivo* led to a concomitant increase in ε-adduct levels[3]. These initial results suggested that oxidative and LPO-derived DNA damage could play a major role in the development of human cancers associated with cancers that have an inflammatory component in their aetiopathogenesis, such as colon cancer associated with inflammatory bowel diseases.

We have developed sensitive and specific methods which allowed detection of ε-DNA adducts *in vivo* and allowed us to study their role in experimental and human carcinogenesis. To further demonstrate a link between DNA damage, LPO and chronic inflammatory processes in human colon cancer, ε-DNA adduct levels were analysed in affected colon epithelium from patients suffering from Crohn's disease (CD), ulcerative colitis (UC) and familial adenomatous polyposis (FAP) and compared with normal colon and sporadic colon cancer. We could demonstrate for the first time an accumulation of miscoding lesions in human colon carcinogenesis, as well as in other organs[13]. This brief review will focus on the detection of ε adducts as lead markers for oxidative stress- and LPO-induced DNA damage and their possible role in human colon carcinogenesis.

RESULTS AND DISCUSSION

Background levels of ε-DNA adducts

The ε-DNA adducts (εdA, εdC) in tissues can be quantitated in small amounts of DNA by an ultrasensitive immunoaffinity/^{32}P-postlabelling procedure[14]. Etheno-bridged nucleosides (εdA) can also be measured in human urine by a quantitative immunoaffinity–HPLC–fluorescence method[15]. Use of the above highly specific, ultrasensitive method, involving immunoaffinity chromatography coupled with ^{32}P-postlabelling, unambiguously and quantitatively revealed the existence of background levels of ε adducts in human liver and other organs from unexposed rodents and humans[14,16,17]. Comparable but variable εdA and εdC levels were detected in DNA of asymptomatic human colon tissue obtained from accident victims[18]. The highly variable background levels of ε adducts in asymptomatic tissues from unexposed humans, and also rodents, support an endogenous pathway of ε-adduct formation by reaction of HNE (via its 2,3-epoxide) with DNA bases[16], as part of a physiological LPO[19] process that the cell can cope with.

Detection of persistent oxidative stress in colon cancer-prone patients, as measured by ε-DNA adducts in colon

We then investigated whether an enhanced level of promutagenic ε-DNA adducts can be detected in human colon epithelium of patients who are predisposed to a higher risk of colon cancer. We analysed ε-DNA adduct levels in affected colon epithelia from FAP, UC and CP patients and compared them with normal human colon. Miscoding ε adducts are one of the lead markers that may reflect this increase of oxidative stress/LPO-derived DNA damage. Therefore, we assume that they contribute to mutations and genomic instability that could drive the inflamed or genetically predisposed (FAP) colon epithelium to malignancy.

Patients with FAP, an inherited disease due to mutations in the *APC* gene, develop multiple adenomatous polyps and later carcinomas in the colon. COX-2 and phospholipase A_2 (sPLA$_2$) are up-regulated in colorectal adenomatous polyps[20], and the activity of xanthine oxidase, which generates free radicals, is increased[21]. It was hypothesized[22] that a 'self-promotion' by *APC* mutations and COX-2 up-regulation takes place in FAP polyps. To discover whether this is also paralleled by an increased load of oxidative stress-related DNA damage, DNA from asymptomatic colon epithelia from accident victims, colonic polyps from FAP patients, and colorectal cancer tissue was analysed for ε-adducts. A statistically significant, about two-fold, increase in εdA and εdC adduct levels in FAP polyps in comparison with controls was observed, whereas the ε-adduct levels were lower in colon cancer tissue, but highly variable in the adjacent non-tumorous colon tissue[18]. A plausible explanation for this increase in DNA damage in FAP polyps could be the chronic overproduction of ROS and subsequently LPO-derived DNA adducts in the precancerous lesion due to COX-2, ʃPlA$_2$ and/or xanthine oxidase up-regulation (Figure 1). Persistent generation of such miscoding lesions may contribute to genetic instability and progression of FAP polyps to malignancy as one of the mechanisms for the postulated self-promotion process. In urethane-induced lung carcinogenesis in mice a two-fold increase

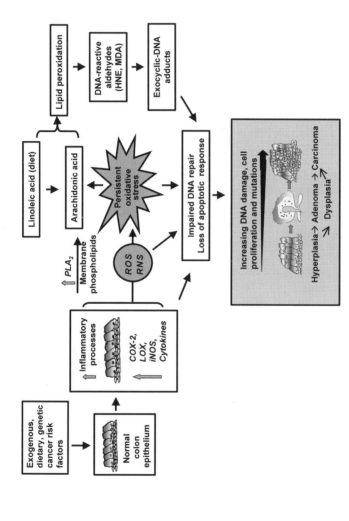

Figure 1 Hypothetical scheme linking linoleic acid/arachidonic acid (AA) metabolism, persistent oxidative stress and DNA damage to multistage colon carcinogenesis. In initiated or preneoplastic cells, sPLA$_2$, COX-2, LOX and iNOS are often overexpressed. This leads to increased release of AA, faster AA oxygenation and to higher levels of reactive oxygen (ROS)/nitrogen species (RNS). These can cause DNA damage and trigger lipid peroxidation (LPO) of polyunsaturated fatty acids in a self-perpetuating process, leading to various forms of exocyclic DNA adducts (e.g. via 4-HNE and MDA). Such DNA damage may accumulate because of impaired DNA repair of oxidatively damaged DNA lesions by NO or inflammatory cytokines, or because of up-regulation of anti-apoptotic signals (see text for details). A tight link between LOX activity and exocyclic DNA adducts during two-stage skin carcinogenesis in mice was recently demonstrated[4]. In rapidly dividing colon cells the resulting genetic changes and disrupted signalling pathways may drive premalignant cells to malignancy. 4-HNE, *trans*-4-hydroxy-2-nonenal; LOX, lipoxygenase; MDA, malonaldehyde; PLA$_2$, phospholipase A$_2$

242

above background in etheno-adduct levels was associated with tumour induction in this organ[12].

Patients with the inflammatory bowel diseases ulcerative colitis (UC) and Crohn's disease (CD) have an elevated risk for developing colon cancer. In the mucosa of these patients, large quantities of ROS were found to be produced that correlated with disease severity. Furthermore, NO generation and iNOS activity were increased in colonic tissue, together with a depletion of antioxidant defence, rendering DNA in colonic epithelium susceptible to ROS/RNS injury[23]. Using the immunoaffinity/^{32}P-postlabelling assay we recently reported[24] that etheno-DNA adducts, especially εdC, were significantly elevated in target colon epithelial cells of cancer-prone CD and UC patients. We conclude that promutagenic etheno-DNA adducts could play a role in the acquisition of mutations during colon carcinogenesis in CD and UC patients. In support of this, colon mucosa in long-standing UC showed a high frequency of K-*ras* mutations[25] and an increased p53 mutation load was observed in this cancer-prone colon tissue, which was higher in regions of UC patients affected by chronic inflammatory conditions than in non-lesional regions[26].

Possible mechanisms for accumulation of promutagenic lesions in target organs

Factors that may influence the steady-state levels of ε-DNA adducts in cancer-prone colon tissues may include: (a) reduced antioxidant levels, (b) variations in detoxifying reactions of HNE by glutathione S-transferases which display genetic polymorphisms, (c) differential or impaired repair of ε-DNA adducts in the inflamed colon and (d) a reduced apoptotic rate. εdA and εdC are removed by different repair enzymes, 3-methyl-adenine-DNA-glycosylase and mismatch-specific thymine-DNA-glycosylase, respectively[27,28]. There is growing support for the inhibition of DNA repair pathways by inflammatory mediators[29]. For example inflammatory cytokines induced DNA damage in a cell line[30] and inhibited DNA repair by an NO-dependent mechanism: global DNA repair was inhibited by 70% when NO was overproduced via iNOS after addition of IL-1β, IFN-γ and TNF-α. A key repair enzyme (hOGG1) responsible for base excision of 8-oxoguanine was inhibited by NO, an inflammatory mediator in a human cholangiocarcinoma cell line[31]. Another study reported that 8-oxoguanine was repaired by only 50% when a human cell line was treated with IL-6; this interleukin inhibits apoptosis through up-regulation of an anti-apoptotic gene *mcl*-1, thus retaining more oxidative DNA lesions[32]. Similar conditions may prevail in inflamed colon of patients with IBD and possibly also in premalignant stages of sporadic colorectal cancers, leading to the inhibition of global and/or specific repair pathways of oxidative and LPO-derived DNA lesions. Recent investigations lend further support to this assumption: the expression of two protein subunits Ku 70 and Ku 86 DNA-dependent protein kinase, which participates in the repair of DNA double-strand breaks, was significantly reduced in human colon carcinomas and more so in adenomas as compared to normal tissue[33].

In conclusion, our results on the significantly increased ε-DNA adduct levels in affected colon epithelium of FAP patients and in UC and CP patients suffering from inflammatory bowel disease lend further support to the hypothesis that persistent oxidative stress is implicated as one of the major events in the development and progression of malignant colon tumours (Figure 1). An increasing load of ROS/LPO-induced DNA damage seems to be triggered by up-regulation/ overexpression of 'emergency enzymes' such as LOX, COX-2 and iNOS reported to occur in early and late stages of the carcinogenic process. Promutagenic etheno-DNA adducts thus represent useful markers for LPO-induced or oxidative DNA damage which, if not efficiently removed due to impaired DNA repair or reduced apoptotic rate (possibly as a consequence of inflammatory mediators), will lead to increased mutations and genomic instability, which could drive cells to a malignant state. Chromosomal instability has been recognized as a common event occurring very early during colorectal neoplasia[34]. If true, this scheme could apply to a number of human tumours that are caused by infectious agents, or which have persistent inflammatory processes as a part of their aetiopathogenesis. Therefore, etheno (and other LPO-derived exocyclic) DNA adducts appear to be promising biomarkers for studying the aetiopathogenesis of human colon carcinogenesis, but more importantly they may serve to measure the efficacy of preventive interventions, e.g. by dietary antioxidants. Our recent results on the presence of powerful antioxidants in olive oil[35–38] should encourage trials to explore the antioxidative and cancer-protective potential by these agents, particularly in patients with inflammatory bowel disease. Our non-invasive assay to measure εdA in urine[15] should facilitate such clinical and molecular epidemiology studies. Its utility has been demonstrated in a recently completed intervention study in Japanese women in northern Japan: urinary excretion of εdA was found to be positively correlated with salt and ω-6 polyunsaturated fatty acid (PUFA) intake[39]. These findings are in keeping with the assumption that chronic inflammatory processes (stimulated by high NaCl intake and *H. pylori* infection, e.g. in the stomach) and a diet rich in ω-6 PUFA, good substrates for LPO, lead to endogenous DNA damage, the aetiological role of which can now be investigated.

Acknowledgements

The authors' research in this area was in part supported by EU contracts ENV4-CT97-0505 and QLRT-RT-2000-00286. The authors acknowledge the work contributed by A. Barbin and K. Schmid, and collaboration with H. G. Beger and P. Dolara. Dr P. Lorenz, University of Essen, Essen, Germany, is thanked for providing the Mab used in these studies. C. Ditrich is thanked for skilled technical assistance and S. Fuladdjusch for excellent secretarial help.

References

1. Potter JD. Colorectal cancer: molecules and populations: Review. J Nat Cancer Inst. 1999; 91:916–32.
2. Stoler DL, Chen N, Basik M *et al*. The onset and extent of genomic instability in sporadic colorectal tumor progression. Proc Natl Acad Sci. 1999;96:15121–6.
3. Nair J, Gal A, Tamir S *et al*. Etheno adducts in spleen DNA of SJL mice stimulated to overproduce nitric oxide. Carcinogenesis. 1998;19:2081–4.
4. Nair J, Fürstenberger G, Bürger F *et al*. Promutagenic etheno-DNA adducts in multistage mouse skin carcinogenesis: correlation with lipoxygenase-catalyzed arachidonic acid metabolism. Chem Res Toxicol. 2000;13:703–9.

5. Ohshima H, Bartsch H. Chronic infections and inflammatory processes as cancer risk factors: possible role of nitric oxide in carcinogenesis. Mutat Res. 1994;305:253–64.

6. Liu RH, Hotchkiss JH. Potential genotoxicity of chronically elevated nitric oxide: a review. Mutat Res. 1995;339:73–89.

7. Ambs S, Bennett WP, Merriam WG et al. Relationship between p53 mutations and inducible nitric oxide synthase expression in human colorectal cancer. J Natl Cancer Inst. 1999;91:86–8.

8. Tamir S, Burney S, Tannenbaum SR. DNA damage by nitric oxide. Chem Res Toxicol. 1996;9:821–7.

9. Bartsch H, Nair J, Owen RW. Dietary polyunsaturated fatty acids and cancer of the breast and colorectum: emerging evidence for their role as risk modifiers. Carcinogenesis. 1999;12:2209–18.

10. Chung F-L, Chen H-JC, Nath RG. Lipid peroxidation as a potential endogenous source for the formation of exocyclic DNA adducts. Carcinogenesis. 1996;17:2105–11.

11. Bartsch H. Exocyclic adducts as new risk markers for DNA damage in man. In: Singer B, Bartsch H, editors. Exocyclic DNA Adducts in Mutagenesis and Carcinogenesis. Lyon: IARC Scientific Publication No. 150, 1999:1–16.

12. Fernando RC, Nair J, Barbin A et al. Detection of 1,N^6-ethenodeoxy adenosine and 3,N^4-ethenodeoxycytidine by immunoaffinity/^{32}P-postlabelling in liver and lung DNA of mice treated with ethyl carbamate (urethane) or its metabolites. Carcinogenesis. 1996;17:1711–18.

13. Bartsch H, Nair J. New DNA-based biomarkers for oxidative stress and cancer chemoprevention studies. Eur J Cancer. 2000;36:1229–34.

14. Nair J, Barbin A, Guichard Y et al. 1,N^6-ethenodeoxyadenosine and 3,N^4-ethenodeoxycytidine in liver DNA from humans and untreated rodents detected by immunoaffinity/32P-postlabelling. Carcinogenesis. 1995;16:613–17.

15. Nair J. Lipid peroxidation-induced etheno-DNA adducts in humans. In: Singer B, Bartsch H, editors. Exocyclic DNA Adducts in Mutagenesis and Carcinogenesis. Lyon: IARC Scientific Publication No. 150, 1999:55–62.

16. Nair J, Barbin A, Velic I et al H. Etheno DNA-base adducts from endogenous reactive species. Mutat Res. 1999;424:59–69.

17. Bartsch H, Barbin A, Marion MJ et al. Formation, detection and role in carcinogenesis of ethenobases in DNA. Drug Metab Rev. 1994;26:349–71.

18. Schmid K, Nair J, Winde G et al. Increased levels of promutagenic etheno-DNA adducts in colonic polyps of FAP patients. Int J Cancer. 2000;87:1–4.

19. El Ghissassi F, Barbin A, Nair J et al. 1,N^6-ethenoadenine and 3,N^4-ethenocytosine by lipid peroxidation products and nucleic acid bases. Chem Res Toxicol. 1995;8:278–83.

20. Eberhart CE, Coffey RJ, Radhika A et al. Up-regulation of cyclooxygenase-2 gene expression in human colorectal adenomas and adenocarcinomas. Gastroenterology. 1994;107:1183–8.

21. Spigelman AD, Farmer KCR, Oliver S et al. Caffeine phenotyping of cytochrome P4501A2, N-acetyltransferase, and xanthine oxidase in patients with familial adenomatous polyposis. Gut. 1995;36:251–4.

22. Prescott SM, White RL. Self-promotion? Intimate connections between APC and prostaglandin H synthase-2. Cell. 1996;87:783–6.

23. Fiocchi C. Inflammatory bowel disease: aetiology and pathogenesis. Gastroenterology. 1998; 115:182–205.

24. Nair J, Schmid K, Winde G et al. Miscoding etheno-DNA adducts in colonic epithelium of patients suffering from Crohn's disease, ulcerative colitis and familial adenomatous polyposis. Proc American Association for Cancer Research. 2000;41:594.

25. Andersen SN, Lovig T, Clausen OPF et al. Villous, hypermucinous mucosa in long standing ulcerative colitis shows high frequency of K-ras mutations. Gut. 1999;45:686–92.

26. Hussain SP, Amstad P, Raja K et al. Increased p53 mutation load in noncancerous colon tissue from ulcerative colitis: a cancer-prone chronic inflammatory disease. Cancer Res. 2000; 60:3333–7.

27. Hang B, Chenna A, Rao S et al. 1,N^6-ethenoadenine and 3,N^4-ethenocytosine are excised by separate human DNA glycosylases. Carcinogenesis. 1996;17:155–7.

28. Saparbaev M, Kleibl K, Laval J. Escherichia coli, Saccharomyces cerevisiae, rat and human 3-methyladenine DNA glycolyases repair 1,N^6-ethenoadenine when present in DNA. Nucl Acids Res. 1995;23:3750–5.

29. Wink DA, Vodovotz Y, Laval J et al. The multifaceted roles of nitric oxide in cancer. Carcinogenesis. 1998;19:711–21.

30. Jaiswal M, LaRusso NF, Burgart LJ et al. Inflammatory cytokines induce DNA damage and inhibit DNA repair in cholangiocarcinoma cells by a nitric oxide-dependent mechanism. Cancer Res. 2000;60:184–90.
31. Jaiswal M, LaRusso NF, Nishioka N, Nakabeppu Y, Gores GJ. Human Ogg1, a protein involved in the repair of 8-oxoguanine, is inhibited by nitric oxide. Cancer Res. 2001;61:6388–93.
32. Lin MT, Juan CY, Chang KJ, Chen WJ, Kuo ML. IL-6 inhibits apoptosis and retains oxidative DNA lesions in human gastric cancer AGS cells through up-regulation of anti-apoptotic gene mcl-1. Carcinogenesis. 2001;22:1947–53.
33. Rigas B, Borgo S, Elhosseiny A et al. Decreased expression of DNA-dependent protein kinase, a DNA repair protein, during human colon carcinogenesis. Cancer Res. 2001;61:8381–4.
34. Shih IM, Zhou W, Goodman SN, Lengauer C, Kinzler KW, Vogelstein B. Evidence that genetic instability occurs at an early stage of colorectal tumorigenesis. Cancer Res. 2001;61:818–22.
35. Owen RW, Mier W, Giacosa A et al. Phenolic compounds and squalene in olive oils: the concentration and antioxidant potential of total phenols, simple phenols, secoiridoids, lignans and squalene. Food Chem Toxicol. 2000;38:647–59.
36. Owen RW, Mier W, Giacosa A et al. Phenolic and lipid components of olive oils: identification of lignans as major components of the phenolic fraction of olive oil. Clin Chem. 2000;46:976–88.
37. Owen RW, Giacosa A, Hull WE et al. The antioxidant/anticancer potential of phenolic compounds isolated from olive oil. Eur J Cancer. 2000;36:1235–47.
38. Owen RW, Giacosa A, Hull WE et al. Olive oil consumption and health: the possible role of antioxidants. Lancet Oncol. 2000;1:107–12.
39. Hanaoka T, Nair J, Takahashi Y et al. Urinary excretion of $1,N^6$-ethenodeoxyadenosine, a marker of oxidative DNA damage in postmenopausal Japanese women participating in a dietary intervention trial in northern Japan. Int J Cancer. 2002;100:71–5.

Section VII
Protective nutritional factors

27
Colon carcinogenesis: phytochemicals

H. K. BIESALSKI, H. MÜHLHÖFER and B. BÜHLER-RITTER

Phytochemicals can be defined as plant-derived substances which exert biological effects on cells and tissues. The number of different phytochemicals exceeds the thousands and up to now less than a hundred have been more or less described. Different families such as carotenoids, flavonoids, phytooestrogens and phytosterols and others exist with different biological effects of selected members. One major effect is the antioxidant activity, which contributes to the antimutagenic and at least anticarcinogenic potency. With respect to cancer, carotenoids and especially β-carotene have been most extensively studied and the results are promising. However, intervention studies failed to demonstrate that a single compound can indeed protect from secondary cancer in selected risk groups or cancer development in patients with polyps. In contrast, from epidemiological data it is evident that vegetables rich in carotenoids, especially β-carotene, may indeed protect from colon cancer. The question arises how the preventive effect can be explained and which recommendations can be drawn. Determination of selected carotenoids in polyps, established cancer and healthy mucosa cells showed a significant difference in concentration. Whether this low antioxidant concentrations promotes cancer formation is not known and is a matter of speculation. One of the very early markers of neoplastic growth is an increased activity of ornithine decarboxylase (ODC), the rate-limiting enzyme of polyamine metabolism. In rectal polyps, a significant higher ODC activity was detected compared to normal tissue. Supplementation with β-carotene resulted in a rapid and transient (during supplementation) decrease of ODC activity. The expression of the ODC is controlled via the redox sensitive transcription factor AP-1, which itself is under the control of retinoic acid (RA). RA can be formed from β-carotene in the colonic mucosa, where the cleavage enzyme 15,15′-dioxygenase was recently detected.

Concerning prevention, a major question is how fat-soluble carotenoids reach the colonic mucosa. Most of the carotenoids are absorbed in the upper intestine and consequently the concentration in the colonic lumen is suspected to be very low. Soluble fibres, however, absorb fat-soluble substances and prevent them from absorption in the upper intestine. As a consequence, these substances reach the colon, where an uptake (not absorption) into the mucosa cells may appear after bacterial fermentation of the fibres. If this is the case, this would also explain why intervention studies with pure fibres failed to demonstrate a preventive effect. To study the preventive potential of carotenoids, they can be packed into fibres (edible coating with pectin). After reaching the colon, the bacteria will metabolize the pectin and, as a consequence, short chain fatty acids, as regulators of cellular growth, and β-carotene as a precursor for RA, will be available. Understanding the fate and metabolism of provitamin A and non-provitamin carotenoids in healthy and neoplastic cells will help to develop new strategies of prevention and at least intervention of colonic cancer.

28
Dietary fibre

M. E. MARTÍNEZ

INTRODUCTION

Significant progress has been made over the last decade in identifying factors that modify risk of colorectal cancer. Large international variation in colorectal cancer incidence and mortality rates and the prominent increases in the incidence of colorectal cancer in groups that migrated from low- to high-incidence areas provide important evidence that lifestyle factors influence the development of this malignancy. It has been estimated that adoption of a healthy diet could prevent up to 50–75% of colorectal cancers[1]. These observations have formed the basis for various hypotheses of lifestyle factors in the aetiology of colorectal neoplasia. The benefits of dietary fibre were first proposed by Dennis Burkitt, who observed that diseases of the bowel, including colon cancer, were rare in Africa, where a high-fibre diet was consumed[2]. Since then, numerous observational, animal and experimental studies have been conducted throughout the world.

The following review summarizes existing evidence from human studies for the role of dietary fibre in the aetiology of colorectal neoplasia. Issues related to assessment of dietary fibre, potential biological mechanisms of action, and study design settings to test hypotheses are first addressed. Finally, existing data from recent observational epidemiological studies and chemoprevention trials are described and interpreted.

ASSESSMENT OF DIETARY FIBRE

Uncertainty related to the role of dietary fibre in cancer aetiology is due to a number of reasons (Table 1); these include the chemical complexity and heterogeneity of dietary fibre, the variety of food sources which themselves have protective capacities other than fibre, and consumption patterns. Primary sources of dietary fibre include fruits, vegetables, grains, seeds, nuts and legumes. Fibre consists of an assorted mixture of complex polysaccharides and non-polysaccharide polymers, mostly made up of plant cell wall carbohydrate and non-starch polysaccharides. Current analytical methods have determined that dietary fibre

Table 1   Issues related to dietary fibre and its interpretation in aetiologic studies of disease risk

---

Definition
Consists of remnants of edible plant cell, polysaccharides, lignin, and associated substances resistant to digestion by the alimentary enzymes

Total dietary fibre
Includes insoluble (cellulose, lignin, hemicellulose present in wheat, grain products and vegetables) and soluble (pectin, gums, mucilages found in fruit, oats, barley, legumes) fibre

Food sources
Fruit, vegetables, legumes, nuts, whole grains

Consumption influenced by
Portion of plant consumed, maturity, storage and processing

---

is made up of several components (e.g. cellulose, hemicellulose, pectin, etc.); biological mechanisms potentially responsible for fibre's protective role in colon carcinogenesis depend on the specific type, as discussed below. Issues related to accurate assessment of dietary fibre include the specific part of the food that is consumed, its maturity, storage and processing. In addition, the physiological effects of dietary fibre also depend on the composition of the rest of the meal or diet and the unique physiology of the individual.

Various dietary instruments exist in order to assess dietary intake. These range from a single 24-h recall to a series of dietary diaries or food records, to more complex food-frequency and dietary history questionnaires. Twenty-four-hour recalls and food records are rarely used in epidemiological studies since the goal in this setting is to assess dietary intake in the distant past. Dietary history and food-frequency questionnaires ascertain intake during a specified period of time (e.g. the previous year) and consist of a list of foods and beverages that are commonly consumed by the target population. In the case of fibre, it is important that the primary source of food items and preparation methods common in the study population are included in the questionnaire. It is important to consider, however, that no method of dietary intake assessment is without flaws. Special attention must be focused on using validated questionnaires, preferably those that have been tested in the population of interest.

BIOLOGICAL MECHANISMS

Numerous biological mechanisms responsible for the protective effects of fibre and its components have been proposed (Table 2). Physiological effects of fibre depend largely on the type of fibre. Although several types of fibre have been identified, they can be generally classified in terms of their water solubility. Soluble fibres are present in fruit, vegetables and certain grains, such as oats; these also include gel-forming fibres such as pectins, gums and mucilages. Soluble fibre undergoes metabolism as bacterial enzymes convert it to products that increase stool size. Pectins, however, mainly absorb water, form gel and increase bulk. Insoluble fibres, present in considerable amounts in bran cereals, such as wheat and rice, affect intestinal function by retaining water in the stool, increasing faecal bulk, and decreasing gastrointestinal transit time. The larger

Table 2   Fiber and colorectal cancer: mechanisms of action

- Increased stool bulk and lower transit time
- Binding or dilution of bile acids and other carcinogens
- Lower faecal pH
- Inhibition of bacterial degradation of food products to potential carcinogens
- Favourable changes in microflora
- High consumption associated with lower intake of deleterious foods/food products and higher intake of protective nutrients/food products

---

bulk resulting from the action of these fibres dilutes carcinogens, especially tumour-promoters such as secondary bile acids.

Mechanisms responsible for the protective effects of fruit and vegetables include inhibition of nitrosamine formation, provision of substrate for formation of antineoplastic agents, dilution and binding of carcinogens, alteration of hormone metabolism, antioxidant effects and the induction of detoxification enzymes by cruciferous vegetables[3]. Vegetables contain several compounds that possess a variety of anticarcinogenic properties[4]. Specifically, the anticarcinogenic properties of cruciferous vegetables have been mainly attributed to the degradation products of glucosionolates (e.g. isothiocyanates and indoles), which induce detoxification enzymes[5]. As discussed later, a possible mechanism of action of isothiocyanates is thought to be through the induction of glutathione S-transferases[6], enzymes involved in the detoxification of carcinogens.

STUDY DESIGNS

The goal of epidemiological studies is to assess the distribution and determinants of disease in human populations. Within this context, various study designs have been used to test diet-related hypotheses in cancer causation; these include: correlational or ecological studies, migrant studies, retrospective or case–control studies, cohort or prospective studies, and clinical trials.

Ecological studies compare *per capita* consumption of foods or nutrients and cancer incidence or mortality rates among different populations, usually based on national data. However, ecological studies are considered among the weakest form of epidemiological evidence. The primary problem of these correlational studies is that many potential determinants of the cancer of interest, other than those under consideration, may vary between areas with high and low incidence rates. Such confounding factors can include genetic predisposition, other dietary factors, or additional environmental or lifestyle practices. For these reasons, ecological studies have been useful, but are not sufficient in providing conclusions regarding relationships between diet and cancer. Correlational studies also provide evidence that environmental factors play an important role by documenting changes in cancer rates over a period of time that occur within a population.

Studies of migrants are probably the strongest form of evidence for environmental versus genetic factors. In these studies, populations migrating between areas with different cancer rates acquire the rate of the host country for a variety of cancers. For example, as migrants move from countries with low rates to those with higher rates of colorectal cancer, they show increased risks similar or close to those of the host country. Thus, results of migrant studies suggest that colorectal cancer is particularly sensitive to changes in environmental factors.

Case–control and cohort studies are the main sources of analytical epidemiological data. Some of the weaknesses of correlational and migrant data are overcome in these analytical studies, where confounding factors are taken into account in the design or analysis phase. In case–control studies, the investigator compares reported past diet as recalled by cancer cases and cancer-free controls. Data on potential confounding factors are also collected in this fashion. Case–control studies are especially appealing for rare diseases or for investigations of special populations, which are usually not addressed in cohort studies. Weaknesses of case–control studies include differential reporting of past diet between cases and controls and limited variation of dietary intake within study populations.

Prospective cohort studies assess diet in cancer-free individuals and correlate specific factors to subsequent cancer occurrence. The prospective study design is considered the strongest form of evidence in observational epidemiology. This is largely due to the overcoming of methodological flaws of other types of studies: participants' diets are assessed prior to the outcome of disease (eliminating differential in reporting), cases and controls arise from the same population, and data on confounding factors are also ascertained at baseline. In addition, biological samples can be collected on all or a subset of the total population prior to disease outcome, which is not possible in case–control studies. This is of particular importance, given that some important biomarkers may be altered after the onset of cancer. One potential problem with these studies is the loss of follow-up of participants. If disease incidence or specific dietary exposures are related to a loss to follow-up, then estimates of risk are biased or associations may not be detected. In addition, the long follow-up period and large number of participants needed to draw meaningful conclusions makes for highly expensive studies; however, it is important to recognize that when several disease end-points can be addressed, cohort studies become cost-effective.

Randomized controlled trials of diet randomly assign individuals to a dietary intervention or placebo (or usual diet) arm. A major strength of the randomized trial is the balance that occurs with respect to confounding factors between the treatment and control arms. If a double-blind design is employed, the evidence becomes even stronger; however, this is not always possible for dietary interventions, such as those that comprise a food or dietary pattern. In spite of their important strengths, trials also carry limitations. Trials that are short in duration may fail to detect an effect due to an insufficient time for the intervention to alter disease outcome. In addition, participants who volunteer for these trials are usually a highly select group of health-conscientious, highly motivated, and educated individuals; thus generalizability of study findings to the general population is questionable.

FIBRE, FRUIT AND VEGETABLES, AND COLORECTAL NEOPLASIA

Observational studies

High consumption of fruit and vegetables has been shown to be associated with a decreased risk of colorectal neoplasia[7]. Results of most published studies have shown an inverse association between intake of vegetables and colon cancer, while data for fruit consumption are less compelling[8-24]. Results of a pooled analysis of six case–control studies[25] showed a high intake of vegetables to be associated with an odds ratio (OR) for colon cancer of 0.48 (95% confidence interval (CI) of 0.41–0.57), and a weaker inverse association with fibre (OR = 0.58 for upper versus lower categories). Foods high in fibre have also been shown to be inversely associated with colon cancer risk in most[10,11,13,17,26-31], but not all[18,32-35] studies. Howe et al.[36] reported a lower risk associated with higher fibre intake (OR = 0.53 for upper versus lower quintile) based on pooled analyses of 13 case–control studies. Conversely, results of large prospective studies have shown weak or non-existent inverse associations for fibre intake and risk of colon cancer[33,37-40]. As with case–control studies, when sources of fibre were examined separately in earlier studies[12-14,16-18,26-29,33,35,39,41-50], a reduced risk also appears to be stronger for vegetable sources than for other fibre components. In a recently published large prospective study of female nurses examining the role of fibre on risk of colorectal neoplasia, Fuchs et al.[38] found no association between fibre intake and risk of colorectal cancer or adenoma. The relative risk (RR) for women in the upper quintile of fibre intake (median of 24.5 g/day) was 0.95 (95% CI = 0.73–1.25) compared with those in the lowest quintile (median of 9.8 g/day). No important associations were observed when analyses were conducted for cereal, fruit or vegetable fibre. Also, no significant associations were shown for fibre intake and colorectal adenoma. In a later publication focused on fruit and vegetable consumption[51], data from the Nurses' Health Study and the Health Professionals Follow-up Study cohorts were combined for a follow-up of over 1 700 000 person-years to yield 937 cases of colon and 244 of rectal cancer. No inverse association was shown for either men or women who reported consuming six or more servings per day of fruit and vegetables compared to those who consumed two or fewer servings per day. More recent results of the Swedish Mammography Screening cohort[52] showed no overall protective effects for fibre and colorectal cancer incidence. However, when the investigators focused on fruit and vegetable consumption, significant inverse associations were observed: women in the upper quartile of fruit and vegetable intake, compared to those in the lower quartile had approximately a 30% lower risk of developing colorectal cancer (RR = 0.73; 95% CI = 0.56–0.96).

Clinical trials

Given the scientific and published health interest related to fruit and vegetable consumption and colorectal cancer risk, Schatzkin et al.[53] conducted a multi-centre trial testing a diet high in fibre, high in fruit and vegetables, and low in fat versus a usual diet. The 1905 participants were followed for approximately four years for adenoma recurrence end-points. Recurrence rates were essentially identical between the two intervention groups (approximately 40%); the RR was 1.00 (95% CI = 0.90–1.12). Based on these results, the authors concluded that adopting a diet low in fat and high in fibre, fruit and vegetables does not influence risk of adenoma recurrence. Likewise, results of a large chemoprevention trial testing the effects of a high- versus low-wheat bran fibre intervention on adenoma recurrence among 1304 participants showed a lack of effect of the intervention on adenoma recurrence[54]. The OR for recurrent adenomas in the high- (13.5 g/day) versus the low- (2 g/day) fibre group was 0.88 (95% CI = 0.70–1.11). Results of a smaller European trial were later published[55], where 665 men and women were randomized to a calcium, fibre or placebo arm; the fibre intervention consisted of 2.5 g of ispaghula husk per day. Although results for the effect of calcium were encouraging, those for the fibre intervention suggest that a higher risk of adenoma recurrence is associated with this treatment arm (OR = 1.67; 95% CI = 1.01–2.76). However, given the challenges presented in the conduct of this trial, leading to low follow-up rates that were possibly different across intervention arms, these results must be interpreted with caution. Given the inherent limitations associated with adenoma recurrence trials, including the timing and relatively short duration of the intervention[56], results of these studies can be interpreted as inconclusive.

SUMMARY AND FUTURE DIRECTIONS

The role of dietary fibre in the aetiology of colorectal neoplasia has been extensively studied. However, the precise nature and magnitude of the relationship between fibre and risk have not been clearly established. Early epidemiological studies found that high consumption of fibre, including fruit and vegetables, was associated with a decreased risk of colorectal cancer. However, large prospective studies have shown weak or null associations. Furthermore, two large adenoma recurrence trials conducted in the United States and a smaller trial conducted in Europe showed a lack of an effect of fibre on the study endpoint. Given the results of these recent observational and intervention studies, doubts have been cast as to the preventive capacities of fibre on colorectal cancer risk. Although conflicting findings exist, when the entire body of evidence from human and animal studies is examined, the overall conclusion supports an inverse association between dietary fibre and intake of colorectal cancer. Ongoing large epidemiological studies, including the ambitious efforts of the 484 042-participant European Prospective Investigation into Cancer and Nutrition (EPIC) study[57] should further clarify this important scientific area.

References

1. Doll R, Peto R. The causes of cancer: quantitative estimates of avoidable risks of cancer in the United States today. J Natl Cancer Inst. 1981;66:1191–308.
2. Burkitt DP. Epidemiology of cancer of the colon and rectum. Cancer. 1971;28:3–13.
3. Steinmetz KA, Potter JD. A review of vegetables, fruit and cancer. I. Epidemiology. Cancer Causes Cont. 1991;2:325–57.
4. Steinmetz KA, Potter JD. Vegetables, fruit, and cancer. II. Mechanisms. Cancer Causes Cont. 1991;2:427–42.
5. Mehta RG, Liu J, Constantinou A et al. Cancer chemopreventive activity of brassinin, a phytoalexin from cabbage. Carcinogenesis. 1995;16:399–404.
6. Hecht SS. Chemoprevention by isothiocyanates. J Cell Biochem Suppl. 1995;22:195–209.
7. World Cancer Research Fund. Food, Nutrition and the Prevention of Cancer: A Global Perspective. The American Institute for Cancer Research, Washington, D.C., 1997:497–500.
8. Benito E, Stiggelbout A, Bosch FX et al. Nutritional factors in colorectal cancer risk: a case-control study in Majorca. Int J Cancer. 1991;49:161–7.

9. Bjelke E. Epidemiology of colorectal cancer, with emphasis on diet. In: Davis W, Harrup KR, Stathopoulos G, eds. Human Cancer. Its Characterization and Treatment. Amsterdam, Congress Series No. 484: Exerpta Medica, Int., 1980:158–74.

10. Graham S, Marshall J, Haughey B et al. Dietary epidemiology of cancer of the colon in western New York. Am J Epidemiol. 1988;128:490–503.

11. Kune GA, Kune S, Watson LF. The nutritional causes of colorectal cancer: An introduction to the Melbourne Study. Nutr Cancer. 1987;9:5–56.

12. Lee HP, Gourley L, Duffy SW, Esteve J, Lee J, Day NE. Colorectal cancer and diet in an Asian population – a case–control study among Singapore Chinese. Int J Cancer. 1989;43:1007–16.

13. Macquart-Moulin G, Riboli E, Cornee J, Charnay B, Berthezene P, Day N. Case–control study on colorectal cancer and diet in Marseilles. Int J Cancer. 1986;38:183–91.

14. Manousos O, Day NE, Trichopoulos D, Gerovassilis F, Tzonou A, Polychronopoulou A. Diet and colorectal cancer: a case–control study in Greece. Int J Cancer. 1983;32:1–5.

15. Mayne ST, Janerich DT, Greenwald P et al. Dietary beta carotene and lung cancer risk in U.S. nonsmokers. J Natl Cancer Inst. 1994;86:33–8.

16. Miller AB, Howe GR, Jain M, Craib KJ, Harrison L. Food items and food groups as risk factors in a case–control study of diet and colo-rectal cancer. Int J Cancer. 1983;32:155–61.

17. Modan B, Barell V, Lubin F, Modan M, Greenberg RA. Low-fiber intake as an etiologic factor in cancer of the colon. J Natl Cancer Inst. 1975;55:15–18.

18. Peters RK, Pike MC, Garabrandt D, Mack TM. Diet and colon cancer in Los Angeles County, California. Cancer Causes Cont. 1992;3:457–73.

19. Phillips RL. Role of life-style and dietary habits in risk of cancer among Seventh-Day Adventists. Cancer Res. 1975;35:3513–22.

20. Steinmetz KA, Kushi LH, Bostick RM, Folsom AR, Potter JD. Vegetables, fruit, and colon cancer in the Iowa Women's Health Study. Am J Epidemiol. 1994;139:1–15.

21. Tuyns AJ, Kaaks R, Haelterman M. Colorectal cancer and the consumption of foods: a case–control study of Belgium. Nutr Cancer. 1988;11:189–204.

22. West DW, Slattery ML, Robison LM et al. Dietary intake and colon cancer: sex and anatomic site-specific associations. Am J Epidemiol. 1989;130:883–94.

23. Young TB, Wolf TB. Case–control study of proximal and distal colon cancer and diet in Wisconsin. Int J Cancer. 1988;42:167–75.

24. Levi F, Pasche C, La Vecchia C, Lucchini F, Franceschi S. Food groups and colorectal cancer risk. Br J Cancer. 1999;79:1283–7.

25. Trock B, Lanza E, Greenwald P. Dietary fiber, vegetables, and colon cancer: critical review and meta-analyses of the epidemiologic evidence. J Natl Cancer Inst. 1990;82:650–61.

26. Benito E, Obrador A, Stiggelbout A et al. A population-based case–control study of colorectal cancer in Majorca. I. Dietary Factors. Int J Cancer. 1990;45:69–76.

27. Gerhardsson de Verdier M, Hagman U, Steineck G et al. Diet, body mass and colorectal cancer: a case-referent study. Int J Cancer. 1990;46:832–8.

28. Meyer F, White E. Alcohol and nutrients in relation to colon cancer in middle-aged adults. Am J Epidemiol. 1993;138:225–36.

29. Slattery ML, Schumacher MC, Smith KR, West DW, Abd-Elghany N. Physical activity, diet, and risk of colon cancer in Utah. Am J Epidemiol. 1988;128:989–99.

30. Whittemore AS, Wu-Williams AH, Lee M et al. Diet, physical activity and colorectal cancer among Chinese in North America and China. J Natl Cancer Inst. 1990;82:915–26.

31. Zaridze D, Filipchenko V, Kustov V et al. Diet and colorectal cancer: results of two case–control studies in Russia. Eur J Cancer. 1993;29A:112–15.

32. Jain M, Cook GM, Davis FG, Grace MG, Howe GR, Miller AB. A case–control study of diet and colorectal cancer. Int J Cancer. 1980;26:757–68.

33. Willett WC, Stampfer MJ, Colditz GA, Rosner BA, Speizer FE. Relation of meat, fat, and fiber intake to the risk of colon cancer in a prospective study among women. N Engl J Med. 1990;323:1664–72.

34. Tuyns AJ, Haelterman M, Kaaks R. Colorectal cancer and the intake of nutrients: oligosaccharides are a risk factor, fats are not. A case–control study in Belgium. Nutr Cancer. 1987;10:181–96.

35. Lyon JL, Mahoney AW, West DW et al. Energy intake: its relationship to colon cancer risk. J Natl Cancer Inst. 1987;78:853–61.

36. Howe GR, Benito E, Castelleto R et al. Dietary intake of fiber and decreased risk of cancers of the colon and rectum: evidence from the combined analysis of 13 case–control studies. J Natl Cancer Inst. 1992;84:1887–96.

37. Bostick RM, Potter JD, Kushi LH *et al.* Sugar, meat, and fat intake, and non-dietary risk factors for colon cancer incidence in Iowa women (United States). Cancer Causes Cont. 1994;5:38–52.
38. Fuchs CS, Giovannucci EL, Colditz GA *et al.* Dietary fiber and the risk of colorectal cancer and adenoma in women. N Engl J Med. 1999;340:169–76.
39. Giovannucci E, Rimm EB, Stampfer MJ, Colditz GA, Ascherio A, Willett WC. Intake of fat, meat, and fiber in relation to risk of colon cancer in men. Cancer Res. 1994;54:2390–7.
40. Goldbohm RA, van den Brandt PA, van't Veer P *et al.* A prospective cohort study on the relation between meat consumption and the risk of colon cancer. Cancer Res. 1994;54:718–23.
41. Bidoli E, Franceschi S, Talamini R, Barra S, La Vecchia C. Food consumption and cancer of the colon and rectum in north-eastern Italy. Int J Cancer. 1992;50:223–9.
42. Dales LG, Friedman GD, Ury HK, Grossman S, Williams SR. A case–control study of relationships of diet and other traits to colorectal cancer in American blacks. Am J Epidemiol. 1979; 109:132–44.
43. Gerhardsson de Verdier M, Hagman U, Peters RK, Steineck G. Meat, cooking methods and colorectal cancer: A case-referent study in Stockholm. Int J Cancer. 1991;49:520–5.
44. Heilbrun L, Nomura A, Hankin J, Stemmermann G. Diet and colorectal cancer with special reference to fiber intake. Int J Cancer. 1989;44:1–6.
45. Hu J, Liu Y, Yu Y *et al.* Diet and cancer of the colon and rectum: a case–control study in China. Int J Epidemiol. 1991;20:362–7.
46. Iscovich JM, L'Abbe KA, Caastellerto R *et al.* Colon cancer in Argentina. II. Risk from fiber, fat and nutrients. Int J Cancer. 1992;51:858–61.
47. Kune S, Kune GA, Watson LF. Case–control study of dietary etiologic factors: the Melbourne Colorectal Cancer Study. Nutr Cancer. 1987;9:21–42.
48. Thun MJ, Calle EE, Namboodiri MM *et al.* Risk factors for fatal colon cancer in a large prospective study. J Natl Cancer Inst. 1992;84:1491–500.
49. Zaridze DG. Environmental aetiology of large-bowel cancer. J Natl Cancer Inst. 1983;70: 389–400.
50. Frudenheim JL, Graham S, Marshall JR *et al.* A case–control study of diet and rectal cancer in western New York. Am J Epidemiol. 1990;131:612–24.
51. Michels K, Giovannucci E, Joshipura KJ *et al.* Prospective study of fruit and vegetable consumption and incidence of colon and rectal cancers. J Natl Cancer Inst. 2000;92:1740–52.
52. Terry P, Giovannucci E, Michels KB *et al.* Fruit, vegetables, dietary fiber, and risk of colorectal cancer. J Natl Cancer Inst. 2001;93:525–33.
53. Schatzkin A, Lanza E, Corle D *et al.* Lack of effect of a low-fat, high-fiber diet on the recurrence of colorectal adenomas. Polyp Prevention Trial Study Group. N Engl J Med. 2000;342:1149–55.
54. Alberts DS, Martinez ME, Roe DJ *et al.* Lack of effect of a high-fiber cereal supplement on the recurrence of colorectal adenomas. N Engl J Med. 2000;342:1156–62.
55. Bonithon-Kopp C, Kronborg O, Giacosa A, Rath U, Faivre J. Calcium and fiber supplementation in prevention of colorectal adenoma recurrence: a randomized intervention trial. European Cancer Prevention Organisation Study Group. Lancet. 2000;356:1300–6.
56. Martínez ME. Hormone replacement therapy and adenoma recurrence: implications for its role in colorectal cancer risk. J Natl Cancer Inst. 2001;93:1764–5.
57. Riboli E. The European Prespective Investigation into Cancer and Nutrition (EPIC): plans and progress. J Nutr. 2001;131:170–5s.

29
Short-chain fatty acids: the magic bullet?

T. MENZEL, H. LÜHRS, R. MELCHER, J. SCHAUBER,
A. GOSTNER, T. KUDLICH and W. SCHEPPACH

During the past 25 years short-chain fatty acids (SFCA) have attracted consider-able interest in human nutrition, physiology and pathophysiology. SCFA are organic acids produced by anaerobic fermentation of undigested carbohydrates within the colonic lumen[1]. SFCA represent the mayor energy source for colono-cytes[2] and may play a role in various types of colitis and in colonic neoplasia[3]. Of these SCFA, butyrate appears to mediate the most profound protective effects of a high-fibre diet[4]. A critical analysis of epidemiological, animal and intervention studies supports the overall conclusion that an inverse association between dietary fibre intake and colorectal cancer risk does exist[5]. Among the SCFAs, butyrate appears to mediate the most profound protective effects of a high-fibre diet.

The mechanisms of the effects of butyrate at the molecular level have been studied extensively, employing various *in-vitro* models. *In vitro*, butyrate has been shown to modulate cell proliferation, differentiation, motility, adhesion and apoptosis[6–13]. In addition, the expression of cell-cycle-regulating genes[14] as well as the hyperacetylation of histone proteins have been shown to be modulated by butyrate[15]. Butyrate is the major luminal source of energy for colonocytes[16]. Colonocytes from patients with UC have reduced capacity to oxidize SCFAs[17]. It has been proposed that chronic inflammation of the intestinal mucosa may result from either the inability to oxidize SCFA (in UC) or from decreased lumi-nal concentrations of SCFA (in diversion colitis)[18,19]. Several controlled[20–22] and uncontrolled[23–25] clinical trials employing SCFA enemas have been published. These data suggest that SCFA can be clinically effective in ameliorating symp-toms, and that chronic inflammation of the intestinal mucosa is controlled effec-tively. Although several potential mechanisms by which SCFA can induce clinical, endoscopic and histologic remission of the inflamed colonic mucosa have been proposed[26–28], the mechanisms of action of SCFA on the inflamma-tory cascade is only partially understood. Recently, several reports described an inhibitory effect of butyrate on NF-κB activation.

Due to space limitations, this paper will focus exclusively on data generated in our own laboratory. The discussed topics will include effects of a butyrate–aspirin combination on human colon cancer cells, the butyrate-mediated modulation of the expression of the transcription factor NF-κB, the endogenous antibiotic peptide LL37, and the adhesion molecule VCAM-1. In addition, data on butyrate effects on high-mobility group proteins will be discussed.

BUTYRATE AND ASPIRIN

Butyrate and aspirin exert antiproliferative effects on colon cancer cells. In order to explore the potentially synergistic effects of a butyrate–aspirin combination, human adenocarcinoma cells were treated with butyrate or aspirin alone or in combination. Both substrates decreased proliferation and induced differentiation and apoptosis. Butyrate reduced mutant p53-expression, whereas aspirin did not affect p53-expression. Butyrate-induced apoptosis correlated with an increase in Bak expression and a decrease in the expression of Bcl-X_L. Aspirin had no effect on the investigated apoptosis-controlling factors. The antiproliferative and pro-apoptotic effects of the butyrate–aspirin combination were markedly enhanced. The combination resulted in a stronger decrease of PCNA expression and cdk2 expression. Our data suggest that the anticancerogenic effect of aspirin might effectively be augmented by a diet high in butyrate-producing fermentable fibre[29].

BUTYRATE-MEDIATED MODULATION OF THE EXPRESSION OF THE TRANSCRIPTION FACTOR NF-κB

Human adenocarcinoma cells (SW480, SW620 and HeLa229) were treated with butyrate for up to 48 h followed by TNFα stimulation. Stimulation with TNFα resulted in rapid phosphorylation and degradation of IκBα followed by NF-κB nuclear translocation. Butyrate pretreatment successfully inhibited NF-κB activation. Pretreatment of adenocarcinoma cells with butyrate is associated with inhibition of TNFα-mediated phosphorylation and degradation of IκBα and effective blocking of NF-κB nuclear translocation. The anti-inflammatory effects of butyrate may at least in part be mediated by an inhibition of IκBα-mediated activation of NF-κB[30].

THE ENDOGENOUS ANTIBIOTIC PEPTIDE LL37

SCFA are known to modulate mucosal immune functions. The antimicrobial cathelicidin LL-37 is expressed by colonocytes and leukocytes. In-vivo, LL-37 expression in healthy mucosa is restricted to differentiated epithelial cells in human colon and ileum. In colonocytes, increased LL-37 expression associated with cell differentiation can be detected in vitro following treatment with butyrate, isobutyrate, propionate and trichostatin A (TSA). Flavone induced LL-37 transcription but did not affect differentiation, while cytokines had no effect. Interestingly, butyrate and TSA downregulate LL-37 expression in PBMC, whereas LL-37 expression was induced in a monocytic cell line. The expression of the cathelicidin LL-37 in colonocytes or immune cells and cellular differentiation is independently modulated by SCFA via distinct signalling pathways (Schauber et al. 2002, unpublished results).

THE VASCULAR ADHESION MOLECULE VCAM-1

Leukocyte recruitment to areas of inflammation depends on integrin–VCAM/ICAM interaction. Blocking the vascular cell adhesion molecule (VCAM-1) and the intracellular adhesion molecule (ICAM-1) may have therapeutic benefit for the acute inflammatory component of inflammatory bowel disease (IBD). Notably, the induction of ICAM and VCAM is mediated by a NF-κB-dependent mechanism. Butyrate is able to modulate the expression of two major cell adhesion molecules, VCAM-1 and ICAM-1, in endothelial cells. This effect is associated with a butyrate-mediated inhibition of NF-κB nuclear translocation. A significant reduction of leukocytes in the lamina propria of patients with ulcerative colitis who had previously been treated with topical butyrate was noted. This may be due to the observed complete inhibition of monocyte adhesion to these endothelial cells in vitro (Menzel et al. 2002, unpublished results).

HIGH-MOBILITY GROUP PROTEINS (HMG)

Butyrate enhances acetylation of core histones, a process directly linked to the formation of active chromatin and gene expression. However, additional chromatin components also contribute to the formation of transcriptionally active chromatin. The high-mobility group protein N2 (HMGN2), a non-histone protein, is involved in chromatin structure modulation. Treatment of HT29 cells with butyrate leads to significant hyperacetylation of HMG-N2. Levels of HMG-N2 protein remained unchanged. Northern blot analysis reveals a significant reduction in HMG-N2 mRNA levels after treatment with butyrate. Analysis of HMG-N2-EGFP-transfected HT29 cells demonstrates that butyrate treatment changes the binding properties of HMG-N2-EGFP to chromatin. In addition, butyrate treatment results in solubilization of endogenous acetylated HMG-N2 into the supernatant of permeabilized cells. Thus, we were able to demonstrate that butyrate treatment is associated with hyperacetylation of HMG-N2 protein in HT29 cells. The modulation of this non-histone chromatin protein resulted in altered binding properties to chromatin. This may represent an additional step in changing chromatin structure and composition with subsequent consequences for transcription and gene expression. Modulation of non-histone chromatin proteins, like the ubiquitous HMG-N2 proteins, may be partly responsible for the wide range of butyrate-associated effects[31].

CONCLUSION

Short-chain fatty acids, in particular butyrate, display a wide array of effects on colon epithelial cells. Butyrate may not be the magic bullet but may be a powerful protective agent in conjunction with other factors. Possible areas of clinical application include cancer chemoprevention, inhibition of inflammation and maintenance of the gut barrier. Notably, most data on the potential molecular mechanisms of butyrate-induced effects are generated *in vitro* employing established colonic adenocarcinoma cell lines. However, it is assumed that the protective effects of SCFA are exerted rather in the early stages of the adenoma–carcinoma sequence. Thus, an *in-vitro* model consisting of cells stemming from a colon adenoma or normal colon cells would be desirable.

References

1. Topping DL, Clifton PM. Short-chain fatty acids and human colonic function: roles of resistant starch and nonstarch polysaccharides. Physiol Rev. 2001;81:1031–64.
2. Livesey G, Elia M. 1995 Short Chain Fatty Acids as an Energy Source in the Colon: Metabolism and Clinical Implications. Cambridge, UK: Cambridge University Press.
3. Cummings JH, Bingham SA. Dietary fibre, fermentation and large bowel cancer. Cancer Surv. 1987;6:601–21.
4. Wargovich MJ, Levin B. Grist for the mill: role of cereal fiber and calcium in prevention of colon cancer. J Natl Cancer Inst. 1996;88:67–9.
5. Kim YI. AGA technical review: impact of dietary fiber on colon cancer occurrence. Gastroenterology. 2000;118:1235–57.
6. Archer SY, Meng S, Shei A, Hodin RA. p21(WAF1) is required for butyrate-mediated growth inhibition of human colon cancer cells. Proc Natl Acad Sci USA. 1998;95:6791–6.
7. Emenaker NJ, Basson MD. Short chain fatty acids differentially modulate cellular phenotype and c-myc protein levels in primary human nonmalignant and malignant colonocytes. Dig Dis Sci. 2001;46:96–105.
8. Emenaker NJ, Calaf GM, Cox D, Basson MD, Qureshi N. Short-chain fatty acids inhibit invasive human colon cancer by modulating upA, TIMP-1, TIMP-2, mutant p53, Bcl-2, Bax, p21 and PCNA protein expression in an in vitro cell culture model. J Nutr. 2001;131:3041–6S.
9. Hague A, Diaz GD, Hicks DJ et al. bcl-2 and bak may play a pivotal role in sodium butyrate-induced apoptosis in colonic epithelial cells; however overexpression of bcl-2 does not protect against bak-mediated apoptosis. Int J Cancer. 1997;72:898–905.
10. Hague A, Elder DJ, Hicks DJ, Paraskeva C. Apoptosis in colorectal tumour cells: induction by the short chain fatty acids butyrate, propionate and acetate and by the bile salt deoxycholate. Int J Cancer. 1995;60:400–6.
11. Mariadason JM, Corner GA, Augenlicht LH. Genetic reprogramming in pathways of colonic cell maturation induced by short chain fatty acids: comparison with trichostatin A, sulindac, and curcumin and implications for chemoprevention of colon cancer. Cancer Res. 2000;60:4561–72.
12. Mariadason JM, Velcich A, Wilson AJ, Augenlicht LH, Gibson PR. Resistance to butyrate-induced cell differentiation and apoptosis during spontaneous Caco-2 cell differentiation. Gastroenterology. 2001;120:889–99.
13. Palmer DG, Paraskeva C, Williams AC. Modulation of p53 expression in cultured colonic adenoma cell lines by the naturally occurring lumenal factors butyrate and deoxycholate. Int J Cancer. 1997;73:702–6.
14. Siavoshian S, Blottiere HM, Cherbut C, Galmiche JP. Butyrate stimulates cyclin D and p21 and inhibits cyclin-dependent kinase 2 expression in HT-29 colonic epithelial cells. Biochem Biophys Res Commun. 1997;232:169–72.
15. Boffa LC, Lupton JR, Mariani MR et al. Modulation of colonic epithelial cell proliferation, histone acetylation, and luminal short chain fatty acids by variation of dietary fiber (wheat bran) in rats. Cancer Res. 1992;52:5906–12.
16. Roediger WE. Role of anaerobic bacteria in the metabolic welfare of the colonic mucosa in man. Gut. 1980b;21:793–8.
17. Roediger WE. The colonic epithelium in ulcerative colitis: an energy-deficiency disease? Lancet. 1980a;2:712–15.
18. Roediger WE, Lawson MJ, Radcliffe BC. Nitrite from inflammatory cells – a cancer risk factor in ulcerative colitis? Dis Colon Rectum. 1990;33:1034–6.
19. Agarwal VP, Schimmel EM. Diversion colitis: a nutritional deficiency syndrome? Nutr Rev. 1989;47:257–61.

20. Scheppach W, Sommer H, Kirchner T et al. Effect of butyrate enemas on the colonic mucosa in distal ulcerative colitis. Gastroenterology. 1992;103:51–6.
21. Vernia P, Cittadini M, Caprilli R, Torsoli A. Topical treatment of refractory distal ulcerative colitis with 5-ASA and sodium butyrate. Dig Dis Sci. 1995a;40:305–7.
22. Senagore AJ, MacKeigan JM, Scheider M, Ebrom JS. Short-chain fatty acid enemas: a cost-effective alternative in the treatment of nonspecific proctosigmoiditis. Dis Colon Rectum. 1992;35:923–7.
23. Breuer RI, Buto SK, Christ ML et al. Rectal irrigation with short-chain fatty acids for distal ulcerative colitis. Preliminary report. Dig Dis Sci. 1991;36:185–7.
24. Steinhart AH, Brzezinski A, Baker JP. Treatment of refractory ulcerative proctosigmoiditis with butyrate enemas. Am J Gastroenterol. 1994;89:179–83.
25. Vernia P, Marcheggiano A, Caprilli R et al. Short-chain fatty acid topical treatment in distal ulcerative colitis. Aliment Pharmacol Ther. 1995b;9:309–13.
26. Kripke SA, Fox AD, Berman JM, Settle RG, Rombeau JL. Stimulation of intestinal mucosal growth with intracolonic infusion of short-chain fatty acids. J Parenter Enteral Nutr. 1989;13:109–16.
27. Kvietys PR, Granger DN. Effect of volatile fatty acids on blood flow and oxygen uptake by the dog colon. Gastroenterology. 1981;80:962–9.
28. Mortensen FV, Nielsen H, Mulvany MJ, Hessov I. Short chain fatty acids dilate isolated human colonic resistance arteries. Gut. 1990;31:1391–4.
29. Menzel T, Schauber J, Kreth F et al. Butyrate and aspirin in combination have an enhanced effect on apoptosis in human colorectal cancer cells. Eur J Cancer Prev. 2002;11:1–11.
30. Luhrs H, Gerke T, Schauber J et al. Cytokine-activated degradation of inhibitory kappaB protein alpha is inhibited by the short-chain fatty acid butyrate. Int J Colorectal Dis. 2001;16:195–201.
31. Luhrs H, Hock R, Schauber J et al. Modulation of HMG-N2 binding to chromatin by butyrate-induced acetylation in human colon adenocarcinoma cells. Int J Cancer. 2002;97:567–73.

30
Flavonoids and their possible role in colon cancer prevention and therapy

U. WENZEL and H. DANIEL

EFFECTS OF INGREDIENTS OF FRUITS AND VEGETABLES ON CANCER DEVELOPMENT

Results obtained in cell cultures or in animal studies have demonstrated significant inhibitory effects of a number of ingredients of fruits and vegetables on cancer cell growth. Amongst these food compounds are the antioxidative vitamins A[1], C[2] and E[3], the carotenoids[4], minerals, such as calcium[5] and selenium[6], dietary fibres[7] and flavonoids[8]. However, human intervention trials investigating the effects of those compounds in colon cancer patients have been more or less disappointing[9–11]. Even more unexpected results were obtained in the CARET[12] study and the ATBC study[13]. Both primary prevention trials were stopped because of a higher lung cancer incidence and mortality in smokers when supplemented with β-carotene. What can be learned from this, is that compounds that are effective growth inhibitors in cancer cells are not necessarily good chemopreventive agents *in vivo*, and *vice versa*. In particular antioxidants are generally regarded as effective chemopreventive agents since they are potent scavengers of reactive oxygen species (ROS). ROS-mediated DNA damage contributes to spontaneous mutagenesis, and cells with impaired repair mechanisms and with low concentrations of protective compounds, including antioxidants, have elevated levels of spontaneous mutations, which might initiate cancer development[14]. On the other hand, ROS may be essential as activators of programmed cell death (apoptosis) to remove cells that have accumulated mutations. It was demonstrated recently that the depletion of antioxidants was able to inhibit tumour growth in a transgenic mouse brain tumour model[15]. Moreover, anti-apoptotic proteins that act as antioxidants, such as bcl-2, are usually upregulated in cancer cells as a mechanism to escape apoptosis[16,17], supporting the notion that a high level of antioxidants could be fatal in allowing transformed cells to resist the cell death signals. What is important to remember is that every compound displays a distinct dose–response relationship. It was shown for lycopene as well as β-carotene in human colonocytes, that protection against

DNA damage occurs only at relatively low concentrations, comparable to those found in the plasma of individuals consuming a carotenoid-rich diet. At higher concentrations, however, both carotenoids may actually increase the extent of DNA damage[18]. On the basis of these results, the enormous popularity of dietary supplements containing carotenoids or (bio)flavonoids is worrisome. It also should be kept in mind that side-effects of certain flavonoids, including immunoallergic acute haemolysis, thrombocytopenia and acute renal failure, have been observed in patients[19].

FLAVONOIDS AND COLONIC CELLS

Flavonoids are low-molecular-weight phenylbenzopyrones that are found in fruits, vegetables, nuts and seeds, as well as tea and wine[20]. They are categorized into the subclasses of flavones, flavonols, flavanones, catechines, anthocyanidines and isoflavones depending on the molecular structure (Figure 1). The core unit of flavonoids consists of a o-heterocyclic ring fused to an aromatic ring with a third ring system attached at either C3 or C4 of the heterocyclic ring. The 6 most common classes differ in their structures only in the position of the ring C with respect to the fused ring system and by the number and positions of hydroxy- or methoxy-group substituents as given in Table 1. Plant flavonoids are frequently found as glycosides[21]. The glycosides appear to be resistant to the endogenous enzymes of the gastrointestinal tract but are cleaved by bacterial

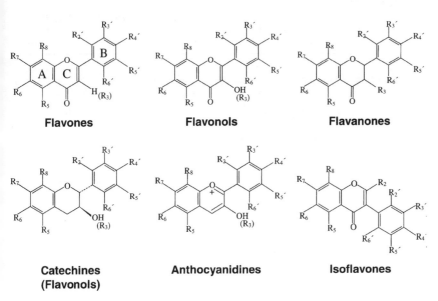

Flavones   **Flavonols**   **Flavanones**

Catechines   **Anthocyanidines**   **Isoflavones**
(Flavonols)

Figure 1 Subclasses of flavonoids. The basic structure of the phenylchromane derivatives consists of an O-heterocyclic ring (C) fused to an aromatic ring (A) and by a carbon–carbon bond to a second aromatic ring (B). Classification is based on variations on the heterocyclic C ring. The various substituents then lead to the different flavonoids as given in Table 1 for the flavone and flavanol subclasses

Table 1 Chemical composition of selected flavonoids of the flavone and flavanol subclasses with reference to Figure 1 and the substituents

	Substituents									
	R3	R5	R6	R7	R8	R2'	R3'	R4'	R5'	R6'
Flavones; flavonoles										
Flavone	H	H	H	H	H	H	H	H	H	H
3-OH-flavon	OH	H	H	H	H	H	H	H	H	H
5-OH-flavon	H	OH	H	H	H	H	H	H	H	H
7-OH-flavon	H	H	H	OH	H	H	H	H	H	H
7,8-(OH)$_2$-flavon	H	H	H	OH	OH	H	H	H	H	H
Apigenin	H	OH	H	OH	H	H	H	OH	H	H
Baicalein	H	OH	OH	OH	H	H	H	H	H	H
Kämpferol	OH	OH	H	OH	H	H	H	OH	H	H
Fisetin	OH	H	H	OH	H	H	OH	OH	H	H
Luteolin	H	OH	H	OH	H	H	OH	OH	H	H
Quercetin	OH	OH	H	OH	H	H	OH	OH	H	H
Morin	OH	OH	H	OH	H	OH	H	OH	H	H
Chrysin	H	OH	H	OH	H	H	H	H	H	H
Myricetin	OH	OH	H	OH	H	H	OH	OH	OH	H
Acacetin	H	OH	H	OH	H	H	H	OCH$_3$	H	H
Diosmin	H	OH	H	Sugar	H	H	OH	OCH$_3$	H	H
Diosmetin	H	OH	H	OH	H	H	OH	OCH$_3$	H	H
Apiin	H	OH	H	-Apiosyl glucoside	H	H	H	OH	H	H
Kämpferide	OH	OH	H	OH	H	H	H	OCH$_3$	H	H
Puerarin (?)										
Tangeretin	H	OH	OH	OH	OH	H	H	OCH$_3$	H	H
Rutin (rhamno-glucoside)	Manno-glucopyranosyl	OH	H	OH	H	H	H	OH	OH	H

enzymes in the large intestine to yield the corresponding aglycons[22]. The absorption of the glycosides in the human small intestine is generally poor[22] but flavonoids that reach the large intestine are easily deglycosylated by the microflora[23], delivering the aglycon directly to colonic cells. However, recent findings suggest that some flavonoids may even be better absorbed in their glycosylated form in the small intestine due to their ability to be transported actively by the intestinal glucose transporter SGLT-1[24].

On average, the daily Western diet provides around 20–50 mg of different flavonoids but with a great variability in intake depending on the food source[25]. Although there is only limited, and inconsistent, information on the extent of intestinal absorption and bioavailability of most flavonoids, the concentrations attained in intestinal epithelial cells should by nature exceed those in circulation, and therefore the analysis of biological effects of flavonoids in human intestinal epithelial cells deserves attention.

BIOLOGICAL FUNCTIONS OF FLAVONOIDS

Flavonoids have a large spectrum of biological activities. In particular, the inhibitory potency of selected compounds on various stages of cancer development

Table 2 Summary of reported biological activities of selected flavonoids

Flavonoid	Receptor ligands		Protein kinase inhibition	Antioxidant	Xenobiotic metabolism	
	Tyrosine kinase-R	Oestrogen-R			Phase I enzymes	Phase II enzymes
Flavones	+					
Kaempferol	+		+	+		+
Baicalein	+			+		
Fisetin	+		+	+		
Quercetin	+		+	+		+
Apigenin			+	+		
Myricetin	+		+	+		+
Substitute flavones						
Acatein				+		
Apiin				+		
Diosmetin				+		
Diosmin				+		
Tangeretin				+	+	+
Flavanones						
Flavanon				+	+	+
Hesperidin				+		
Hesperetin		+		+		
Naringenin		+		+		
Bavachinin				+		
Isoflavones						
Biochanin A		+		+		
Genistein	+	+		+		+
Genistin	+	+		+		
Daidzein		+	+	+		+

has attracted much attention[25–27]. Apart from the antioxidative properties of most, but not all, flavonoids, they also display a multitude of other biological functions which might be relevant in cancer prevention and therapy. Table 2 summarizes their functions as receptor ligands, protein kinase inhibitors and effectors of phase I and phase II enzymes in xenobiotic metabolism.

A large number of flavonoids was screened for their effects on cell proliferation and their potential cytotoxicity in human colon cancer cell lines, such as Caco-2 and HT-29. Studies on the dose-dependent effects of the flavonoids showed antiproliferative activity of all compounds with EC_{50} values ranging between 20 and 250 µmol/L. In almost all cases, growth inhibition of the flavonoids occurred in the absence of cytotoxicity. There was no obvious structure–activity relationship in the antiproliferative effects either on the basis of the subclasses (i.e. isoflavones, flavones, flavonols, flavanones) or with respect to kind or position of substituents within a class[8].

Most flavonoids are potent antioxidants and inhibition of cell growth might therefore depend on the capacity of the compounds to serve as free-radical scavengers. It has been described that flavonoids with 4–6 OH groups act as strong antioxidants in an aqueous milieu, whereas those with more or fewer OH groups show low or no antioxidant activities[26]. Moreover, it was found that OH groups in the ortho-position at ring B as well as the double bond between C2 and C3, together with the carbonyl function in ring C, are important structural determinants for the antioxidant effects of flavonols[27]. One might therefore expect that flavonoids with lower antioxidative properties also possess less antiproliferative activities. This is indeed the case with flavones carrying only 1 or 2 OH groups. However, some flavanones and isoflavones with one or two OH groups also display surprisingly high antiproliferative potencies[8].

Cancer cells differ from normal cells not only by increased cell proliferation but also by blunted differentiation responses and reduced apoptosis rates. Apopain, a caspase-3 protease, is considered to represent a specific and early marker in the apoptotic pathway in normal and transformed intestinal cells[28,29] and a variety of flavonoids that possess antiproliferative effects (i.e. baicalein, genistein, bavachinin, flavon and myricetin) are also able to increase apopain activity in intestinal cancer cell lines but not in renal or breast cancer cells[8]. In particular, flavone turned out to be a very potent apoptosis inducer in colonic cancer cells with the additional capability to promote cell differentiation. The alterations of apoptosis in cancer cells by flavonoids appears to be mediated by quite different molecular mechanisms. For instance, the flavonoid flavopiridol inhibits various cyclin-dependent kinases (CDK), which are crucial for transition of a cell through the cell cycle[30]. As a consequence, a growth arrest in human breast carcinoma cells was observed. The catechin EGCG[31], the isoflavone genistein[32], the flavonol quercetin[33] and flavone[34,35] were shown to induce the gene expression of the CDK inhibitor, p21. Expression of p21 is usually associated with a cell-cycle arrest that allows other proteins to control and repair the replicated DNA. The *p21* gene is also a major transcriptional target of the tumour-suppressor protein, p53[36]. As *p53* is mutated in almost 50% of all human cancers, one consequence of its loss of function is the inability to induce p21 expression. This causes a key problem in cell-cycle control and the reduced expression of p21[37] is consequently associated with the development of sporadic tumours. On the other hand, expression of p21 is documented to inhibit the proliferation of malignant cells *in vitro* and *in vivo*[38]. As shown for human lung and colon adenocarcinoma cells[35,39], flavone in particular can induce efficiently the expression of p21 independent of the tumour suppressor p53 which makes this flavonoid a promising therapeutic agent.

Analysing in more detail the mechanisms by which flavone induces apoptosis in p53 mutant cells, it was observed that the mRNA levels of the anti-apoptotic factors, NF-κB and bcl-X$_L$, and of cyclo-oxygenase-2 (COX-2) were downregulated by the compound[39]. The ability of the transcription factor NF-κB to inhibit apoptosis in cancer cells contributes significantly to their chemoresistance[40] and therefore flavone might also be helpful as an adjuvant in cancer therapy. The downregulation of bcl-X$_L$ by flavone could also provide a benefit in cancer therapy since bcl-X$_L$ seems to play a major role in colorectal tumorigenesis and disease progression[41]. Overexpression of the COX-2 gene is consistently found during neoplastic development in a variety of tissues, and prostaglandins formed along the dysregulated COX pathways have been shown to mediate tumour promotion in various animal models. However, prostaglandins may also play a role in other processes of tumour growth, such as angiogenesis, metastasis and immunosuppression[42]. Consequently, COX-2 has become a prime target of pharmacotherapy, especially in the prevention and therapy of colorectal cancers[43]. Inhibition of COX-2 enzyme activity is mainly achieved by non-steroidal anti-inflammatory drugs, including newly developed COX-2-specific inhibitors, whereas flavone prevents the gene expression of the enzyme in colonic tumour cells. Figure 2 summarizes some of the observed effects of flavone at the molecular level in cancer cells as identified so far.

Besides an effective induction of apoptosis by cancer therapeutics, a major goal is to achieve a high selectivity for transformed cells in order to reduce the number and severity of side-effects by damage of normal cells. The limited selectivity of classical apoptosis-inducing anti-tumour drugs in the treatment of colorectal cancers frequently leads to mucosal damage and, moreover, increased apoptosis rates in the non-transformed cells that can be accompanied by neoplastic transformation[44,45]. Therefore, the effects of flavone have been compared to those of camptothecin in normal colonic cells isolated and cultivated from colonic crypts of healthy mice[39]. Whereas camptothecin proved to be a strong growth inhibitor of the non-transformed colonocytes, flavone was without effect on the proliferation rates of the normal murine cells. The growth inhibition caused by camptothecin seemed to be mediated by enhanced apoptosis rates since caspase-3 activity was increased about 7-fold. In contrast, flavone did not possess any significant effects on apoptosis and showed no cytotoxicity in normal murine colonocytes, suggesting that it could have only minor side-effects. Such a cell-selective growth-inhibitory activity and significant apoptosis-inducing effect in cancer cells has also been demonstrated for the green tea polyphenol, EGCG[46]. The constitutive expression of NF-κB and the binding of NF-κB to DNA-*cis*-regulatory elements was inhibited by EGCG at much lower concentrations in the cancer cells than in the non-transformed cells[47]. Moreover, the activation of NF-κB by stress stimuli, such as tumour necrosis factor-α (TNF-α) or lipopolysaccharide (LPS), was also inhibited by EGCG more prominently in cancer cells than in normal cells[47]. Certain flavonoids, therefore, possess both a high potency and a high selectivity towards transformed cells to reduce their growth by apoptosis. Figure 3 summarizes the effects of flavone in transformed and non-transformed colonocytes.

Flavonoids, including those that do not possess any antioxidant activity, have been shown to be potent inhibitors of cancer cell growth *in vitro* and in animal models. Although epidemiology suggests that flavonoid intake could be associated with reduced colon cancer development, there is no direct proof of this function from human studies. A growing market of dietary supplements containing more or less unspecified preparations of 'bioflavonoids' with proposed health-promoting activities might therefore be considered as a field test on their safety and efficiency.

Biochemical studies, however, demonstrate that certain flavonoids have a multitude of effects on the biology of normal and transformed cells. The key problem is that only a very few compounds of the more than 5000 flavonoids have been characterized with regard to biological activity, and, moreover, there is no obvious structure–function relationship allowing predictions on their biology. Similar to other dietary constituents, most flavonoids have a high antioxidative

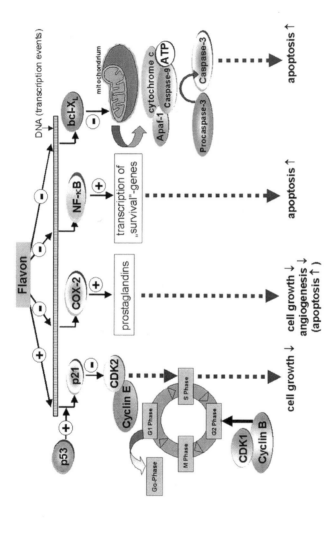

Figure 2 Molecular effects of flavone identified in colonic cancer cells. Flavone increases the transcription of the cyclin-dependent-kinase (CDK)-inhibitor, p21. The p21 protein is usually induced by the tumour suppressor p53 but induction of p21 by flavone occurs independently on p53 activity. Increased p21 levels inhibit the CDK2–cyclin E complex that is crucial for S-phase entry of the cell cycle. As a consequence of increased p21 expression and reduced expression of cyclins[32], flavone leads to a cell-cycle arrest. Growth inhibition may be exerted by flavone also through a diminished cyclooxygenase-2 (COX-2) expression. COX-2 is responsible for the synthesis of prostaglandins, which have been shown to be involved in stimulation of cell growth and inhibition of apoptosis but may also play a role in angiogenesis and metastasis. The reduced mRNA levels of NF-κB observed by flavone exposure may inhibit the transcription of survival genes and thereby allow apoptotic signals to prevail. Flavone moreover reduces the transcript levels of bcl-X$_L$, a mitochondrial antiapoptotic factor that inhibits the release of cytochrome c from mitochondria. Cytochrome c together with the apoptotic-protease-activating factor-1 (Apaf-1), ATP and caspase-9 forms the so-called apopto-some that triggers the activation of the executioner protease caspase-3. Therefore, the flavone-induced inhibition of bcl-X$_L$ expression causes an increased apopto-sis rate. The symbols + and − represent stimulation or inhibition, respectively

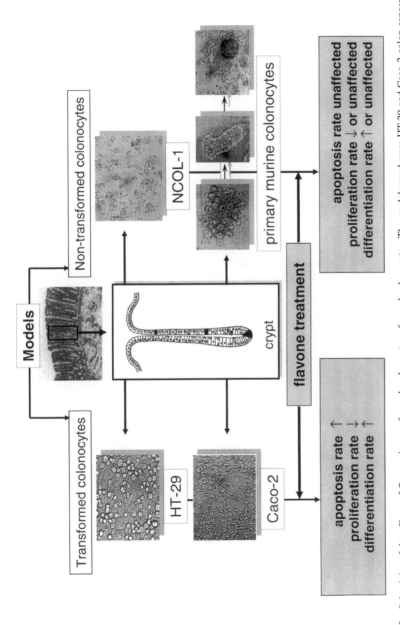

Figure 3 Selectivity of the effects of flavone in transformed and non-transformed colonocytes. The models used were HT-29 and Caco-2 colon cancer cells for transformed cells and NCOL-1 cells, derived from a non-transformed human colon biopsy specimen as well as primary murine colonocytes as non-transformed cell cultures. ↑, ↓ indicate the changes observed after flavone treatment in the different cellular models

271

capacity and are consequently perceived as effective chemopreventive agents. However, even the high intake of antioxidants for tumour prevention and therapy seems currently a bit like a dance on the edge of a sword.

As shown in various *in-vitro* studies, flavonoids such as ECCG or flavone possess very interesting activities that target specifically hyperproliferating tissues and cells in the transformation process. These compounds could by their multifunctional bioactivity turn out to be especially beneficial in the prevention and treatment of tumours either alone or in combination with other antitumour agents. Such a combinatorial therapy has proven its effectiveness in the prevention of colorectal adenomas in mice using inhibitors of the epidermal growth factor and of COX-signalling pathways[48]. This synergistic action of compounds needs to be exploited systematically in cancer therapy, in particular towards modulating the 'threshold' for apoptosis[49]. Clinical trials currently being carried out with individual flavonoids should show whether these agents are effective also in humans[50-52].

References

1. Lee MO, Han SY, Jiang S, Park JH, Kim SJ. Differential effects of retinoic acid on growth and apoptosis in human colon cancer cell lines associated with the induction of retinoic acid receptor beta. Biochem Pharmacol. 2000;59:485–96.
2. Rao CV, Rivenson A, Kelloff GJ, Reddy BS. Chemoprevention of azoxymethane-induced colon cancer by ascorbylpalmitate, carbenoxolone, dimethylfumarate and p-methoxyphenol in male F344 rats. Anticancer Res. 1995;15:1199–204.
3. Chinery R, Brockman JA, Peeler MO, Shyr Y, Beauchamp RD, Coffey RJ. Antioxidants enhance the cytotoxicity of chemotherapeutic agents in colorectal cancer: a p53-independent induction of p21WAF1/CIP1 via C/EBPbeta. Nat Med. 1997;3:1233–41.
4. Narisawa T, Fukaura Y, Hasebe M, Nomura S, Oshima S, Inakuma T. Prevention of N-methylnitrosourea-induced colon carcinogenesis in rats by oxygenated carotenoid capsanthin and capsanthin-rich paprika juice. Proc Soc Exp Biol Med. 2000;224:116–22.
5. Wargovich MJ, Jimenez A, McKee K *et al.* Efficacy of potential chemopreventive agents on rat colon aberrant crypt formation and progression. Carcinogenesis. 2000;21:1149–55.
6. Redman C, Xu MJ, Peng YM *et al.* Involvement of polyamines in selenomethionine induced apoptosis and mitotic alterations in human tumor cells. Carcinogenesis. 1997;18:1195–202.
7. Avivi-Green C, Polak-Charcon S, Madar Z, Schwartz B. Apoptosis cascade proteins are regulated in vivo by high intracolonic butyrate concentration: correlation with colon cancer inhibition. Oncol Res. 2000;12:83–95.
8. Kuntz S, Wenzel U, Daniel H. Comparative analysis of the effects of flavonoids on proliferation, cytotoxicity, and apoptosis in human colon cancer cell lines. Eur J Nutr. 1999;38:133–42.
9. Cascinu S, Ligi M, Del Ferro E *et al.* Effects of calcium and vitamin supplementation on colon cell proliferation in colorectal cancer. Cancer Invest. 2000;18:411–16.
10. McKeown-Eyssen G, Holloway C, Jazmaji V, Bright-See E, Dion P, Bruce WR. A randomized trial of vitamins C and E in the prevention of recurrence of colorectal polyps. Cancer Res. 1988;48:4701–5.
11. Greenberg ER, Baron JA, Tosteson TD *et al.* A clinical trial of antioxidant vitamins to prevent colorectal adenoma. Polyp Prevention Study Group. N Engl J Med. 1994;331:141–7.
12. Omenn GS, Goodman GE, Thornquist MD *et al.* Risk factors for lung cancer and for intervention effects in CARET, the Beta-Carotene and Retinol Efficacy Trial. J Natl Cancer Inst. 1996;88:1550–9.
13. Blumberg J, Block G. The alpha-tocopherol, beta-carotene cancer prevention study in Finland. Nutr Rev. 1994;52:242–5.
14. Volkert MR, Elliott NA, Housman DE. Functional genomics reveals a family of eukaryotic oxidation protection genes. Proc Natl Acad Sci. 2000;97:14530–5.
15. Salganik RI, Albright CD, Rodgers J *et al.* Dietary antioxidant depletion: enhancement of tumor apoptosis and inhibition of brain tumor growth in transgenic mice. Carcinogenesis. 2000;21:909–14.

16. Hockenbery DM, Oltvai ZN, Yin XM, Milliman CL, Korsmeyer SJ. Bcl-2 functions in an antioxidant pathway to prevent apoptosis. Cell. 1993;75:241–51.
17. Frommel TO, Zarling EJ. Chronic inflammation and cancer: potential role of Bcl-2 gene family members as regulators of cellular antioxidant status. Med Hypoth. 1999;52:27–30.
18. Lowe GM, Booth LA, Young AJ, Bilton RF. Lycopene and beta-carotene protect against oxidative damage in HT29 cells at low concentrations but rapidly lose this capacity at higher doses. Free Rad Res. 1999;30:141–51.
19. Jaeger A, Walti M, Neftel K. Side effects of flavonoids in medical practice. Prog Clin Biol Res. 1988;280:379–94.
20. Middleton E, Kandaswami C. The impact of plant flavonoids on mammalian biology: implications for immunity, inflammation and cancer. In: Harborne JB (ed) The Flavonoids: Advances in Research since 1986. London: Chapman & Hall, 1993:619–52.
21. Hempel J, Böhm H. Quality and quantity of prevailing flavonoid glycosides of yellow and green french beans (*Phaseolus vulgaris* L.). J Agric Food Chem. 1996;44:2114–16.
22. Hollman PC, van Trijp JM, Buysman MN *et al.* Relative bioavailability of the antioxidant flavonoid quercetin from various foods in man. FEBS Lett. 1997;418:152–6.
23. Winter J, Moore LH, Dowell VR, Bokkenheuser VD. C-ring cleavage of flavonoids by human intestinal bacteria. Appl Environ Microbiol. 1989;55:1203–8.
24. Wolffram S, Block M, Ader P. Quercetin-3-glucoside is transported by the glucose carrier SGLT1 across the brush border membrane of rat small intestine. J Nutr. 2002;132:630–5.
25. Linseisen J, Radtke J, Wolfram G. Flavonoid intake of adults in a Bavarian subgroup of the national food consumption survey. Z Ernährungswiss. 1997;36:403–12.
26. Rice-Evans CA, Miller NJ, Bolwell PG, Bramley PM, Pridham JP. The relative antioxidant activities of plant-derived polyphenolic flavonoids. Free Rad Res. 1995;22:375–83.
27. Bors W, Heller W, Michel C, Saran M. Flavonoids as antioxidants: determination of radical-scavenging efficiencies. Meth Enzymol. 1990;186:343–55.
28. Grossmann J, Mohr S, Lapentina EG, Fiocchi C, Levine AD. Sequential and rapid activation of select caspases during apoptosis of normal intestinal epithelial cells. Am J Physiol. 1998;274: G1117–24.
29. Shao RG, Shimizu T, Pommier Y. 7-Hydroxystaurosporine (UCN-01) induces apoptosis in human colon carcinoma and leukemia cells independently of p53. Exp Cell Res. 1998;234: 388–97.
30. Caltagirone S, Rossi C, Poggi A *et al.* Flavonoids apigenin and quercetin inhibit melanoma growth and metastatic potential. Int J Cancer. 2000;87:595–600.
31. Carlson BA, Dubay MM, Sausville EA, Brizuela L, Worland PJ. Flavopiridol induces G1 arrest with inhibition of cyclin-dependent kinase (CDK) 2 and CDK4 in human breast carcinoma cells. Cancer Res. 1996;56:2973–8.
32. Liang YC, Lin-Shiau SY, Chen CF, Lin JK. Inhibition of cyclin-dependent kinases 2 and 4 activities as well as induction of Cdk inhibitors p21 and p27 during growth arrest of human breast carcinoma cells by (−)-epigallocatechin-3-gallate. J Cell Biochem. 1999;75:1–12.
33. Kuzumaki T, Kobayashi T, Ishikawa K. Genistein induces p21(Cip1/WAF1) expression and blocks the G1 to S phase transition in mouse fibroblast and melanoma cells. Biochem Biophys Res Commun. 1998;251:291–5.
34. Iwao K, Tsukamoto I. Quercetin inhibited DNA synthesis and induced apoptosis associated with increase in c-fos mRNA level and the upregulation of p21WAF1CIP1 mRNA and protein expression during liver regeneration after partial hepatectomy. Biochim Biophys Acta. 1999;1427:112–20.
35. Bai F, Matsui T, Ohtani-Fujita N, Matsukawa Y, Ding Y, Sakai T. Promoter activation and following induction of the p21/WAF1 gene by flavone is involved in G1 phase arrest in A549 lung adenocarcinoma cells. FEBS Lett. 1998;437:61–4.
36. Pellegata NS, Antoniono RJ, Redpath JL, Stanbridge EJ. DNA damage and p53-mediated cell cycle arrest: a reevaluation. Proc Natl Acad Sci. 1996;93:15209–14.
37. Sinicrope FA, Roddey G, Lemoine M *et al.* Loss of p21WAF1/Cip1 protein expression accompanies progression of sporadic colorectal neoplasms but not hereditary nonpolyposis colorectal cancers. Clin Cancer Res. 1998;4:1251–61.
38. Yang ZY, Perkins ND, Ohno T, Nabel EG, Nabel GJ. The p21 cyclin-dependent kinase inhibitor suppresses tumorigenicity in vivo. Nat Med. 1995;1:1052–6.
39. Wenzel U, Kuntz S, Brendel MD, Daniel H. Dietary flavone is a potent apoptosis inducer in human colon carcinoma cells. Cancer Res. 2000;60:3823–31.

40. Wang CY, Cusack JC, Liu R, Baldwin AS. Control of inducible chemoresistance: enhanced anti-tumor therapy through increased apoptosis by inhibition of NF-kappaB. Nat Med. 1999;5:412–17.
41. Maurer CA, Friess H, Buhler SS et al. Apoptosis inhibiting factor Bcl-xL might be the crucial member of the Bcl-2 gene family in colorectal cancer. Dig Dis Sci. 1998;43:2641–8.
42. Marks F, Furstenberger G. Cancer chemoprevention through interruption of multistage carcinogenesis. The lessons learnt by comparing mouse skin carcinogenesis and human large bowel cancer. Eur J Cancer. 2000;36:314–29.
43. Elder DJ, Paraskeva C. COX-2 inhibitors for colorectal cancer. Nat Med. 1998;4:392–3.
44. Van Huyen JP, Bloch F, Attar A et al. Diffuse mucosal damage in the large intestine associated with Irinotecan (CPT-11). Dig Dis Sci. 1998;43:2649–51.
45. Sinicrope FA, Roddey G, McDonnell TJ, Shen Y, Cleary KR, Stephens LC. Increased apoptosis accompanies neoplastic development in the human colorectum. Clin Cancer Res. 1996;2: 1999–2006.
46. Ahmad N, Feyes DK, Nieminen AL, Agarwal R, Mukhtar H. Green tea constituent epigallocatechin-3-gallate and induction of apoptosis and cell cycle arrest in human carcinoma cells. J Natl Cancer Inst. 1997;89:1881–6.
47. Ahmad N, Gupta S, Mukhtar H. Green tea polyphenol epigallocatechin-3-gallate differentially modulates nuclear factor kappaB in cancer cells versus normal cells. Arch Biochem Biophys. 2000;376:338–46.
48. Torrance CJ, Jackson PE, Montgomery E et al. Combinatorial chemoprevention of intestinal neoplasia. Nat Med. 2000;6:1024–8.
49. Wilson WH, Sorbara L, Figg WD et al. Modulation of clinical drug resistance in a B cell lymphoma patient by the protein kinase inhibitor 7-hydroxystaurosporine: presentation of a novel therapeutic paradigm. Clin Cancer Res. 2000;6:415–21.
50. Senderowicz AM. Flavopiridol: the first cyclin-dependent kinase inhibitor in human clinical trials. Invest New Drugs. 1999;17:313–20.
51. Senderowicz AM, Sausville EA. Response: re: preclinical and clinical development of cyclin-dependent kinase modulators. J Natl Cancer Inst. 2000;92:1185.
52. Shapiro G et al. A phase II trial of flavopiridol in patients with stage IV non-small cell lung cancer (Abstract). Proc ASCO. 1999;18:522A.

31
Selenium in cancer prevention: optimization of selenoprotein expression or specific functions of selenium compounds?

R. BRIGELIUS-FLOHÉ, C. MÜLLER, S. FLORIAN and
K. MÜLLER-SCHMEHL

HISTORY

Selenium was discovered in 1817 by Jöns Jacob Berzelius and has since undergone a varied history. For a long time it was only considered as toxic, causing major health problems in livestock and humans, as reviewed in ref. 1. Its image changed when Schwarz and Foltz[2] in 1957 recognized selenium to be an essential trace element for mammals. Selenium-deficiency symptoms were identified such as white muscle disease in cattle, mulberry heart disease in pigs, and exudative diathesis in poultry (reviewed in ref. 3). In China two major human diseases were found to be associated with insufficient selenium supply: Keshan disease, which is a fatal cardiomyopathy; and Kashin-Beck disease, a disabling chondronecrosis (reviewed in ref. 4). In view of the growing awareness of nutrition in health care a suboptimal alimentary selenium supply is now being discussed in accelerated ageing, development of cardiovascular diseases and cancer, impaired immune response, and function of the endocrine system, as well as in male reproduction.

MAMMALIAN SELENOPROTEINS

Selenoproteins contain selenium as selenocysteine which is incorporated as the 21st amino acid in the peptide chain. Selenocysteine is encoded by TGA, which usually stands for stop. Thus, organisms had to develop a mechanism to differentiate between TGA meaning stop and TGA meaning selenocysteine. This mechanism is complex. It has been elucidated for prokaryotes in elegant studies by the

275

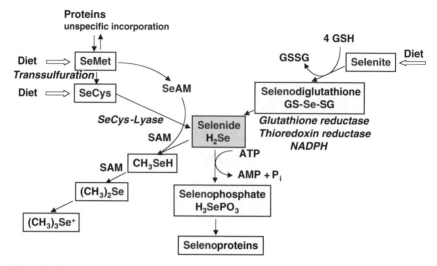

Figure 1 Scheme of utilization of alimentary selenium compounds. SeMet: selenomethionine; SeCys: selenocysteine; S(Se)AM: S(Se)adenosylmethionine; GSH: glutathione; GSSG: glutathione disulphide; CH₃SeH: methylselenide

group of Böck (reviewed in ref. 5). It is similar but not identical in eukaryotes. The reader is referred to recent reviews, since a description of selenoprotein biosynthesis is beyond the scope of this chapter[6,7]. It should only be mentioned that the incorporation of selenium into selenocysteine requires hydrogen selenide, which is transferred into selenophosphate that is used for the synthesis of selenocysteine in the form of a selenocysteyl-tRNA. Thus, only selenium compounds whose metabolism leads to hydrogen selenide production can serve as precursors for selenoprotein biosynthesis (Figure 1). Knockout of the tRNA gene specifically incorporating selenocysteine into proteins is lethal, which indicates that at least one of the mammalian selenoproteins is of vital importance[8].

So far 19 selenoproteins have been characterized, at least by sequence and from less than 10 is the function known (reviewed in refs 9–12). Among those whose function is known, at least in part, four are glutathione peroxidases: the classical one (cGPx or GPx-1), the phospholipid hydroperoxide GPx (PHGPx or GPx-4), the plasma GPx (pGPx or GPx-3), and the gastrointestinal GPx (GI-GPx or GPx-2) (see refs 13 and 14 for reviews). The redundancy of glutathione peroxidases strongly suggests that they may have functions which are different from those of merely reducing hydroperoxides. This has been convincingly demonstrated for PHGPx, which was shown to build the mitochondrial capsule in spermatozoa by crosslinking either with itself or with other protein(s)[15]. The exclusive expression of GI-GPx in the gastrointestinal system gave rise to the assumption that its function is to prevent absorption of hydroperoxides. Experimental evidence supports this hypothesis[16]; however, other functions may also be possible, as discussed below.

Mammalian selenoproteins are not supplied equally with selenium when it becomes limiting; they are rather provided according to a ranking called the hierarchy of selenoproteins[13,17]. Those which rank low in this hierarchy rapidly disappear in selenium-limiting conditions. Their mRNA is also degraded. Those which rank high in the hierarchy remain stable under a moderate decrease in selenium supply and the mRNA is not degraded even in severe selenium deficiency. On the other hand, stable selenoproteins are preferentially synthesized upon refeeding with selenium, whereas unstable selenoproteins recover only after others have been repleted. This phenomenon led to the conclusion that stable selenoproteins may have more important functions than those which are unstable. Examples for both types can be found in the family of glutathione peroxidases. Whereas GI-GPx and PHGPx are among those selenoproteins ranking highest in the hierarchy, cGPx is one of the most unstable selenoproteins identified so far. pGPx behaves rather like cGPx. Maximum plasma GPx and erythrocyte cGPx activities are therefore used as biomarkers for optimal selenium status. The high ranking of GI-GPx has been demonstrated by an extraordinarily stable mRNA in selenium deficiency, and by a rapid reoccurrence of the GI-GPx protein upon repletion of selenium[18]. Both effects were observed in cultured cells and in rats.

SELENIUM AND CANCER

A link between low selenium intake and increased cancer incidence was first described by Shamberger and Frost in 1969[19], who compared the average selenium content of forage crops in different parts of the United States with the corresponding cancer death rate. Since then, evidence for the anticarcinogenic effects of selenium compounds has been derived from numerous epidemiological and experimental animal studies, as well as from clinical trials (reviewed in ref. 20). However, only one large-scale prospective, placebo-controlled trial has been completed to date[21]. This study failed to meet its primary endpoint, recurrence of skin carcinoma, but revealed a 50% reduction in total cancer incidence, and an approximately 50% reduction in cancers from prostate, colon and lung. Participants received 200 μg selenium from selenium-enriched yeast per day. This is an amount about 3 times higher than the recommended daily allowance (RDA) of 1 μg per kg body weight per day, which was recommended at that time, and 4 times higher than the dietary reference intake (DRI) of 50 μg recently agreed upon[22]. It is also far in excess of the amount of selenium required to bring cGPx activity to an optimum. It is therefore doubtful whether optimization of selenoprotein(s) is responsible for the observed effects of selenium.

SELENIUM COMPOUNDS WITH ANTICANCEROGENIC EFFECTS

In most of the studies undertaken to prove the anticarcinogenic properties of selenium in experimental animals, selenite or selenomethionine applied as selenium-enriched yeast was used. As a rule the dosages required for an anticarcinogenic effect exceeded the dosage required for optimizing the activity of, for example, cGPx. This may be for various reasons:

1. Optimizing selenoprotein expression is not sufficient to prevent chemically induced carcinogenesis, or the responsible selenoprotein has not yet been identified. If so, this selenoprotein should rank low in the hierarchy, and is synthesized only with excess availability of selenium. The only selenoprotein shown so far to respond to supranutritional selenium supply is thioredoxin reductase[23]. This, however, does not rank particularly low in the hierarchy and is also not particularly irrelevant for survival.

2. Not a selenoprotein but, instead, an intermediate of selenite or selenomethionine metabolism could be effective (Figures 1 and 2). During the reduction of selenite to selenide selenodiglutathione is produced[24], which has been found to be potently anticarcinogenic[25]. Selenomethionine metabolism also ends in selenide production. Selenomethionine must, however, first enter the trans-sulphuration pathway to be converted to selenocysteine (see Figure 1). Selenocysteine is then cleaved into selenide, pyruvate and ammonia by a β-lyase[26]. In addition, selenomethionine is incorporated into proteins as such, since the tRNA specific for methionine does not discriminate between methionine and selenomethionine. Due to this mechanism, selenomethionine supplementation leads to higher tissue selenium concentrations than selenite, but may also contribute to its lower toxicity[27], and to its lower anticarcinogenic effect[28,29].

3. In the most effective selenium compounds the selenium is alk(en)ylated. This now becomes evident from elegant studies performed by the groups of Ip and Ganther. They clearly showed that methylated selenium compounds exceeded the efficacy of both selenite and selenomethionine. Particularly efficient were: Se-methylselenocysteine[30,31], methylseleninic acid[32], Se-propylselenocysteine and Se-allylselenocysteine[33]. Se-methylselenocysteine and γ-glutamyl-Se-methylselenocysteine are the major compounds present in selenium-enriched garlic[34], which proved to have better anticarcinogenic properties than selenium-enriched yeast[35] in which selenomethionine is the prominent selenium compound[36]. Alk(en)ylated selenium compounds are metabolized to alk(en)ylated selenides by the β-lyase. Alk(en)ylated selenides are now believed to be responsible for the anticarcinogenic effects.

POSSIBLE ANTICARCINOGENIC MECHANISMS
(summarized in Figure 2)

Antioxidative effects

For a long time the lower incidence of cancer in selenium-adequate subjects has been attributed to an optimal glutathione peroxidase activity. The hypothesis is based on the often-observed DNA damage induced by hydroperoxides which, in turn, are removed by glutathione peroxidases. Two lines of evidence argue against the assumption that selenium simply acts as a source for antioxidative enzymes: (a) anticarcinogenic effects of selenium compounds require higher dosages than required for optimizing cGPx and pGPx activity, the other two

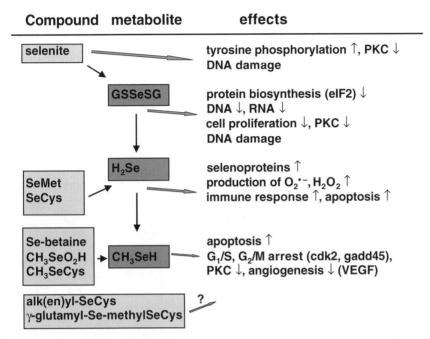

Figure 2 Potential impact of low molecular weight selenium compounds on parameters related to carcinogenesis

glutathione peroxidases being active in moderate selenium limitation anyway; and (b) cGPx knockout mice grow and develop normally[37]; they die earlier than controls only when stressed with oxidants[38]. However, it has not so far been reported that they develop cancer.

Induction of apoptosis

A pro-apoptotic effect has been observed with selenium compounds producing superoxide radicals by redox cycling. These are, for example, selenide, methylselenol, selenite, selenium dioxide, selenocysteine, selenocystamine and methylseleninic acid[39].

These observations are in favour of an oxidatively induced apoptosis. Selenium compounds can, however, trigger apoptosis independently from DNA damage and a functional p53. Thus mechanisms distinct from oxidative damage might also be involved[40–43].

Cytostatic effects

In most cultured cells a concentration above 100 μM selenite is toxic and the cells die[44]. This effect may also be triggered by redox cycling of H_2Se, or methylselenol[24]. Whether tumour cells are more efficiently killed than other cells remains to be investigated.

Antiproliferative activity

Moderate concentrations of selenium compounds do not kill cells but rather retard cell growth. Part of this effect may be related to the ability of some compounds to produce DNA damage, as has been shown for selenite, and to trigger programmed cell death[25,45,46]. Selenium may, however, also alter the activity of enzymes involved in the regulation of proliferation and cell cycle, such as protein kinase C, cyclin-dependent kinase 2 or gadd 45[47-49].

Modulation of transcription factor activity

By still-undefined oxidative processes, NFκB is activated in the cytoplasm, but needs to be maintained at a reduced level in the nucleus for adequate DNA binding[50]. Thus, factors either influencing cytoplasmic oxidation and/or nuclear reduction modify NFκB activation. Inhibition of NFκB activation has been shown for selenite[51], overexpression of cGPx[52], or PHGPx[53]. On the other hand, the DNA-binding capacity of NFκB is maintained by keeping cysteine 62 in the p50 subunit in the reduced state by means of thioredoxin, which in turn is provided with reduction equivalents from NADPH catalysed by the selenoenzyme thioredoxin reductase[54]. Whether these regulatory phenomena play a role in the anticarcinogenic effects of selenium compounds remains to be elucidated.

Optimization of the immune system

The interplay of glutathione peroxidases and possibly other selenoproteins with the immune system has often been demonstrated; for example, antibody formation[1,55], activity of cytotoxic T lymphocytes and natural killer cells[56] were increased and the IL-2 receptor induced[57-60] with high dosages of selenium. The molecular mechanisms of these findings remain elusive.

Inhibition of angiogenesis

Increased selenium intake as Se-enriched garlic, selenite, or Se-methylselenocysteine was reported to suppress expression of the vascular growth factor VEGF in rats. Prevention of vascularization was thus suggested to be one of the mechanisms by which selenium can inhibit cancer promotion[61].

Alteration in DNA methylation and polyamine biosynthesis

Se-methylselenocysteine and others were shown to inhibit the activity of ornithine decarboxylase in colon cancer cells[62,63]. Apart from association with polyamines, gene activity is regulated by DNA methylation. DNA hypomethylation was observed in selenium-deficient Caco-2 cells, which could be reversed by supplementation with selenite[64]. Since these findings were also observed in the liver and colon of rats, alteration of DNA methylation was implicated in enhanced tumorigenesis under dietary selenium deficiency, but not considered for the chemoprotective effect of supranutritional intakes of selenium.

Modification of protein thiols

Interference of selenium compounds with protein thiols is an attractive hypothesis and would link global effects exerted by selenium compounds to defined signalling cascades and thus render selenium compounds specific. Thioredoxin reductase has been proposed as target[65], and a modification of protein kinase C was demonstrated[66]. Whether more targets can be identified, and whether this might be a common mechanism for many selenium compounds, awaits investigation.

Potential impact of poorly characterized selenoproteins

A 15 kDa selenoprotein is expressed in the endoplasmic reticulum in a complex with UDP-glucose:glycoprotein glucosyltransferase[67]. The latter is believed to be involved in the surveillance of correct folding of secreted proteins. Based on gene polymorphism studies, a relationship with the incidence of certain cancers is also discussed in ref. 68. The second selenoprotein associated with cancer is the gastrointestinal glutathione peroxidase.

GASTROINTESTINAL GLUTATHIONE PEROXIDASE

Detected in the gastrointestinal system and liver[69,70], GI-GPx was originally believed to prevent hydroperoxide absorption. GI-GPx, however, was also detected in oestrogen-negative breast tumour cell lines and tissues[71], where it could be induced by retinoic acid treatment[72]. A GI-GPx promoter analysis revealed several GATA sites[73] which have been shown to be implicated in growth and differentiation of intestinal epithelial cells[74]. The GI-GPx gene maps to chromosome14q24.1[75] close to the colon cancer susceptibility locus Ccs1[76]. Finally, a correlation between GI-GPx mRNA levels and resistance against dimethylhydrazine-induced colon cancer in rats was described[77]. These observations do not speak in favour of a simple barrier function.

GI-GPx is one of the most stable selenoproteins known to date. It is difficult to completely deplete GI-GPx protein by selenium deprivation in cultured cell lines[18]. Its mRNA is stable in selenium deficiency, and in some cells is even increased. The speed of its resynthesis upon selenium repletion exceeds by far the speed at which cGPx is resynthesized. It prevents cell damage by hydroperoxides in selenium deficiency[16] but does not prevent alterations in lipid metabolism caused either by linoleic acid hydroperoxide or its reduction product hydroxy-linoleic acid[78]. GI-GPx was not uniformly distributed in the epithelial layer of the small intestine and colon in humans[79]. In the ileum it was preferentially expressed in Paneth cells, which are not involved in absorption, again casting doubt on its function as a mere barrier against hydroperoxides. In the colon GI-GPx was found to be organized in distinct structures apically capping the nuclei of luminal epithelial cells[79]. Although reminiscent of Golgi vesicles, a co-localization with known Golgi markers was not achieved, leaving the nature of the vesicular structures unidentified. A comparison of healthy tissue and early and advanced stages of malignant transformation in the colon of patients with adenocarcinoma showed an increase of GI-GPx protein in these structures in early stages, but a disruption of the structures and spreading of GI-GPx protein over the entire cytoplasm in advanced stages[79]. These observations are confirmed by an increase of GI-GPx mRNA in human colorectal carcinomas[80]. The link to malignant transformation being unknown, these findings at least classify GI-GPx as a potential marker.

CONCLUSIONS

The precise role of selenium in cancer prevention remains unknown. Early epidemiological studies suggesting an increased deficiency have often been interpreted to unravel the mutagenic potential of peroxides that have to be eliminated by selenium-containing peroxidases. However, the vast majority of animal studies, as well as clinical studies, demonstrate that only selenium dosages beyond those optimizing the levels of glutathione peroxidases and other known selenoproteins are effective in the prevention of cancer. Significant differences in cancer prevention between different low molecular weight selenium compounds were also observed, which is not paralleled by their potency in improving selenoprotein synthesis. Instead of a summary, three still-unresolved questions emerge from the accumulated knowledge:

1. Does impaired hydroperoxide metabolism due to selenium deficiency really increase the risk of cancer initiation?
2. Is there any selenoprotein to be discovered that requires a higher selenium supply for optimal activity than, for example, cGPx or pGPx, and that is relevant to initiation or progression of malignancies?
3. Or has the efficacy of certain selenium compounds, that has amply been demonstrated in experimental carcinogenesis, to be considered as a pharmacodynamic characteristic of its own that is unrelated to physiological selenium metabolism?

Acknowledgement

This work was supported by the Deutsche Forschungsgemeinschaft (SPP 1087, Br 778/5-1).

References

1. Combs JGF, Combs SB. The Role of Selenium in Nutrition. Orlando, FL: Academic Press, 1986.
2. Schwarz K, Foltz CM. Selenium as an integral part of factor 3 against dietary necrotic liver degeneration. J Am Chem Soc. 1957;79:3292–3.
3. Lockitch G. Selenium: clinical significance and analytical concepts. Crit Rev Clin Lab Sci. 1989;27:483–541.
4. Yang G, Ge K, Chen J, Chen X. Selenium-related endemic diseases and the daily selenium requirement of humans. World Rev Nutr Diet. 1988;55:98–125.
5. Böck A. Selenium metabolism in bacteria. In: Hatfield LD, editor. Selenium: its Molecular Biology and Role in Human Health. Boston: Kluwer, 2001: 7–22.
6. Mansell JB, Berry MJ. Towards a mechanism for selenocysteine incorporation in eukaryotes. In: Hatfield DL, editor. Selenium: its Molecular Biology and Role in Human Health. Boston: Kluwer, 2001:69–80.
7. Lescure A, Fagegaltier D, Carbon P, Krol A. Protein factors mediating selenoprotein synthesis. Curr Protein Peptide Sci. 2002;3:143–51.

8. Bosl MR, Takaku K, Oshima M, Nishimura S, Taketo MM. Early embryonic lethality caused by targeted disruption of the mouse selenocysteine tRNA gene (Trsp). Proc Natl Acad Sci USA. 1997;94:5531–4.

9. Köhrle J, Brigelius-Flohé R, Böck A, Gärtner R, Meyer O, Flohé L. Selenium in biology: facts and medical perspectives. Biol Chem. 2000;381:849–64.

10. Flohé L, Andreesen JR, Brigelius-Flohé R, Maiorino M, Ursini F. Selenium, the element of the moon, in life on earth. IUBMB Life. 2000;49:411–20.

11. Gladyshev VN. Identity, evolution and function of selenoproteins and selenoprotein genes. In: Hatfield LD, editor. Selenium: its Molecular Biology and Role in Human Health. Boston: Kluwer, 2001:99–114.

12. Brigelius-Flohé R, Maiorino M, Ursini F, Flohé L. Selenium: An antioxidant? In: Cadenas E, Packer L, editors. Handbook of Antioxidants. New York: Marcel Dekker, 2001:633–64.

13. Brigelius-Flohé R. Tissue-specific functions of individual glutathione peroxidases. Free Radic Biol Med. 1999;27:951–65.

14. Flohé L, Brigelius-Flohé R. Selenoproteins of the glutathione system. In: Hatfield DL, editor. Selenium: its Molecular Biology and Role in Human Health. Boston: Kluwer, 2001:157–78.

15. Ursini F, Heim S, Kiess M et al. Dual function of the selenoprotein PHGPx during sperm maturation. Science. 1999;285:1393–6.

16. Wingler K, Müller C, Schmehl K, Florian S, Brigelius-Flohé R. Gastrointestinal glutathione peroxidase prevents transport of lipid hydroperoxides in Caco-2 cells. Gastroenterology. 2000;119:420–30.

17. Behne D, Kyriakopoulos A. Effects of dietary selenium on the tissue concentrations of type I iodothyronine 5'-deiodinase and other selenoproteins. Am J Clin Nutr. 1993;57:310–12S.

18. Wingler K, Böcher M, Flohé L, Kollmus H, Brigelius-Flohé R. mRNA stability and selenocysteine insertion sequence efficiency rank gastrointestinal glutathione peroxidase high in the hierarchy of selenoproteins. Eur J Biochem. 1999;259:149–57.

19. Shamberger RJ, Frost DV. Possible protective effect of selenium against human cancer. Can Med Assoc J. 1969;100(14):682.

20. Combs GF, Gray WP. Chemopreventive agents: selenium. Pharmacol Ther. 1998;79:179–92.

21. Clark LC, Combs GF, Tumbuli BW et al. Effects of selenium supplementation for cancer prevention in patients with carcinoma of the skin. J Am Med Assoc. 1996;25:1957–85.

22. Levander OA. Evolution of human dietary standards for selenium. In: Hatfield LD, editor. Selenium: its Molecular Biology and Role in Human Health. Boston: Kluwer, 2001:299–312.

23. Berggren MM, Mangin JF, Gasdaka JR, Powis G. Effect of selenium on rat thioredoxin reductase activity: increase by supranutritional selenium and decrease by selenium deficiency. Biochem Pharmacol. 1999;57:187–93.

24. Spallholz JE. On the nature of selenium toxicity and carcinostatic activity. Free Radic Biol Med. 1994;17:45–64.

25. Poirier KA, Milner JA. Factors influencing the antitumorigenic properties of selenium in mice. J Nutr. 1983;113:2147–54.

26. Soda K, Esaki N, Nakamura T, Karai N, Chocat P, Tanaka H. Selenocysteine beta-lyase: a novel pyridoxal enzyme. Prog Clin Biol Res. 1984;144A:319–28.

27. Whanger PD, Butler JA. Effects of various dietary levels of selenium as selenite or selenomethionine on tissue selenium levels and glutathione peroxidase activity in rats. J Nutr. 1988;118:846–52.

28. Ip C, White G. Mammary cancer chemoprevention by inorganic and organic selenium: single agent treatment or in combination with vitamin E and their effects on *in vitro* immune functions. Carcinogenesis. 1987;8:1763–6.

29. Ip C, Hayes C. Tissue selenium levels in selenium-supplemented rats and their relevance in mammary cancer protection. Carcinogenesis. 1989;10:921–5.

30. Ip C, Ganther HE. Activity of methylated forms of selenium in cancer prevention. Cancer Res. 1990;50:1206–11.

31. Ip C, Hayes C, Budnick RM, Ganther HE. Chemical form of selenium, critical metabolites, and cancer prevention. Cancer Res. 1991;51:595–600.

32. Ip C, Thompson HJ, Zhu Z, Ganther HE. *In vitro* and *in vivo* studies of methylseleninic acid: evidence that a monomethylated selenium metabolite is critical for cancer chemoprevention. Cancer Res. 2000;60:2882–6.

33. Ip C, Zhu Z, Thompson HJ, Lisk D, Ganther HE. Chemoprevention of mammary cancer with Se-allylselenocysteine and other selenoamino acids in the rat. Anticancer Res. 1999;19:2875–80.
34. Kotrebai M, Birringer M, Tyson JF, Block E, Uden PC. Identification of the principal selenium compounds in selenium-enriched natural sample extracts by ion-pair liquid chromatography with inductively coupled plasma- and electrospray ionization-mass spectrometric detection. Anal Commun. 1999;36:249–52.
35. Ip C, Birringer M, Block E et al. Chemical speciation influences comparative activity of selenium-enriched garlic and yeast in mammary cancer prevention. J Agric Food Chem. 2000; 48:2062–70.
36. Kotrebai M, Birringer M, Tyson JF, Block E, Uden PC. Selenium speciation in enriched and natural samples by HPLC-ICP-MS and HPLC-ESI-MS with perfluorinated carboxylic acid ion-pairing agents. Analyst. 2000;125:71–8.
37. Ho YS, Magnenat JL, Bronson RT et al. Mice deficient in cellular glutathione peroxidase develop normally and show no increased sensitivity to hyperoxia. J Biol Chem. 1997;272:16644–51.
38. Cheng WH, Ho YS, Valentine BA, Ross DA, Combs GF Jr, Lei XG. Cellular glutathione peroxidase is the mediator of body selenium to protect against paraquat lethality in transgenic mice. J Nutr. 1998;128:1070–6.
39. Spallholz JE, Shriver BJ, Reid TW. Dimethyldiselenide and methylseleninic acid generate superoxide in an in vitro chemiluminescence assay in the presence of glutathione: implications for the anticarcinogenic activity of L-selenomethionine and L-Se-methylselenocysteine. Nutr Cancer. 2001;40:34–41.
40. Sundaram N, Pahwa AK, Ard MD, Lin N, Perkins E, Bowles AP Jr. Selenium causes growth inhibition and apoptosis in human brain tumor cell lines. J Neurooncol. 2000;46:125–33.
41. Zhu Z, Jiang W, Ganther HE, Ip C, Thompson HJ. In vitro effects of Se-allylselenocysteine and Se-propylselenocysteine on cell growth, DNA integrity, and apoptosis. Biochem Pharmacol. 2000;60:1467–73.
42. Shen H, Yang C, Liu J, Ong C. Dual role of glutathione in selenite-induced oxidative stress and apoptosis in human hepatoma cells. Free Radic Biol Med. 2000;28:1115–24.
43. Thompson HJ, Wilson A, Lu J et al. Comparison of the effects of an organic and an inorganic form of selenium on a mammary carcinoma cell line. Carcinogenesis. 1994;15:183–6.
44. Brigelius-Flohé R, Lötzer K, Maurer S, Schultz M, Leist M. Utilization of selenium from different chemical entities for selenoprotein biosynthesis by mammalian cell lines. Biofactors. 1995;5:125–31.
45. Lu J, Jiang C, Kaeck M et al. Dissociation of the genotoxic and growth inhibitory effects of selenium. Biochem Pharmacol. 1995;50:213–19.
46. Cho DY, Jung U, Chung AS. Induction of apoptosis by selenite and selenodiglutathione in HL-60 cells: correlation with cytotoxicity. Biochem Mol Biol Int. 1999;47:781–93.
47. Sinha R, Medina D. Inhibition of cdk2 kinase activity by methylselenocysteine in synchronized mouse mammary epithelial tumor cells. Carcinogenesis. 1997;18:1541–7.
48. Sinha R, Kiley SC, Lu JX et al. Effects of methylselenocysteine on PKC activity, cdk2 phosphorylation and gadd gene expression in synchronized mouse mammary epithelial tumor cells. Cancer Lett. 1999;146:135–45.
49. Kaeck M, Lu J, Strange R, Ip C, Ganther HE, Thompson HJ. Differential induction of growth arrest inducible genes by selenium compounds. Biochem Pharmacol. 1997;53:921–6.
50. Flohé L, Brigelius-Flohé R, Saliou C, Traber MG, Packer L. Redox regulation of NF-kappa B activation. Free Radic Biol Med. 1997;22:1115–26.
51. Makropoulos V, Bruning T, Schulze-Osthoff K. Selenium-mediated inhibition of transcription factor NF-kappa B and HIV- 1 LTR promoter activity. Arch Toxicol. 1996;70:277–83.
52. Kretz-Remy C, Mehlen P, Mirault ME, Arrigo AP. Inhibition of I kappa B-alpha phosphorylation and degradation and subsequent NF-kappa B activation by glutathione peroxidase overexpression. J Cell Biol. 1996;133:1083–93.
53. Brigelius-Flohé R, Friedrichs B, Maurer S, Schultz M, Streicher R. Interleukin-1-induced nuclear factor kappa B activation is inhibited by overexpression of phospholipid hydroperoxide glutathione peroxidase in a human endothelial cell line. Biochem J. 1997;328:199–203.
54. Matthews JR, Wakasugi N, Virelizier JL, Yodoi J, Hay RT. Thioredoxin regulates the DNA binding activity of NF-kappa B by reduction of a disulphide bond involving cysteine 62. Nucl Acids Res. 1992;20:3821–30.

55. Spallholz JE, Martin JL, Gerlach ML, Heinzerling RH. Enhanced immunoglobulin M and immunoglobulin G antibody titers in mice fed selenium. Infect Immun. 1973;8:841–2.
56. Kiremidjian-Schumacher L, Roy M, Wishe HI, Cohen MW, Stotzky G. Supplementation with selenium augments the functions of natural killer and lymphokine-activated killer cells. Biol Trace Elem Res. 1996;52:227–39.
57. Kiremidjian-Schumacher L, Roy M, Wishe HI, Cohen MW, Stotzky G. Regulation of cellular immune responses by selenium. Biol Trace Elem Res. 1992;33:23–35.
58. Kiremidjian-Schumacher L, Roy M, Wishe HI, Cohen MW, Stotzky G. Supplementation with selenium and human immune cell functions. II. Effect on cytotoxic lymphocytes and natural killer cells. Biol Trace Elem Res. 1994;41:115–27.
59. Roy M, Kiremidjian-Schumacher L, Wishe HI, Cohen MW, Stotzky G. Effect of selenium on the expression of high affinity interleukin 2 receptors. Proc Soc Exp Biol Med. 1992;200: 36–43.
60. Roy M, Kiremidjian-Schumacher L, Wishe HI, Cohen MW, Stotzky G. Supplementation with selenium and human immune cell functions. I. Effect on lymphocyte proliferation and inter-leukin 2 receptor expression. Biol Trace Elem Res. 1994;41:103–14.
61. Jiang C, Jiang W, Ip C, Ganther H, Lu J. Selenium-induced inhibition of angiogenesis in mam-mary cancer at chemopreventive levels of intake. Mol Carcinogen. 1999;26:213–25.
62. McGarrity TJ, Peiffer LP, Hartle RJ. Effect of selenium on growth, S-adenosylmethionine and polyamine biosynthesis in human colon cancer cells. Anticancer Res. 1993;8:811–15.
63. Thompson HJ, Ip C, Ganther HE. Changes in ornithine decarboxylase activity and polyamine levels in response to eight different forms of selenium. J Inorg Biochem. 1991;44:283–92.
64. Davis CD, Uthus EO, Finley JW. Dietary selenium and arsenic affect DNA methylation in vitro in Caco-2 cells and in vivo in rat liver and colon. J Nutr. 2000;130:2903–9.
65. Ganther HE. Selenium metabolism, selenoproteins and mechanisms of cancer prevention: complexities with thioredoxin reductase. Carcinogenesis. 1999;20:1657–66.
66. Gopalakrishna R, Gundimeda U, Chen ZH. Cancer-preventive selenocompounds induce a specific redox modification of cysteine-rich regions in Ca(2+)-dependent isoenzymes of protein kinase C. Arch Biochem Biophys. 1997;348:25–36.
67. Korotkov KV, Kumaraswamy E, Zhou Y, Hatfield DL, Gladyshev VN. Association between the 15-kDa selenoprotein and UDP-glucose : glycoprotein glucosyltransferase in the endoplasmic reticulum of mammalian cells. J Biol Chem. 2001;276:15330–6.
68. Gladyshev VN, Diamond AM, Hatfield DL. The 15 kDa selenoprotein (Sep15): functional studies and a role in cancer etiology. In: Hatfield DL, editor. Selenium: its Molecular Biology and Role in Human Health. Boston: Kluwer, 2001:147–55.
69. Chu FF, Esworthy RS. The expression of an intestinal form of glutathione peroxidase (GSHPx-GI) in rat intestinal epithelium. Arch Biochem Biophys. 1995;323:288–94.
70. Brigelius-Flohé R, Wingler K, Müller C. Estimation of individual types of glutathione peroxi-dases. Methods Enzymol. 2002;347:101–12.
71. Esworthy RS, Swiderek KM, Ho YS, Chu FF. Selenium-dependent glutathione peroxidase-GI is a major glutathione peroxidase activity in the mucosal epithelium of rodent intestine. Biochem Biophys Acta. 1998;1381:213–26.
72. Chu FF, Esworthy RS, Lee L, Wilczynski S. Retinoic acid induces Gpx2 gene expression in MCF-7 human breast cancer cells. J Nutr. 1999;129:1846–54.
73. Kelner MJ, Bagnell RD, Montoya MA, Lanham KA. Structural organization of the human gastrointestinal glutathione peroxidase (GPX2) promoter and 3'-nontranscribed region: transcriptional response to exogenous redox agents. Gene. 2000;248:109–16.
74. Gao X, Sedgwick T, Shi YB, Evans T. Distinct functions are implicated for the GATA-4, -5, and -6 transcription factors in the regulation of intestine epithelial cell differentiation. Mol Cell Biol. 1998;18:2901–11.
75. Chu FF, Rohan de Silva HA, Esworthy RS et al. Polymorphism and chromosomal localization of the GI-form of human glutathione peroxidase (GPX2) on 14q24.1 by in situ hybridization. Genomics. 1996;32:272–6.
76. Jacoby RF, Hohman C, Marshall DJ et al. Genetic analysis of colon cancer susceptibility in mice. Genomics. 1994;22:381–7.
77. Chu FF, Esworthy RS, Ho YS, Bermeister M, Swiderek K, Elliott RW. Expression and chromo-somal mapping of mouse Gpx2 gene encoding the gastrointestinal form of glutathione peroxi-dase, GPX-GI. Biomed Environ Sci. 1997;10:156–62.

285

78. Müller C, Friedrichs B, Wingler K, Brigelius-Flohé R. Perturbation of lipid metabolism by linoleic acid hydroperoxide in CaCo-2 cells. Biol Chem. 2002;383:637–48.
79. Florian S, Wingler K, Schmehl K *et al.* Cellular and subcellular localization of gastrointestinal glutathione peroxidase in normal and malignant human intestinal tissue. Free Rad Res. 2001; 35:655–63.
80. Mörk H, Al-Taie OH, Bähr K *et al.* Inverse mRNA expression of the selenocysteine-containing proteins GI-GPx and SeP in colorectal adenomas compared with adjacent normal mucosa. Nutr Cancer. 2000;37:108–16.

32
Calcium: a protective agent against colorectal cancer?

J. H. KLEIBEUKER, E. G. E. DE VRIES and R. VAN DER MEER

INTRODUCTION

For a long time dietary composition has been considered to be a major contributing factor in the aetiology of colorectal cancer. A diet high in fat was repeatedly perceived as an especially important risk factor[1]. It was generally assumed that a high-fat diet affected colorectal cancer risk mainly through the process of promotion, in particular by increasing epithelial cell proliferative activity. Both in animals and in humans a high fat intake has been shown to induce an increase of proliferative activity of the colorectal epithelium[2,3]. Hyperproliferation makes cells more susceptible to adverse mutations and in addition stimulates outgrowth of (pre)malignant cells into tumours. Colonic epithelial hyperproliferation has been found by many investigators to be increased in subjects with an increased risk of colon cancer[4]. One of the mechanisms through which a high intake of fat induces an increase of epithelial proliferation might be that it causes an increase of concentrations of fatty acids and bile acids in the colonic contents. Both fatty acids and bile acids have been shown experimentally to be cytotoxic to colonic epithelial cells and to stimulate compensatory mitotic activity. Direct stimulation of the mitotic process may also be involved, through stimulating protein kinase C activity in the epithelial cells by fatty acids and bile acids, and especially by diacylglycerol[5].

CALCIUM AND COLORECTAL CANCER

A hypothesis

In 1984 Newmark et al.[6] published a hypothesis on the interactions of fatty and bile acids, calcium and phosphate in relation to colon cancer. They suggested that calcium might have beneficial effects on colonic epithelium by binding the fatty and bile acids in the colonic lumen, thus forming insoluble soaps that would be harmless to the colonic mucosa. In this way increased oral calcium intake might help in exerting a proliferation-inhibiting effect on colonic epithelium, and might protect against the development of colon cancer. The authors further hypothesized that phosphate would compete for calcium in the colon, to produce insoluble calcium phosphate. The proposed protective effect of calcium might thus be opposed by an excess of phosphate. This hypothesis has led to a large number of investigations into the possible role of calcium as a protective agent against the development of colorectal neoplasms. A concise review of these studies will be presented in this chapter.

Epidemiology

Many studies have been performed to evaluate the association of the level of daily calcium intake from food and/or supplements with the risk for developing colorectal adenomas and/or cancer. A quantitative summary[7] of the early studies did not yield support for a preventive effect of calcium. At the same time, results of two large prospective cohort studies, i.e. the (male) Health Professionals Follow-up Study[8] and the (female) Nurses' Health Study[9], similarly indicated that calcium intake did not substantially affect colorectal cancer risk. Subsequent studies[10–14], however, mostly showed a modest protective effect of a high calcium intake, though not all studies could confirm this[15]. In one study[16] even a protective effect of a low calcium intake was found in a subset of persons, carrying a specific polymorphism in the vitamin D receptor gene. Recently the association between calcium consumption and colon cancer risk was re-examined in the cohorts of the Health Professionals Follow-up Study and the Nurses' Health Study[17]. This time an inverse association between higher total calcium intake and distal colon cancer was found, both in women (RR 0.73) and in men (RR 0.58). For proximal cancer no such association was found. Surprisingly, the incremental benefit of additional calcium intake beyond approximately 700 mg/day appeared to be minimal.

In vitro studies

Calcium is an important mediator of many cellular biological processes, including cell proliferation. An increased intake of calcium might thus affect cell proliferative activity through a direct effect of calcium. Contradictory results have been obtained in this respect, when incubating human colorectal biopsies with increasing concentrations of calcium: one study showing a decrease of cell proliferation[18]; another showed no effect[19]. In a third study[20] the role of the Ca^{2+}-sensing receptor in mediating effects of extracellular Ca^{2+} on cellular proliferation was investigated in Caco-2 cells, a human colon adenocarcinoma-derived cell line. Activation of this receptor by either calcium or a specific agonist, Gd3+, inhibited cell replication. Both normal colonic epithelium and carcinomatous lesions of the colon revealed cells positive for this receptor by immunostaining. Though these data are provocative, it remains questionable whether a high calcium intake affects the colonic epithelium through a direct effect of calcium on the epithelial cells.

Other *in-vitro* studies have focused on the interactions of calcium with fatty acids, bile acids and other cytotoxic substances. The binding of calcium to fatty and bile acids to form insoluble soaps is a well-known phenomenon. However, the supposed role of phosphate in this process, as formulated by Newmark et al.[6], was purely hypothetical. In a series of *in-vitro* studies it has now been shown that bile acids are not precipitated by soluble Ca^{2+}, but that phosphate is a requisite for this[21-23]. This precipitation is an almost unique property of freshly formed, amorphous calcium phosphate, and is rarely observed with aged, more crystalline calcium phosphates and with other insoluble calcium salts. The mechanism of this precipitation is by hydrophobic aggregation of bile acid monomers at the surface of the amorphous calcium phosphate[23]. As fatty acids and bile acids are thought to promote colon carcinogenesis at least in part through their cytotoxic effects on colorectal epithelial cells it was studied whether calcium could counteract these effects. Soluble Ca^{2+} did not reduce the cytotoxic effect of bile acids *in vitro*, whereas calcium phosphate almost abolished it, as measured in a haemolysis assay[24]. Calcium phosphate also potently reduced the cytolytic effects of fatty acids and of the highly lytic mixed micelles, formed by the addition of small amounts of bile acids to fatty acids[25]. In slight contrast to these results it was shown by other investigators[26] that $CaCl_2$ could inhibit the hyperproliferative effect of deoxycholic acid on colonic crypt cells in a short-term culture system of colonic biopsies.

Recent studies indicate that the association between dietary fat intake and colorectal cancer risk is not as strong as presumed for many years[27]. As a part of the fat intake is due to meat consumption, attention shifted to the relationship between cancer risk and meat intake. A systematic review of prospective cohort studies[28] showed a significant positive association, in particular with the intake of red meat and of processed meat. From these results we hypothesized that haem might be the offending component in red meat. Feeding rats a haem-supplemented diet did cause an increase in cytolytic activity of faecal water and colonic epithelial cell hyperproliferation (see below). When adding freshly formed, amorphous calcium phosphate to faecal water of haem-fed rats its cyto-toxicity was completely abolished, suggesting that calcium might mediate its protective effect by preventing the harm induced by the haem in red meat[29].

Studies in animals

Studies in rodents have repeatedly shown that a high calcium intake causes a reduction of epithelial cell proliferation in the colon, whether induced by increased colonic concentrations of fatty and/or bile acids or not[4]. In one study calcium supplementation was found to increase apoptosis in the distal murine colonic epithelium[30]. Several studies have indicated that tumorigenesis is inhibited by calcium supplementation[4], and a similar effect was found on colon aberrant crypt formation[31]. With regard to the mechanism of the effect of calcium, studies by our group in rats have shown the following. First it was determined whether insoluble calcium phosphate is formed *in vivo* in the intestine of rats. Intestinal and faecal samples of rats, fed low and high calcium phosphate purified diets, were analysed[32]. It was found that calcium and phosphate already precipitated in the small intestine and were almost completely precipitated in colon and faeces. In addition, it was observed that the solubility of faecal calcium and phosphate is determined by the pH of its solubility product, analogous to that observed for amorphous calcium phosphate *in vitro*[33]. Thus, the amount of soluble Ca^{2+} is low, whereas that of amorphous calcium phosphate is high in the colon. The colonic interactions between calcium, phosphate, and bile acids and their effects on colonic epithelial parameters were studied in rats fed a Western high-risk control diet, containing a low amount of calcium (20 μmol/g)[34]. This control diet simulates a human calcium intake of about 400 mg/day (10 mmol/ day). The amount of calcium phosphate in this diet was increased to 180 μmol/g by supplementing the diet with milk mineral. Faecal water was isolated to quantitate the physiologically relevant cytolytic surfactants, as only soluble surfactants are lytic. Supplementation of the low-calcium control diet with calcium phosphate drastically decreased the concentration of bile acids and fatty acids in faecal water and inhibited its cytolytic activity, measured with the same haemolysis bioassay mentioned above. Milk mineral also inhibited epitheliolysis, measured as the release of the epithelial cell marker alkaline phosphatase, as well as colonic epithelial proliferation. In other experiments the proposed inhibitory effects of dietary phosphate[32], and the effects of different types of dietary calcium[34], were studied. Taken together, these experiments confirm earlier studies that have shown that dietary calcium inhibits colonic epithelial proliferation. They extend these studies by showing that this effect is not inhibited by phosphate and that milk calcium has at least a similar protective effect. In addition, they show that the protective effect of calcium is mediated by a decrease in solubility of colonic surfactants, e.g. bile acids and fatty acids, and an inhibition of luminal cytolytic activity, epithelial cell damage and proliferation. It was found that cytolytic activity of faecal water, as well as epitheliolysis, were correlated with colonic epithelial proliferation ($r = 0.97$ and 0.88, respectively), suggesting cause and effect relationships.

As mentioned above, recently the effects of haem supplementation on risk factors for colonic cancer in rats were studied. Supplementing the diet with haem induced a marked increase in cytotoxicity of faecal water and colonic epithelial cell proliferative activity[35]. This effect was not due to the singular components of haem, i.e. porphyrin and iron. Additional experiments showed that the hyperproliferative effect of haem was slightly lower on a low-fat diet, compared to a high-fat diet[36]. Based on the finding that cytotoxicity of faecal water could be abolished by the addition of freshly formed, amorphous calcium phosphate, it was then studied whether calcium, added to the food, could counteract the effects of haem supplementation on cytolytic activity[29]. This proved to be the case, adding further strength to the supposition that calcium may protect against colon cancer, at least in part through binding haem-derived cytotoxic substances in the colon.

Studies in humans

In 1985 Lipkin and Newmark[37] published their study on the effect of calcium supplementation on rectal epithelial cell proliferation in subjects at increased risk for colorectal cancer. They showed that increasing oral calcium intake by about 1200 mg/day was associated with a marked decrease of epithelial proliferation. This study prompted a series of studies by other investigators on the effect of calcium in high-risk subjects. Most of the early studies were not placebo-controlled. Almost invariably they showed a decrease of rectal cell proliferation after a supplementation period of 1 or more months[4]. Only in one study[38] were biopsies for determination of proliferation taken proximal to the rectum, namely from the sigmoid colon. Surprisingly, in that study, proliferative activity increased during calcium supplementation. More recently the results of a number of randomized studies have become available. About half of these studies were small and comprised 30 subjects or less. Four were carried out in patients who had had sporadic adenomas removed in the past. Two of the studies[39,40] were placebo-controlled crossover studies, both showing a reduction of rectal epithelial proliferation. The other two[41,42] were placebo-controlled parallel group studies. In one of these[41] biopsies were taken from the sigmoid, not from the rectum. Neither of the two yielded any significant effect of calcium. The other studies were carried out in patients with familial adenomatous polyposis groups an effect was one[43] showing a reduction of proliferative activity, the other[44] not; in patients operated on for colon cancer[45] or with ulcerative colitis[46]: in neither of the two observed; and one in first-degree family members of patients with hereditary nonpolyposis colorectal cancer[46–47]. In this latter study biopsies were taken from the rectum, sigmoid and descending colon. Calcium slightly but significantly lowered labelling with bromodeoxyuridine in the upper crypt compartment of the rectal epithelium, without an effect on total crypt labelling, whereas no effect was observed in the sigmoid or descending colon. Six placebo-controlled studies[48–53] comprised more than 50 subjects each; all studies were performed in sporadic adenoma patients. Only in one of these[52] was calcium supplementation associated with a decrease in epithelial proliferative activity in the whole crypts, whereas in two[48,52], including the former one, such a decrease was observed in the upper part of the crypts. In another of these six studies[53], epithelial proliferative activity was measured not only in the rectum, but also in the caecum and in the transverse and sigmoid colon. No effect of calcium was observed in these parts of the colon either. In the study[52] showing an effect on total and upper crypt proliferative activity a lower fat and a higher carbohydrate, fibre or fluid intake were each found to interact with the calcium supplementation to decrease proliferation.

Two studies addressed the effect of dairy products on rectal epithelial cell proliferation. In the first[54], a randomized, single-blind controlled study, a significant lowering effect on proliferative activity in total crypts and their upper parts was observed. In addition, beneficial effects were seen on some differentiation markers. In the other[55], a randomized, single-blind crossover trial, no differences between the two interventions were apparent. It is apparent from all this that calcium supplementation may induce some beneficial change in proliferative indices of the rectal epithelium, but that no major conclusions with respect to a cancer-preventive effect can be drawn.

With regard to the mechanisms through which calcium might affect colorectal carcinogenesis, our group has performed a number of studies. To ascertain the relevance of the results of our biochemical and animal studies for human physiology we first studied the intestinal association of calcium, phosphate and bile acids[22]. Because in human diets phosphate is far in excess of calcium, supplemental dietary calcium (without phosphate) may stimulate complexation with phosphate and/or bile acids. This increased complexation can be measured only as an increase in faecal excretion of phosphate and bile acids, provided that the intake of phosphate is maintained constant. In healthy subjects supplemental calcium carbonate increased the faecal excretion of both phosphate and bile acids, which indicates the intestinal formation of an insoluble complex of calcium, phosphate and bile acids. Also in humans the solubility of faecal calcium and phosphate is determined by the solubility product of amorphous calcium phosphate[56]. Using the calcium chelator EDTA, we found that resolubilization of calcium resulted in an increase of soluble phosphate and of soluble bile acids[22]. This shows that calcium, phosphate and bile acids are present in faeces as an insoluble complex. We also studied the effects of calcium on duodenal bile acid composition[22], and showed that calcium decreased the proportions of the hydrophobic and cytolytic dihydroxy bile acids chenodeoxycholate and deoxycholate, and increased that of the hydrophilic, less cytolytic trihydroxy bile acid cholate. These results suggest that calcium lowers the cytolytic activity of the soluble bile acids in the intestinal lumen. In line with this we found that calcium decreased the concentration of hydrophobic surfactants in faecal water and inhibited the cytolytic activity of faecal water[56]. Similar effects of supplemental calcium on faecal bile acid excretion, duodenal bile acid composition and cytolytic activity of faecal water were obtained in patients with colonic adenomas[57].

These effects of calcium supplementation of the diet prompted us to study whether calcium in the habitual diet has similar protective effects on the luminal metabolic risk factors. In a typical Western diet about 70% of dietary calcium is derived from milk and dairy products. Therefore we studied the effects of habitual dietary calcium in a double-blind crossover experiment using specially prepared milk products[58]. During the experimental period of 2 weeks the male volunteers consumed a constant habitual diet in which all liquid dairy products were replaced by either placebo milk/yogurt or regular, high-calcium-containing milk/yogurt. These products differed only in calcium content and provided 3 and 30 mmol of Ca^{2+}/day for the placebo and calcium period, respectively. At the end of each period the faeces were quantitatively collected for 3 days and urine for 1 day. Minerals were measured in faeces and urine to determine whether the total daily output was in accordance with the designed intake of nutrients. Faecal water was prepared by centrifugation of homogenized faeces and its composition determined by standard procedures. Cytolytic activity was measured as lysis of erythrocytes by faecal water. The measured total excretion of calcium differed by 27 mmol/day, which is exactly the difference in calcium content of the supplied placebo and calcium milk products. Milk calcium significantly increased faecal pH and the faecal excretion of phosphate, bile acids, and fatty acids, indicating intestinal calcium phosphate formation and precipitation of bile acids and fatty acids. Calcium about halved the concentration of bile acids and fatty acids in faecal water, which implies that it precipitates these lipids. Neutral steroids and phospholipids are probably solubilized by hydrophobic bile acids and thus also precipitated by calcium. To quantitate the effects on hydrophobicity of bile acids we also determined their composition in faecal water by capillary gas chromatography. On placebo milk, faecal water bile acids consist mainly (about 80%) of the secondary bile acids deoxycholate and lithocholate. Only the concentration of these bile acids was significantly decreased by milk calcium. Our in-vitro work shows that these hydrophobic secondary bile acids have very severe cytolytic effects[24]. In line with these in-vitro results we found that milk calcium drastically inhibited the cytolytic activity of faecal water. Other investigators[59] have confirmed the faecal water cytotoxicity-lowering effect of a diet rich in dairy products.

As mentioned earlier, a high-fat intake might also stimulate proliferation by increasing the activity of protein kinase C by fat-derived substances such as diacylglycerol. Studies in patients with an intestinal bypass for morbid obesity have shown that these subjects have an increased rectal epithelial cell proliferative activity[60] and have very high diacylglycerol concentrations in their faeces[61], both of which are reduced by calcium supplementation, suggesting an association between the two. The precipitation of fatty acids and bile acids by calcium might also be involved in the reduction of cell proliferation in these cases.

Taken together, the studies in humans indicate that calcium supplementation strongly reduces several metabolic risk factors in the colonic lumen but, on the other hand, does not appreciably affect colonic epithelial cell proliferative activity. In addition, from the epidemiological studies, a modest protective effect was the best that could be derived. So the expectations for the large-scale studies on the effect of calcium on adenoma recurrence after endoscopic polypectomy were not high. Notwithstanding these low expectations, calcium was shown to reduce the number of new adenomas, and it is the first agent that was shown to do so in a large-scale randomized controlled trial: in 832 evaluable patients 1200 mg elemental calcium daily reduced the number of subjects with recurrent adenomas by almost 20% and the number of new adenomas by almost 25% after 3 years, compared to placebo[62]. Two smaller studies[63,64] yielded results in accordance with those mentioned above, but lacked power to provide statistical significance. Further analysis of the data from the first of these studies suggests that calcium especially protects against the occurrence of advanced adenomas[65].

CONCLUSION

Calcium supplementation would be a very attractive option to prevent colorectal cancer in high-risk subjects. It is easy to administer, well tolerable and non-toxic. It may easily be incorporated into the diet by increasing the consumption of dairy products. Concerning possible adverse effects, only interference with iron absorption has been well documented[66,67]. Biochemical studies and metabolic studies in animals and humans are all in accordance with each other, and indicate that calcium precipitates luminal cytolytic substances such as bile acids, fatty acids and haem-derived compounds, thus reducing luminal cytolytic activity. In rats this reduction nicely correlates with reduction of parameters of intestinal epitheliolysis and colonic cell proliferation. In addition colonic tumorigenesis is generally inhibited by calcium in animal models. Studies on the effects of calcium on human colorectal epithelium are not as uniform in their conclusions. Nevertheless, calcium is the first agent indisputably shown to be able to reduce adenoma recurrence after polypectomy. Whether this really means that calcium protects against colorectal cancer remains to be proven. This question should be included in cancer-prevention studies whenever possible.

Acknowledgements

This work was supported by the Dutch Cancer Society (grants GUKC 89-08, RUG 94-785) and the Netherlands Organization of Scientific Research, Medical Sciences (grants NWO 900-562-078, NWO 904-62-167).

References

1. Potter JD, Slattery ML, Bostick RM, Gapstur SM. Colon cancer: a review of the epidemiology. Epidemiol Rev. 1993;15:499–545.
2. Bird RP, Medline A, Furrer R, Bruce WR. Toxicity of orally administered fat to the colonic epithelium of mice. Carcinogenesis. 1985;6:1063–6.
3. Stadler J, Stern HS, Yeung KS et al. Effect of high fat consumption on cell proliferation activity of colorectal mucosa and on soluble faecal bile acids. Gut. 1988;29:1326–31.
4. Kleibeuker JH, Cats A, Van der Meer R, Lapré JA, De Vries EGE. Calcium supplementation as prophylaxis against colon cancer? Dig Dis. 1994;12:85–97.
5. Morotomi M, Guillem JG, LoGerfo P et al. Production of diacylglycerol, an activator of protein kinase C, by human intestinal microflora. Cancer Res. 1990;50:3595–9.
6. Newmark HL, Wargovich MJ, Bruce WR. Colon cancer and dietary fat, phosphate, and calcium: a hypothesis. J Natl Cancer Inst. 1984;72:1323–5.
7. Bergsma-Kadijk JA, Van 't Veer P, Kampman E, Burema J. Calcium does not protect against colorectal neoplasia. Epidemiology. 1996;7:590–7.
8. Kearney J, Giovannucci E, Rimm EB et al. Calcium, vitamin D and dairy foods and the occurrence of colon cancer in men. Am J Epidemiol. 1996;143:907–17.
9. Martínez ME, Giovannucci EL, Colditz GA et al. Calcium, vitamin D, and the occurrence of colorectal cancer among women. J Natl Cancer Inst. 1996;88:1375–82.
10. Zheng W, Anderson KE, Kushi LH et al. A prospective cohort study of intake of calcium, vitamin D, and other micronutrients in relation to incidence of rectal cancer among postmenopausal women. Cancer Epidemiol Biomarkers Prev. 1998;7:221–5.
11. Hyman J, Baron JA, Dain BJ et al. Dietary and supplemental calcium and the recurrence of colorectal adenomas. Cancer Epidemiol Biomarkers Prev. 1998;7:291–5.
12. Pietinen P, Malila N, Virtanen M et al. Diet and risk of colorectal cancer in a cohort of Finnish men. Cancer Causes Control. 1999;10:387–96.
13. Whelan RL, Horvath KD, Gleason NR et al. Vitamin and calcium supplement use is associated with decreased adenoma recurrence in patients with a previous history of neoplasia. Dis Colon Rectum. 1999;42:212–17.
14. Kampman E, Slattery ML, Caan B, Potter JD. Calcium, vitamin D, sunshine exposure, dairy products and colon cancer risk (United States). Cancer Causes Control. 2000;11:459–66.
15. Jarvinen R, Knekt P, Hakulinen T, Aromaa A. Prospective study on milk products, calcium and cancers of the colon and rectum. Eur J Clin Nutr. 2001;55:1000–7.
16. Kim HS, Newcomb A, Ulrich CM et al. Vitamin D receptor polymorphism and the risk of colorectal adenomas: evidence of interaction with dietary vitamin D and calcium. Cancer Epidemiol Biomarkers Prev. 2001;10:869–74.
17. Wu K, Willett WC, Fuchs CS, Colditz GA, Giovannucci EL. Calcium intake and risk of colon cancer in women and men. J Natl Cancer Inst. 2002;94:437–46.
18. Lipkin M, Friedman E, Winawer SJ et al. Colonic epithelial cell proliferation in responders and nonresponders to supplemental dietary calcium. Cancer Res. 1989;49:248–54.
19. Bartram H-P, Scheppach W, Schmid H et al. Proliferation of human colonic mucosa as an intermediate biomarker of carcinogenesis: effects of butyrate, deoxycholate, calcium, ammonia, and pH. Cancer Res. 1993;53:3283–8.
20. Kallay E, Bajna E, Wrba F, Kriwanek S, Peterlik M, Cross HS. Dietary calcium and growth modulation of human colon cancer cells: role of the extracellular calcium-sensing receptor. Cancer Detect Prev. 2000;24:127–36.
21. Van der Meer R, De Vries HT. Differential binding of glycine- and taurine-conjugated bile acids to insoluble calcium phosphate. Biochem J. 1985;229:265–8.
22. Van der Meer R, Welberg JWM, Kuipers F et al. Effects of supplemental dietary calcium on the intestinal association of calcium, phosphate, and bile acids. Gastroenterology. 1990;99:1653–9.
23. Govers MJAP, Termont DSML, Van Aken GA, Van der Meer R. Characterization of the adsorption of conjugated and unconjugated bile acids to insoluble, amorphous calcium phosphate. J Lipid Res. 1994;35:741–8.
24. Van der Meer R, Termont DSML, De Vries HT. Differential effects of calcium ions and calcium phosphate on cytotoxicity of bile acids. Am J Physiol. 1991;260:G142–7.
25. Lapré JA, Termont DSML, Groen AK, Van der Meer R. Lytic effects of mixed micelles of fatty acids and bile acids. Am J Physiol. 1992;263:G333–7.

26. Bartram HP, Kasper K, Dusel G *et al.* Effects of calcium and deoxycholic acid on human colonic cell proliferation *in vitro.* Ann Nutr Metab. 1997;41:315–23.
27. Willett WC. Diet and cancer: one view at the start of the millennium. Cancer Epidemiol Biomarkers Prev. 2001;10:3–8.
28. Sandhu MS, White IR, McPherson K. Systematic review of the prospective cohort studies on meat consumption and colorectal cancer risk. A meta-analytical approach. Cancer Epidemiol Biomarkers Prev. 2001;10:439–46.
29. Sesink AL, Termont DS, Kleibeuker JH, Van der Meer R. Red meat and colon cancer: dietary haem-induced colonic cytotoxity and epithelial hyperproliferation are inhibited by calcium. Carcinogenesis. 2001;22:1653–9.
30. Penman ID, Liang QL, Bode J, Eastwoord MA, Arends MJ. Dietary calcium supplementation increases apoptosis in the distal murine colonic epithelium. J Clin Pathol. 2000;53:302–7.
31. Wargovich MJ, Jimenez A, McKee K *et al.* Efficacy of potential chemopreventive agents on rat colon aberrant crypt formation and progression. Carcinogenesis. 2000;21:1149–55.
32. Govers MJAP, Van der Meer R. Effects of dietary calcium and phosphate on the intestinal interactions between calcium, phosphate, fatty acids, and bile acids. Gut. 1993;34:365–70.
33. Lapré JA, De Vries HT, Van der Meer R. Dietary calcium phosphate inhibits intestinal cytotoxicity. Am J Physiol. 1991;261:G907–12.
34. Govers MJAP, Termont DSML, Van der Meer R. The mechanism of the antiproliferative effect of milk mineral and other calcium supplements on colonic epithelium. Cancer Res. 1994;54: 95–100.
35. Sesink AL, Termont DS, Kleibeuker JH, Van der Meer R. Red meat and colon cancer: the cytotoxic and hyperproliferative effects of dietary heme. Cancer Res. 1999;15:5704–9.
36. Sesink AL, Termont DS, Kleibeuker JH, Van der Meer R. Red meat and colon cancer: dietary haem, but not fat, has cytotoxic and hyperproliferative effects on rat colonic epithelium. Carcinogenesis. 2000;21:1909–15.
37. Lipkin M, Newmark H. Effect of added dietary calcium on colonic epithelial cell proliferation in subjects at high risk for familial colonic cancer. N Engl J Med. 1985;313:1381–4.
38. Kleibeuker JH, Welberg JWM, Mulder NH *et al.* Epithelial cell proliferation in the sigmoid colon of patients with adenomatous polyps increases during oral calcium supplementation. Br J Cancer. 1993;67:500–3.
39. Wargovich MJ, Isbell MJ, Shabot M *et al.* Calcium supplementation decreases rectal epithelial cell proliferation in subjects with sporadic adenoma. Gastroenterology. 1992;103:92–7.
40. Barsoum GH, Hendrickse C, Winslet MC *et al.* Reduction of mucosal crypt cell proliferation in patients with colorectal adenomatous polyps by dietary calcium supplementation. Br J Surg. 1992;79:581–3.
41. Bostick RM, Potter JD, Fosdick L *et al.* Calcium and colorectal epithelial cell proliferation: a preliminary randomized, double-blinded, placebo-controlled clinical trial. J Natl Cancer Inst. 1993;85:132–41.
42. Weisgerber UM, Boeing H, Owen RW, Waldherr R, Raedsch R, Wahrendorf J. Effect of longterm placebo controlled calcium supplementation on sigmoidal cell proliferation in patients with sporadic adenomatous polyps. Gut. 1996;38:396–402.
43. Thomas MG, Thomason JPS, Williamson RCN. Oral calcium inhibits rectal epithelial cell proliferation in familial adenomatous polyposis. Br J Surg. 1993;80:499–501.
44. Stern HS, Gregoire RC, Kashtan H, Stadler J, Bruce RW. Long-term effects of dietary calcium on risk markers for colon cancer in patients with familial polyposis. Surgery. 1990;108:528–33.
45. Gregoire R, Stern HS, Yeung KS *et al.* Effect of calcium supplementation on mucosal cell proliferation in high risk patients for colon cancer. Gut. 1989;30:376–82.
46. Bostick RM, Boldt M, Darif M, Wood JR, Overn P, Potter JW. Calcium and colorectal epithelial cell proliferation in ulcerative colitis. Cancer Epidemiol Biomarkers Prev. 1997;6:1021–7.
47. Cats A, Kleibeuker JH, Van der Meer R *et al.* Randomized double-blinded, placebo-controlled intervention study with supplemental calcium in families with hereditary nonpolyposis colorectal cancer. J Natl Cancer Inst. 1995;87:598–603.
48. Bostick RM, Fosdick L, Wood JR *et al.* Calcium and colorectal epithelial cell proliferation in sporadic adenoma patients: a randomized double-blinded placebo-controlled clinical trial. J Natl Cancer Inst. 1995;87:1307–15.
49. Armitage NC, Rooney PS, Gifford K-A, Clark PE, Hardcastle JD. The effect of calcium supplements on rectal mucosal proliferation. Br J Cancer. 1995;71:186–90.

50. Baron JA, Tosteson TD, Wargovich MJ *et al*. Calcium supplementation and rectal mucosal proliferation: a randomized controlled trial. J Natl Cancer Inst. 1995;87:1303–7.
51. Alberts DS, Einspahr J, Ritenbaugh C *et al*. The effect of wheat bran fiber and calcium supplementation on rectal mucosal proliferation rates in patients with resected adenomatous colorectal polyps. Cancer Epidemiol Biomarkers Prev. 1997;6:161–9.
52. Rozen P, Lubin F, Papo N *et al*. Calcium supplements interact significantly with long-term diet while suppressing rectal epithelial proliferation of adenoma patients. Cancer. 2001;91:833–40.
53. Van Gorkom BAP, Karrenbeld A, Van der Sluis T *et al*. Calcium or resistant starch do not affect colonic epithelial cell proliferation throughout the colon in adenoma patients: a randomized controlled trial. Nutr Cancer. 2002;43:31–8.
54. Holt PR, Atillasoy EO, Gilman J *et al*. Modulation of abnormal colonic epithelial cell proliferation and differentiation by low-fat dairy foods. J Am Meet Assoc. 1998;280:1074–9.
55. Karagas MR, Tosteson TD, Greenberg ER *et al*. Effects of milk and milk products on rectal mucosal cell proliferation in humans. Cancer Epidemiol Biomarkers Prev. 1998;7:757–66.
56. Lapré JA, De Vries HT, Termont DSML, Kleibeuker JH, De Vries EGE, Van der Meer R. Mechanism of the protective effects of supplemental dietary calcium on cytolytic activity of fecal water. Cancer Res. 1993;53:248–53.
57. Welberg JWM, Kleibeuker JH, Van der Meer R *et al*. Effects of oral calcium supplementation on intestinal bile acids and cytolytic activity of fecal water in patients with adenomatous polyps of the colon. Eur J Clin Invest. 1993;23:63–8.
58. Govers MJ, Termont DS, Lapré JA, Kleibeuker JH, Vonk RJ, Van der Meer R. Calcium in milk products precipitates intestinal fatty acids and secondary bile acids and thus inhibits colonic cytotoxicity in humans. Cancer Res. 1996;15:3270–5.
59. Glinghammar B, Venturi M, Rowland IR, Rafter JJ. Shift from a dairy product-rich to a dairy product-free diet: influence on cytotoxicity and genotoxicity of fecal water – potential risk factors for colon cancer. Am J Clin Nutr. 1997;66:1277–82.
60. Steinbach G, Lupton J, Reddy BS, Kral JG, Holt PR. Effect of calcium supplementation on rectal epithelial hyperproliferation in intestinal bypass subjects. Gastroenterology. 1994;106:1162–7.
61. Steinbach G, Morotomi M, Nomoto K *et al*. Calcium reduces the increased fecal 1,2-*sn*-diacylglycerol content in intestinal bypass patients: a possible mechanism for altering colonic hyperproliferation. Cancer Res. 1994;54:1216–19.
62. Baron JA, Beach M, Mandel JS *et al*. Calcium supplements for the prevention of colorectal adenomas. N Engl J Med. 1999;340:101–7.
63. Hofstad B, Almendingen K, Vatn M *et al*. Growth and recurrence of colorectal polyps: a double-blind 3-year intervention with calcium and antioxidants. Digestion. 1998;59:148–56.
64. Bonithon-Kopp C, Kronborg O, Giacosa A, Räth U, Faivre J, for the European Cancer Prevention Organisation Study Group. Calcium and fibre supplementation in prevention of colorectal adenoma recurrence: a randomised intervention trial. Lancet. 2000;356:1300–6.
65. Wallace K, Baron JA, Cole BF, Karagas MR, Beach ML. Calcium carbonate chemoprevention in the large bowel: effects on hyperplastic polyps, tubular adenomas, and more advanced lesions. Proc Am Assoc Cancer Res. 2002;43:163–4.
66. Cook JD, Dassenko SA, Whittaker P. Calcium supplementation: effect on iron absorption. Am J Clin Nutr. 1991;53:106–11.
67. Hallberg L, Brune M, Erlandsson M *et al*. Calcium: effect of different amounts on nonheme- and heme-iron absorption in humans. Am J Clin Nutr. 1991;53:112–19.

Section VIII
Summary

33
Dietary recommendations for prevention of colorectal cancer

J. L. ROMBEAU

INTRODUCTION

The role of food as either a cause of or prophylaxis for colorectal cancer is of major interest to both the scientific community and lay public. The putative effects of red meat, saturated fat, alcohol, inactivity and obesity are discussed in other chapters of this volume. This report reviews the following: (1) the effect of nutritional intervention on the reduction of adenomatous polyps in the colon and rectum, (2) an evaluation of dietary interventional studies and colorectal cancer and (3) dietary recommendations for the prevention of colorectal cancer despite the lack of definitive data.

THE EFFECTS OF DIETARY INTERVENTION ON THE REDUCTION OF ADENOMATOUS POLYPS OF THE COLON AND RECTUM

The adenomatous polyp is an important marker and precursor for the development of colorectal cancer. It is estimated that it takes 5 years for normal colonic mucosa to develop into a polyp and an additional 5 years for the polyp to transform into a malignancy[1]. This prolonged interval provides an opportunity for dietary intervention and prophylaxis as exemplified in controlled clinical trials. A complete discussion of these trials is beyond the scope of this report. Several nutrients and lifestyle patterns have been selected for discussion because of their particular relevance to this topic. These include dietary fibre, low-fat foods, supplemental calcium, and the combination of diet and lifestyle patterns.

Dietary fibre purportedly protects against the development of colorectal cancer by decreasing colonic transit time, altering bile acid adsorption, diluting faecal carcinogens, decreasing colonic pH, and increasing the production of short-chain fatty acids such as butyrate[2]. Several trials have examined the effect of dietary fibre on reducing colorectal adenomatous polyps.

A prospective study[3] was conducted of approximately 89 000 women, including a large cohort undergoing colonoscopy, to determine associations between fibre intake and risk of colorectal adenoma. The relative risk (RR) for the highest quintile group as compared with the lowest quintile group with respect to fibre intake was 0.95 (95% confidence interval (CI) = 0.73–1.25). No significant association between fibre intake and the risk of colorectal adenoma was found. In an earlier study, by the same group[4], a modest reduced risk of distal colon adenoma was observed with increasing intake of fibre from fruit ($p = 0.03$) but not cereals or vegetables. Moreover, soluble fibre, but not insoluble fibre, had a stronger inverse correlation on distal adenomas. A randomized trial[5], conducted in 1400 subjects recruited to a supervised programme of dietary supplementation with wheat bran, attempted to show reduced rates of recurrence of colorectal adenomas. Dietary supplements of either low amounts (2 g/day) or high amounts (13.5 g/day) of wheat bran fibre were investigated. The multivariate adjusted odds ratio for recurrent adenoma in the high-fibre group, as compared with the low-fibre group, was 0.88 (95% CI = 0.70–1.11; $p = 0.28$). The RR of recurrence according to the number of adenomas in the high-fibre group as compared to the low-fibre group was 0.99 (95% CI = 0.71–1.36; $p = 0.93$). It was concluded that dietary supplement of wheat bran fibre does not protect against recurrent colorectal adenomas.

A population-based non-colonoscopic case–control study[6] was conducted in three states to identify components of plant foods which may account for their association with colon cancer. Interviewer-administered questionnaires were obtained from nearly 2000 cases and 2400 controls. Higher intakes of vegetables (for highest relative to lowest quintile of intake) were associated inversely with colon cancer risk: odds ratio 0.7 for both men (95% CI = 0.5–0.9) and women (CI = 0.5–1.0). Associations were stronger among those with proximal tumours. Adjustment of plant foods for nutrients found in plant foods or for supplement use did not appreciably alter the observed associations between plant foods and colon cancer.

High-fat diets have been implicated in the pathogenesis of colorectal cancer, providing a rationale to investigate the potential benefits of low-fat diets. These diets have often been administered with high-fibre foods. In a study sponsored by the National Cancer Institute[7] over 2000 subjects were randomized to receive either their standard diet or a low-fat diet (20% of total calories) high in fibre (18 g dietary fibre/1000 kcal) and fruits and vegetables (3.5 servings per 1000 kcal). In an intention-to-treat analysis there was no significant reduction in the rate of recurrence of colorectal adenomas in subjects ingesting a low-fat, high-fibre diet when compared to controls. Of the 958 subjects in the intervention group and the 947 in the control group who completed the study, 39.7% and 39.5%, respectively, had at least one recurrent adenoma; the unadjusted RR was 1.00 (95% CI = 0.90–1.12). Among subjects with recurrent adenomas the mean ($\pm$ SE) number of such lesions was 1.85 ± 0.08 in the intervention group and 1.84 ± 0.07 in the control group. The Australian Polyp Prevention Project[8] investigated combined effects of low fat (25% total calories), wheat bran supplement (25 g/day) and beta-carotene (20 mg/day). There was no statistically significant prevention of total new adenomas with any of the interventions. Patients on the combined intervention of low fat and added wheat bran had no large adenomas at both 24 and 48 months ($p = 0.03$).

Calcium binds bile acids in the bowel lumen, inhibiting their proliferative and carcinogenic effects[9]. (Kleibeuker provides an in-depth discussion of this topic in Chapter 32 of this volume). A recent trial[10] investigated whether calcium supplementation would reduce the risk of recurrent colorectal adenomas as well as decrease the total number of adenomas. The randomized, double-blind trial examined the effect of supplementation with calcium carbonate on the recurrence of colonic adenomatous polyps. Nine hundred and thirty subjects were randomized to receive either calcium carbonate (3 g (1200 mg of elemental calcium) daily) or placebo. Colonoscopies were performed at 1 and 4 years, respectively. The subjects in the calcium group had a modest but significantly lower risk of recurrent adenomas. The adjusted RR for any recurrence of adenoma with calcium as compared to placebo was 0.85 (95% CI = 0.74–0.98; $p = 0.03$). The effect of calcium was independent of initial dietary fat and calcium intake. In another study[11] the association between calcium intake and colon cancer risk was investigated in two prospective cohorts, the Nurses' Health Study (NHS) and Health Professionals Follow-up Study (HPFS). The study population included nearly 88 000 women in the NHS and 47 000 men in the HPFS. In women and men considered together there was an inverse association between higher total calcium intake (>1250 mg/day vs ≤500 mg/day) and distal colon cancer (women: multivariate RR = 0.73, 95% CI = 0.41–1.27; men: RR = 0.58, 95% CI = 0.32–1.05; pooled RR = 0.65, 95% CI = 0.43–0.98). The incremental benefit of additional calcium intake beyond approximately 700 mg/day appeared to be minimal.

A unique way of examining the effects of diet on the development of colorectal cancer is to examine patterns of dietary intake in relation to variations in lifestyle. Although this approach is less specific than supplemental nutrients or chemoprotective studies it is perhaps more relevant to the lifestyles of today. Moreover, dietary patterns may be more strongly associated with disease processes than investigations of specific foods or nutrients. This approach was used in the studies[12,13] of subjects from Northern California, Utah and Minnesota as described previously by Slattery et al.[6] Through factor analysis, detailed dietary intake data from 1993 cases (diagnosed in 1991–1994) and 2410 controls were grouped into factors that were evaluated for relations with lifestyle characteristics and colon cancer risk. Five dietary patterns emerged: 'Western', 'prudent', 'high fat/sugar dairy', 'substituters', and 'drinkers'. The 'Western' dietary pattern was associated with a higher body mass index and a greater intake of total energy and dietary cholesterol. The 'prudent' pattern was associated with higher levels of vigorous leisure-time physical activity, smaller body size, and higher intakes of dietary fibre and folate. Persons who had high scores on the 'drinker' pattern were also more likely to smoke cigarettes. The 'Western' dietary pattern was associated with an increased risk of colon cancer in both men and women. The association was strongest among people diagnosed prior to age 67 years (for men, odds ratio (OR) = 1.96, 95% CI = 1.22–3.15; for women, OR = 2.02, 95% CI = 1.21–3.36) and among men with distal tumours (OR = 2.25, 95% CI = 1.47–3.46). The 'prudent' diet was protective, with the strongest associations being observed among people diagnosed prior to age 67 years (men: OR = 0.63, 95% CI = 0.43–0.92; women: OR = 0.58, 95% CI = 0.38–0.87); associations with this dietary pattern were also strong among persons with proximal tumours (men: OR = 0.55, 95% CI = 0.38–0.80; women: OR = 0.64, 95% CI = 0.45–0.92). Although 'substituters' (people who substituted low-fat dairy products for high-fat dairy products, margarine for butter, poultry for red meat, and whole grains for refined grains) were at reduced risk of colon cancer, the observed reduction in risk was not significant. These data support the hypothesis that overall dietary intake pattern is associated with colon cancer, and that the dietary pattern associated with the greatest increase in risk is the one which typifies a Western-type diet.

Thus, diets high in fibre and low in fat do not significantly decrease the short-term risk of colorectal adenoma formation. Whether fibre-enhanced diets will prevent the later stages of development of colorectal cancer is not known. Calcium intake in amounts greater than 700 mg/day appears to be protective. Increasing the daily intake of calcium by up to 1200 mg via low-fat dairy food in subjects at risk for colonic neoplasia reduces proliferative activity of colonic epithelial cells and restores markers of normal cellular differentiation[14]. Investigations of dietary patterns in relation to changes in lifestyle behaviour may be more relevant than studies of specific foods or nutrients. The 'Western' diet of increased calories and dietary cholesterol intake combined with a sedentary lifestyle is associated with a significantly increased risk of colorectal cancer in both men and women.

EVALUATION OF DIETARY INTERVENTIONAL STUDIES AND COLORECTAL CANCER

When compared to the controlled laboratory environment, nutrition-interventional studies are difficult to conduct and interpret. The prolonged time needed to produce nutrient-induced effects, difficulties in measurement of dietary compliance and the logistical issues associated with food-frequency questionnaires are just a few of the investigative problems in this area of research. Despite these concerns, diet remains an important determinant of health and disease, and is particularly relevant to the colon.

It is important to review the study designs within the context of the pathogenesis of colorectal cancer to optimally interpret the aforementioned studies. As noted, adenomatous colorectal polyps are unequivocal precursors for cancer; however, not all adenomatous polyps have an equal propensity for developing into a discrete malignancy with cancer present in only 0–4%[15]. Adenomatous polyps are common. In autopsy series adenomas are present in 34–52% of males and 29–45% of females over 50 years of age[16]. Most adenomas (87–89%) are <1 cm in size[15]. The extent of villous component, size of the polyp, and increasing age of the patient are independent risk factors for malignancy. Adenomatous polyps are histologically classified as to the amount of their tubular and villous components: tubular (0–25%), tubullovillous (25–75%) and villous (75–100%). Tubular adenomas account for 75% of all neoplastic polyps, tubullovillous adenomas 15% and villous adenomas 10%[17]. When compared to tubular adenomas, polyps with villous components have a greater propensity to evolve into cancers. Many of the nutrition–polyp studies record the number of polyps; however, their histological characteristics are not always completely described. In the Alberts et al. study[5] only 12.9% of polyps had villous features. Additionally, the size of the polyp directly correlates with its premalignant

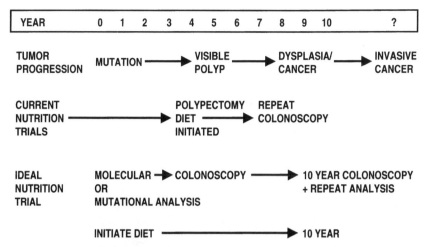

Figure 1 Longitudinal comparisons of polyp–cancer sequence, current nutrition interventional trial and 'ideal' nutrition trial

potential. Polyps <1 cm in length rarely become cancerous. In the National Polyp Study in the United States[18] only 25% of adenomas were >1 cm. In the Polyp Prevention Trial[7] only 16.4% of polyps were >1 cm. Greater emphasis should be directed to the effects of nutrients and chemoprotective agents on the progression of large polyps >1 cm).

Colonoscopy is the 'gold standard' examination to detect colorectal polyps; however, repeated examinations at intervals of 3 years are probably too short to detect new polyps. It is now recommended that persons at average risk for colorectal cancer should have a colonoscopy every 10 years[19]. Moreover, virtual colonoscopy may be a more acceptable screening technique because it is relatively safe and minimally invasive[20].

Most of the nutritional interventional trials have examined colonoscopic findings at 1 and 4 years, respectively. This is probably too short a duration to detect significant changes in appearance and growth of adenomatous polyps[21] (Figure 1). In one study[22] polyps were left *in situ* for 3 years to determine the effects of dietary nutrients on the growth of polyps. No significant effects on growth were observed.

Thus, the difficulty of objectively measuring dietary intake, the paucity of villous polyps, the difficulty in monitoring large polyps, the limited duration of most clinical trials, and the presumed length of time for nutrients to produce either prophylactic or therapeutic effects all underscore the difficulty in interpreting the nutritional interventional trials.

DIETARY RECOMMENDATIONS FOR THE PREVENTION OF COLORECTAL CANCER DESPITE THE LACK OF DEFINITIVE DATA

There is no irrefutable evidence that strict compliance with a specific dietary regimen will either prevent or ameliorate colorectal cancer. Moreover, this issue will probably never be resolved. Despite the absence of definitive data in the aforementioned trials, the health-care provider in 2002 is still confronted with the issue of how best to advise his or her patient as to optimal dietary intake. Significant adverse associations support the recommendations for decreased intakes of total calories[23], red meat[24], and refined grains[25]. Despite the lack of confirmative data to demonstrate diet-induced reduction of colorectal cancer, there is compelling evidence that a prudent diet improves other medical conditions. The increased dietary intake of fish, fresh fruits and vegetables reduces the incidence of arteriosclerotic cardiovascular disease[26], hypertension[27], non-insulin-dependent diabetes mellitus[28] and diverticulosis[29]. Moreover, the ingestion of three to five daily servings of fresh fruit may have the most pronounced effect on reducing colorectal adenomas[4,30].

Studies in modification of dietary intake, such as weight-reduction diets, show that long-term compliance is minimal. This is exemplified by the widespread prevalence and increasing degree of obesity despite widespread public knowledge that obesity kills. To enhance compliance, strategies are needed to make diets palatable and culturally acceptable. In today's society of dual-income households, a 50% divorce rate, joint child custody, decreased family time, computers, beepers, cell phones and decreased time for meal preparation, it is increasingly more difficult to provide a balanced, healthful and palatable diet. For example, it is nearly impossible to convince a teenager to substitute whole grains and fibre for high intakes of sugar and refined grains. It is simply not going to happen. These societal changes lend credence to the increased use of dietary supplements and chemopreventive agents in conjunction with a prudent diet. A detailed discussion of this topic can be found in Chapter 28 of this volume.

CONCLUSIONS

There is no irrefutable evidence that strict compliance with a particular dietary regimen will reduce the risk for colorectal cancer. Most of the nutritional interventional issues will probably never be resolved because of difficulties in conducting and interpreting clinical trials in this area. The proven benefits of diet in medical conditions besides colorectal cancer support the ingestion of increased amounts of fish, whole grains, fresh fruits and vegetables, dietary fibre and calcium. The addition of a chemopreventive regimen, coupled with a healthful diet and moderate exercise, may reduce colorectal cancer and increase longevity.

References

1. Morson BC. The polyp–cancer sequence in the large bowel. Proc R Soc Med. 1974;67:451–7.
2. Kritchevsky D. Epidemiology of fibre, resistant starch and colorectal cancer. Eur J Cancer Prev. 1995;4:345–52.
3. Fuchs CS, Giovannucci EL, Colditz GA et al. Dietary fiber and the risk of colorectal cancer and adenoma in women. N Engl J Med. 1999;340:169–76.
4. Platz EA, Giovannucci E, Rimm EB et al. Dietary fiber and distal colorectal adenoma in men. Cancer Epidemiol Biomarkers Prev. 1997;6:661–70.
5. Alberts DL, Martinez ME, Roe DJ et al. Lack of effect of a high-fiber cereal supplement on the recurrence of colorectal adenomas. N Engl J Med. 2000;342:1156–207.

6. Slattery ML, Potter JD, Coates A *et al*. Plant food and colon cancer: an assessment of specific foods and their related nutrients (United States). Cancer Causes Control. 1997;8:575–90.
7. Schatzkin A, Lanza E, Corle D *et al*. Lack of effect of a low-fat, high-fiber diet on the recurrence of colorectal adenomas. NEngl J Med. 2000;342:1149–55.
8. MacLennan R, Macrae F, Bain C *et al*. Randomized trial of intake of fat, fiber, and beta carotene to prevent colorectal adenomas. J Natl Cancer Inst. 1995;87:1760–6.
9. Newmark HL, Wargovich MJ, Bruce WR. Colon cancer and dietary fat, phosphate and calcium: a hypothesis. J Natl Cancer Inst. 1984;72:1323–5.
10. Baron JA, Beach M, Mandel JS *et al*. Calcium supplements for the prevention of colorectal adenomas. N Engl J Med. 1999;340:101–7.
11. Wu K, Willet WC, Fuchs CS, Colditz GA, Giovannucci EL. Calcium intake and risk of colon cancer in women and men. J Natl Cancer Inst. 2002;94:437–46.
12. Slattery ML, Boucher KM, Caan BJ, Potter JD, Ma K-N. Eating patterns and risk of colon cancer. Am J Epidemiol. 1998;148:4–16.
13. Slattery ML, Edwards SL, Boucher KM, Anderson K, Caan BJ. Lifestyle and colon cancer: an assessment of factors associated with risk. Am J Epidemiol. 1999;150:869–77.
14. Holt PR, Atillasoy EO, Gilman J *et al*. Modulation of abnormal colonic epithelial cell proliferation by low-fat dairy foods. J Au Med Assoc. 1998;280:1074–79.
15. Williams AR, Balasooriya BAW, Day DW. Polyps and cancer of the large bowel: a necropsy study in Liverpool. Gut. 1982;23:835–42.
16. Rickert RR, Averbach O, Garfinkel L, Hammond EC, Frasca JM. Adenomatous lesions of the large bowel: an autopsy survey. Cancer. 1979;43:1847–57.
17. O'Brien MJ. Colorectal adenomas: concepts and controversies. Semin Colon Rectal Surg. 1992;3:195–206.
18. O'Brien MJ, Winawer SJ, Zauber AG *et al*. The National Polyp Study. Patient and polyp characteristics associated with high-grade dysplasia in colorectal adenomas. Gastroenterology. 1990;98:371–9.
19. Ransohoff DF, Sandler RS. Screening for colorectal cancer. N Engl J Med. 2002;346:40–4.
20. Fenlon HM, Nunes DP, Schroy PC, Barish MA, Clarke PD, Ferrucci JT. A comparison of virtual and conventional colonoscopy for the detection of colorectal polyps. N Engl J Med. 1999;341:1496–503.
21. Kinzler KW, Vogelstein B. Lessons from hereditary colorectal cancer. Cell. 1996;87:159–70.
22. Hofstad B, Almendingen K, Vatn M *et al*. Growth and recurrence of colorectal polyps: a double-blind 3 year intervention with calcium and antioxidants. Digestion. 1998;59:148–56.
23. Potter JD, Slattery ML, Bostick RM, Gapstur SM. Colon cancer: a review of the epidemiology. Epidemiol Rev. 1993;15:499–545.
24. Goldbohm RA, Van den Brandt PA, Van't Veer P *et al*. A prospective study on the relation between meat consumption and the risk of colon cancer. Cancer Res. 1994;54:718–23.
25. Jacobs DR, Meyer KA, Kushi LH, Folsom AR. Is whole grain intake associated with reduced total and cause-specific death rates in older women? The Iowa Women's Health Study. Am J Public Health. 1999;89:322–9.
26. Albert CM, Campos H, Stampfer MJ *et al*. Blood levels of long-chain n-3 fatty acids and the risk of sudden death. N Engl J Med. 2002;346:1113–18.
27. Appel LJ, Moore TJ, Obarzanek E *et al*. A clinical trial of the effects of dietary patterns on blood pressure. N Engl J Med. 1997;336:1117–24.
28. Salmeron J, Manson JE, Stampfer MJ, Colditz GA, Wing AL, Willett WC. Dietary fiber, glycemic load, and risk of non-insulin-dependent diabetes mellitus in women. J Am Med Assoc. 1997;277:472–7.
29. Aldoori WH. A prospective study of diet and the risk of symptomatic diverticular disease in men. Am J Clin Nutr. 1994;60:757–64.
30. Brown J, Byers T, Thompson K, Eldridge B, Doyle C, Williams AM. Nutrition during and after cancer treatment: a guide for informed choices by cancer survivors. CA Cancer J Clin. 2001;51:153–87.

34
Pharmacological chemoprevention of colorectal cancer

R. S. BRESALIER

Colorectal cancer is a major cause of cancer-associated mortality in Europe, North America and other regions where life-styles and dietary habits are similar. Globally it is the fourth most common cancer in males and third most common in females with mortality paralleling incidence. Chemoprevention involves the use of natural or synthetic agents to reverse, suppress, or prevent the occurrence of cancer. The most studied pharmacological agents for chemoprevention of colorectal cancer are nonsteroidal anti-inflammatory drugs (NSAIDS). Clinical case–control and cohort studies have shown a 40–50% reduction in colorectal cancer-related mortality in individuals taking aspirin and other NSAIDS on a regular basis compared with those not taking these agents. Animal and laboratory studies indicate that this effect is biologically plausible. The precise mechanism for cancer protection is unknown but appears to relate to altered synthesis of arachidonic acid metabolites that include prostaglandins, thromboxanes, leukotrienes, and hydroxyeicosatetranoic acids. These compounds modulate signal transduction pathways that effect cellular adhesion, growth and differentiation. Cyclooxygenase (COX or prostaglandin endoperoxide synthase) oxidizes arachidonic acid to prostaglandin G_2, reduces prostaglandin G_2 to prostaglandin H_2 and is the key enzyme responsible for production of prostaglandins and other eicosanoids. The COX-2 isoform is induced by cytokines, mitogens, and growth factors and its levels are elevated in 85% to 95% of colorectal cancers and in experimental colorectal tumors. COX-2 inhibition leads to prevention of cancer development during both the initiation and promotion/progression stages of carcinogenesis. Knockout of COX-2 through genetic manipulation or through the use of specific inhibitors reduces tumor formation in animal models. A potential mechanism includes inhibition of gene activation by the nuclear hormone receptor peroxisone-proliferator-activated receptor δ (PPAR). PPARδ activates genes involved in cellular growth, differentiation and apoptosis after exposure to a variety of ligands including eicosanoids. COX-2 inhibition also leads to alterations in cellular adhesion to extracellular matrix proteins, inhibition of angiogenesis, reduction in carcinogen activation, and increases in programmed cell death (apoptosis). Preclinical studies of COX-2 inhibitors in animal models of familial adenomatous polyposis (FAP) such as the Apc$^{\Delta716}$ mouse demonstrate significant dose-dependent reductions in polyp number and size, alterations in polyp morphology and accompanying reductions in proliferation, membrane-bound vascular endothelial growth factor (VEGF) and angiogenesis at blood levels achieved in humans with a clinical anti-inflammatory drug dose (rofecoxib).

Human clinical trials in patients with FAP have shown significant reductions in adenoma number in patients treated with the NSAID sulindac and the COX-2 inhibitor celecoxib, leading to approval of the latter by the U.S. Food and Drug Administration as an adjunct to usual care in this group. Prospective clinical trials of NSAIDS and specific COX-2 inhibitors for prevention of adenoma recurrence in patients with sporadic adenomas are in progress. Data from a large randomized prospective trial using aspirin in this group will soon be reported. There is growing evidence that NSAIDS including COX-2 inhibitors may be effective chemopreventive agents for adenomas and cancer occurrence in the colon, either alone or in combination with other agents. Assessment of their full potential awaits additional trials designed to further elucidate their mechanisms of action and to confirm their efficacy in both average and high-risk groups.

35
Cancer prevention – public health aspects

J. H. WEISBURGER

The twentieth century has provided revolutionary developments in knowledge of diseases that affect mankind worldwide. The infectious diseases such as smallpox or poliomyelitis have been controlled by vaccination or other effective means of prevention. Nutritional deficiency diseases such as scurvy, pellagra and beriberi have been wiped out in most parts of the world through nutritional improvements. Venereal diseases such as syphilis and gonorrhoea have a lower incidence in mortality because of preventive approaches and also the development of antibiotic drugs. A new infectious disease, caused by HIV leading to AIDS, is a relatively new development in the past 25 years, associated with improper sexual practices, mainly failure to use protective condoms and, in part, associated with intravenous addictive drug use, depressing the immune competence, also accounting for a rise in tuberculosis.

The field of geographic pathology provides important information on differences in the worldwide occurrence of specific chronic diseases. Certainly the introduction of manufactured cigarettes at the beginning of the twentieth century led to an epidemic increase in lung cancer in many countries, albeit there are modifying factors by other aspects of lifestyle. For example, there are more smokers now in Japan, but the incidence of lung cancer is lower because of dietary factors such as a lower-fat diet, and frequent intake of protective fish, soy products and green tea[1]. In the USA smoking rates have decreased in men from 70% smokers in 1950 to 22% in the year 2000, with a consequent decline of heart disease and the smoking-associated cancers, including cancer in the lung, kidney, bladder and pancreas. Regrettably, 28% of women now smoke in the USA, and more women died of lung cancer than of breast cancer in the past 5 years.

Geographic pathology also provides important leads on aetiological factors associated with colorectal cancer, the main topic of this timely Symposium[2]. The term colorectal cancer really represents three distinct diseases with different causative and modulating elements. Proximal, right-sided colon cancer has a moderate incidence in many countries of the world, and the aetiological factors are not well known. It would seem that the regular intake of soy products, as practised in the Orient, may lower the risk somewhat.

There are some differences in intake of specific foods between Germany and the USA (Table 1). The major neoplasm associated with Western dietary habits is distal and sigmoid colon cancer, and the risk factors have been reasonably well delineated through biomedical research in many institutions in the world[3]. There is a high cost associated with their clinical management[2–4] (Tables 2–4). Rectal cancer has similar risk factors, with the addition that regular intake of alcoholic beverages increases the risk. The associated dietary habits are intake of mixed fats at about 35–40% of calories, leading to increased formation of bile acids secreted in the bile and having an enhancing effect on colon cancer by promotion, increasing the rate of cell duplication. This has been observed in humans as well as in animal models (cf. B.S. Reddy, Chapter 14 in this volume). Not all fats have identical promoting properties. Monounsaturated oils such as olive oil, and in North America canola oil, do not promote colon cancer, or incidentally other associated Western nutritionally linked cancers such as in the breast, prostate and pancreas[4]. The associated genotoxic carcinogens are most likely the heterocyclic amines formed during cooking, and possibly also reactive oxygen species, (S.R. Tannenbaum, Chapter 21 in this volume)[5]. The Mediterranean

Table 1 Consumption of selected food items per person in kilograms per year for the years 1965–1995

Food	1965	1970	1975	1980	1985	1990	1995
Vegetables							
USA	—	152.2	153.2	153.0	162.7	175.6	181.0
Germany	55.1	55.1	75.2	73.0	80.7	81.0	84.8
Fruit							
USA	57.8	55.9	55.2	56.5	57.5	60.4	64.8
Germany	102.4	111.8	124.1	102.0	1093	124.3	114.0
Red meat (beef, veal, pork, lamb)							
USA	64.7	87.5	82.3	81.8	80.3	73.9	75.9
Germany	54.9	69.5	76.5	81.5	83.5	80.8	72.5
Milk							
USA	117.6	125.0	118.8	111.6	109.5	106.1	102.6
Germany	97.2	91.2	85.4	85.2	87.7	91.2	91.4
Butter and margarine							
USA	7.5	7.4	7.0	7.1	7.1	7.0	7.7
Germany	16.9	16.3	15.3	15.4	15.4	14.4	14.1
Cheese							
USA	4.3	5.2	6.5	8.0	19.2	11.2	12.2
Germany	8.4	9.0	12.3	14.1	15.8	18.4	19.7
Vegetable oil							
USA	6.4	7.0	8.1	9.6	11.0	10.1	11.0
Germany	2.8	3.3	3.9	5.8	5.9	6.6	10.0
Animal fats and oil							
USA	2.9	2.1	1.5	1.2	0.8	0.9	0.8
Germany	4.4	4.8	5.3	4.4	4.3	4.4	4.1

From ref. 29.

Table 2 Annual expenditures in the USA for cancer

	Total ($ billion)
All cancers (2001)[a]	156.7[c]
Colorectal cancers (1998)[b]	4.9[d]
Colorectal cancers (2000)[b]	4.3
Liver cancer (1998)[b]	1.3
Pancreas cancers (1998)[b]	1.2
Diverticulosis (1998)[b]	2.5

[a] NIH data, provided by the American Cancer Society, Atlanta, GA, in billions of dollars.
[b] AGA data, provided by Deborah Zimmer, Managing Editor, *Gastroenterology*. A summary of results, 'The burden of GI disease' has appeared in the May 2002 issue of *Gastroenterology*, 2002; 122(5):1500–1511.
[c] Direct costs $56.4 billion, indirect $100.3 billion.
[d] Direct costs $4.8 billion, indirect $0.106 billion.

Table 3 Expenditures, 1998 (US$)

Physician's	1,093 billion
Hospital outpatients	310 million
Hospital inpatients	3,062 billion
Drugs	19.5 million
Home care	75.2 million
Nursing home	171.2 million
Hospice	94.6 million

Table 4 Statistics on colorectal cancer, 1998

Physician's office visits	1 787 879
Emergency room visits	50 049
Outpatient visits	350 975
Diagnosis in hospital	172 938
Inpatient stays in hospital	267 104

dietary habits involve use of olive oils, plus a regular intake of fruits and vegetables. Furthermore, there is a lower exposure to heterocyclic amines, because the favourite meat, veal, is not browned very much. It follows that the Western-style Mediterranean type of diet should be favoured. One recent development is the increasing Westernization of the diet in Japan, typical of habits acquired from the USA[6]. As a consequence there is an increasing incidence of distal but not proximal colon cancer, an excellent argument for the adverse effects in colon cancer, as well as other Western types of cancer and heart disease related to the dietary traditions prevailing in the USA. In Japan people appear to be switching from green tea, protective in heart disease and many types of cancer, to other beverages. Men, but less so women, are regular consumers of alcoholic beverages, and for that reason they display a higher risk of rectal cancer, despite their former traditional low-fat, soy and fish-related diet[7]. Incidentally, men who smoke and drink have a higher risk of cancer of the oesophagus.

Another area of the world where geographic pathology has provided key leads on dietary habits that are protective is Finland, particularly rural Finland. The Finns used to have a high incidence and mortality from heart disease, mainly because they were extensive consumers of milk, where the underlying risk factor seems to be lactose[3]. Dairy products without lactose, such as yogurt, do not display such adverse effects. Yet the incidence of distal colon cancer in Finland, and incidentally of postmenopausal breast cancer, is quite low. This represents a contrast between the risk for heart disease and colon cancer. The underlying explanation is the regular consumption of Finnish high-bran rye bread. This type of bread, providing sizeable amounts of insoluble bran cereal fibre that increases stool bulk, leads to a dilution of risk factors such as the intestinal bile acids[8–10]. In addition, the Finns' extensive milk intake is a source of calcium that has been found to be protective in colon cancer. Metabolic studies show that the Finns excrete daily about 250 g of stool. In contrast, people in Denmark or the USA usually have a stool weight of 50–80 g (when people are not constipated). Burkitt made the same observation while he was a resident surgeon in Kampala, Uganda[11] (Figure 1). The British people in his care displayed many intestinal diseases, including colon cancer. In contrast he rarely observed colon cancer

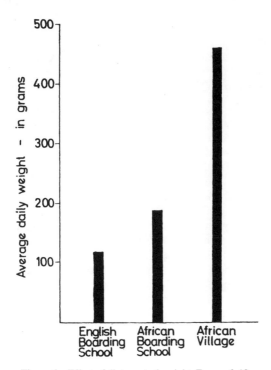

Figure 1 Effect of diet on stool weight. From ref. 10

Table 5   Dietary recommendations intended to reduce the incidence of colorectal cancer

---

Vegetables and whole-grain cereals should be consumed in large amounts and should be a major component of diet
Consumption of fish and poultry should be preferred to red meat
Alcohol consumption should not exceed the equivalent of 20 g of pure alcohol per day
Physical activity should be maintained and excessive energy intake avoided

---

From ref. 13.

among the local African people. The latter were extensive consumers of high-fibre foods, leading to a daily excretion of up to 400 g of stool in one or several passes. Soluble fibres, as found in vegetables and fruits, are also desirable, but for different reasons. They do not increase stool bulk, and are therefore less effective in lowering the risk of colorectal cancer.

Thus, the field of geographic pathology has provided key information on nutritional traditions associated with colon and rectal cancer. These are the intake of heavily fried and browned meat, sources of heterocyclic amines, and also a fairly high calories (30–40%) in total fat, and a limited intake of protective fruits and vegetables, and bran cereal fibre. In much of the Western world there is inadequate intake of foods containing calcium. This mineral decreases the cell duplication rates in the intestinal tract and therefore decreases the development of cancer[12]. A relatively low intake of calcium also represents a risk of osteoporosis.

Therefore, health promotion and disease prevention would be based on recommendations to avoid, for the most part, foods with high risk of colon and rectal cancer, and to adopt a lifelong new wholesome, tasty and health-promoting nutritional tradition. Professor Scheppach and colleagues[13] made similar recommendations on behalf of WHO (Table 5).

1. Heterocyclic amines seem to be associated with a risk for colon cancer. Their formation during the cooking of meat can be decreased by a number of methods. Our research has shown that application of antioxidants, synthetic ones such as butylated hydroxyanisale (BHA), or from foods, such as soy or tea, decreased the formation of heterocyclic amines during cooking[3]. The antioxidants would also be protective in the formation of reactive oxygen species. One key ingredient associated with the production of heterocyclic amines is creatinine. The group of Felton[14] has observed that brief microwave cooking on a heated platter with a groove permitting the collection of juices that run off the heated food leads to the elimination of much of the creatinine, and also some fats. Then, the frying or broiling of such pretreated meat would minimize the formation of heterocyclic amines.

2. Fish and fish oils contain health-promoting ω-3-polyunsaturated oils[15]. Fish is also a source of excellent proteins. Colon cancer is lower in regular fish-eaters, three to six portions per week.

3. Salt provides an essential nutrient as sodium and, with raw sea salt, other desirable minerals. However, only 1–2 g per day are needed. Total salt intake over 10–15 g can increase the risk of hypertension and of stomach cancer, the latter especially in carriers of *Helicobacter pylori*[16–18].

4. Dietary habits including 30–40% of calories in fat promote the development of colon cancer, mainly through the increased formation of bile acids, acting as promoters[4]. Olive oil and related monounsaturated oils do not show adverse effects and would be preferred. Oils and fats are calorie-dense, and intake at about 20–25% of calories would help avoid obesity.

5. Bran cereal fibre in whole-grain breads or breakfast cereals is most desirable[19]. The actual amount of fibre would be about 20 g per day. A good marker for adequate fibre intake is the absence of constipation and a daily stool bulk of about 200–300 g. Food high in resistant starch is likewise beneficial[4]. Worldwide, the use of white bread should be discontinued and replaced by whole-grain bread with bran cereal fibre. Other intestinal diseases such as diverticulosis and even ulcerative colitis are less frequent in lifelong users of whole-grain bread[11,20]. Soy milk with added calcium should be preferred to cow or goat milk, since lactose is a risk factor for coronary heart disease[3,21]. Bran fibre also generates butyrate in the gut, that assists in controlling intestinal diseases[4].

6. Vegetables, legumes and fruits are recommended for many reasons to avoid chronic diseases. In the USA nutritional bodies and government agencies suggest a daily intake of five to ten such foods, preferably the higher level[21,22]. They are excellent sources of antioxidants and plant proteins. Lifelong vegetarians display less distal colon cancer[23].

7. Adequate intake of fluids is important, including the fact that bran cereal fibre needs to be diluted out and provide stool bulk with a proper aqueous phase. Adults should consume, with their total foods and beverages, 2–3 liters of fluids a day[3,24–26]. Fluids rich in antioxidants, such as soy milk and especially green or black tea, are preferred[26]. Data show that eight to ten cups of tea a day lower the risk of heart disease and many types of cancer, including colon cancer. A limited intake, of one or two glasses of wine or beer is fine, and may contribute to health promotion.

8. Children should be conditioned to like and enjoy such wholesome foods and drinks, in proportion to their body weight (except alcoholic beverages). Children through puberty will need dairy products, including milk, to obtain the necessary nutritional factors for growth and development.

9. Regular exercise is part of a healthy lifestyle. This includes walking, sports of many types and other activities that provide bodily mobilities. The risk of colon cancer is lower in individuals with regular exercise, compared to a sedentary population. Exercise also assists in controlling body weight. Obesity can increase the risk of colon cancer.

10. Healthy lifestyle also involves having a regular physical examination by qualified medical staff. This includes gastroenterologists, to perform sigmoidoscopies, or better, colonoscopies after age 40–50, to detect and remove any early lesions in the intestinal tract.

11. Individuals who have displayed a somewhat higher risk by evidence of the presence of polyps in the intestinal tract need to be even more careful to adjust their lifestyle to a lower risk tradition. Even genetically prone individuals with familial polyposis would benefit to some extent from appropriate lifestyle adjustments[20].

12. Prevention of any disease is much less expensive than the high cost of disease care when an avoidable condition has affected a patient[3,10,27,28]. In the USA, and no doubt also in Europe, the annual cost of medical care is very high[29] (Tables 2–4). Therefore, adjusting lifestyle to a lower-risk situation for most chronic diseases is good for the individual, the family, the insurance carriers and government, and may permit reaching old age without debilitating diseases.

Acknowledgements

I am indebted to the Falk Foundation e.V. for a travel fellowship, to the Friends Against Cancer Team for support of research, and to Ms Nancy Rivera for excellent administrative support.

References

1. Weisburger JH, Chung F-L. Mechanisms of chronic disease causation by nutritional factors and tobacco products and their prevention by tea polyphenols. Food Chem Toxicol. 2002;40:1145–54.
2. Stewart HL. Geographic pathology of cancer of the colon and rectum. Cancer. 1971;28:25–8.
3. Weisburger JH. Eat to live, not live to eat. Nutrition. 2000;16:767–73.
4. Weisburger JH. Dietary fat and risk of chronic disease: mechanistic insights from experimental studies. J Am Diet Assoc. 1997;97(Suppl. 7):S16–23.
5. Nagao M, Ushijima T, Watanabe N et al. Studies on mammary carcinogenesis induced by a heterocyclic amine, 2-amino-1-methyl-6-phenylimidazo[4,5-b]pyridine, in mice and rats. Environ Mol Mutagen. 2002;39:158–64.
6. Tominaga S, Kuroishi T. An ecological study on diet/nutrition and cancer in Japan. Int J Cancer. 1997(Suppl. 10):2–6.
7. Seitz HK, Simanowski UA, Garzon FT et al. Possible role of acetaldehyde in ethanol-related rectal cocarcinogenesis in the rat. Gastroenterology. 1990;98:406–13.
8. Reddy BS, Engle A, Katsifis S et al. Biochemical epidemiology of colon cancer: effect of types of dietary fiber on fecal mutagens, and acid and neutral sterols in healthy subjects. Cancer Res. 1989;49:4629–35.
9. Trock B, Lanza E, Greenwald P. Dietary fiber, vegetables, and colon cancer: Critical review and metaanalyses of the epidemiologic evidence. J Natl Cancer Inst. 1990;82:650–61.
10. Burkitt DP. Epidemiology of cancer of the colon and rectum. Cancer. 1971;28:6–13.
11. Scheppach W, Luehrs H, Menzel T. Beneficial health effects of low-digestible carbohydrate consumption. Br J Nutr. 2001;85(Suppl. 1):S23–30.
12. Lipkin M, Reddy B, Newmark H, Lamprecht SA. Dietary factors in human colorectal cancer. Annu Rev Nutr. 1999;19:545–86.
13. Scheppach W, Bingham S, Boutron-Ruault MC et al. WHO consensus statement on the role of nutrition in colorectal cancer. Eur J Cancer Prev. 1999;8:57–62.
14. Felton JS, Gentile JM. Mutagenic/carcinogenic N-substituted aryl compounds. Mutat Res. 1997;376:1.
15. Caygill CPJ, Charlett A, Hill MJ. Fat, fish, fish oil and cancer. Br J Cancer. 1996;74:159–64.
16. Howson CP, Hiyama T, Wynder EL. Decline of gastric cancer: epidemiology of an unplanned triumph. Epidemiol Rev. 1986;8:1–27.
17. Joossens J, Kesteloot H. Salt and stomach cancer. In: Reed PI, Hill MJ, editors. Gastric Carcinogenesis. Amsterdam: Excerpta Medica, 1988:26.
18. Hwang H, Dwyer J, Russell RM. Diet, Helicobacter pylori infection, food preservation and gastric cancer risk: are there new roles for preventative factors? Nutr Rev. 1994;52:75–83.
19. Reddy BS. Role of dietary fiber in colon cancer: an overview. Am J Med. 1999;106:16–19S.
20. DeCosse JJ, Miller HH, Lesser ML. Effect of wheat fiber and vitamins C and E on rectal polyps in patients with familial adenomatous polyposis. J Natl Cancer Inst. 1989;81:1290–7.
21. Ziegler RG. Vegetables, fruits, and carotenoids and the risk of cancer. Am J Clin Nutr. 1991;53:251–9S.

22. Dwyer JT. Health aspects of vegetarian diets. Am J Clin Nutr. 1988;48:712–38.
23. Frentzel-Beyme R, Chang-Claude J. Vegetarian diets and colon cancer: the German experience. Am J Clin Nutr. 1994;59:1143–52S.
24. Fujiki H, Guganuma M, Okabe S *et al*. Mechanistic findings of green tea as cancer prevention for humans. Proc Soc Exp Biol Med. 1999;220:225–8.
25. Dashwood RH, Xu M, Hernaez JF, Hasaniya N, Youn K, Razzuk A. Cancer chemopreventive mechanisms of tea against heterocyclic amine mutagens from cooked meat. Proc Soc Exp Biol Med. 1999;220:239–43.
26. Messina M. Modern applications for an ancient bean: soy-beans and the prevention and treatment of chronic disease. J Nutr. 1995;125(Suppl. 3):567–9S.
27. Greenwald P. Science, medicine, and the future: cancer chemoprevention. Br Med J. 2002; 324:714–18.
28. Rimer BK. Cancer control research 2001. Cancer Causes Control. 2000;11:257–70.
29. Becker N, Muscat JE, Wynder EL. Cancer mortality in the United States and Germany. J Cancer Res Clin Oncol. 2001;127:293–300.

Index

317

Falk Symposium Series

43. Reutter W, Popper H, Arias IM, Heinrich PC, Keppler D, Landmann L, eds.: *Modulation of Liver Cell Expression*. Falk Symposium No. 43. 1987   ISBN: 0-85200-677-2*
44. Boyer JL, Bianchi L, eds.: *Liver Cirrhosis*. Falk Symposium No. 44. 1987   ISBN: 0-85200-993-3*
45. Paumgartner G, Stiehl A, Gerok W, eds.: *Bile Acids and the Liver*. Falk Symposium No. 45. 1987   ISBN: 0-85200-675-6*
46. Goebell H, Peskar BM, Malchow H, eds.: *Inflammatory Bowel Diseases – Basic Research & Clinical Implications*. Falk Symposium No. 46. 1988   ISBN: 0-7462-0067-6*
47. Bianchi L, Holt P, James OFW, Butler RN, eds.: *Aging in Liver and Gastrointestinal Tract*. Falk Symposium No. 47. 1988   ISBN: 0-7462-0066-8*
48. Heilmann C, ed.: *Calcium-Dependent Processes in the Liver*. Falk Symposium No. 48. 1988   ISBN: 0-7462-0075-7*
50. Singer MV, Goebell H, eds.: *Nerves and the Gastrointestinal Tract*. Falk Symposium No. 50. 1989   ISBN: 0-7462-0114-1
51. Bannasch P, Keppler D, Weber G, eds.: *Liver Cell Carcinoma*. Falk Symposium No. 51. 1989   ISBN: 0-7462-0111-7
52. Paumgartner G, Stiehl A, Gerok W, eds.: *Trends in Bile Acid Research*. Falk Symposium No. 52. 1989   ISBN: 0-7462-0112-5
53. Paumgartner G, Stiehl A, Barbara L, Roda E, eds.: *Strategies for the Treatment of Hepatobiliary Diseases*. Falk Symposium No. 53. 1990   ISBN: 0-7923-8903-4
54. Bianchi L, Gerok W, Maier K-P, Deinhardt F, eds.: *Infectious Diseases of the Liver*. Falk Symposium No. 54. 1990   ISBN: 0-7923-8902-6
55. Falk Symposium No. 55 not published
55B. Hadziselimovic F, Herzog B, Bürgin-Wolff A, eds.: *Inflammatory Bowel Disease and Coeliac Disease in Children*. International Falk Symposium. 1990 ISBN 0-7462-0125-7
56. Williams CN, eds.: *Trends in Inflammatory Bowel Disease Therapy*. Falk Symposium No. 56. 1990   ISBN: 0-7923-8952-2
57. Bock KW, Gerok W, Matern S, Schmid R, eds.: *Hepatic Metabolism and Disposition of Endo- and Xenobiotics*. Falk Symposium No. 57. 1991   ISBN: 0-7923-8953-0
58. Paumgartner G, Stiehl A, Gerok W, eds.: *Bile Acids as Therapeutic Agents: From Basic Science to Clinical Practice*. Falk Symposium No. 58. 1991   ISBN: 0-7923-8954-9
59. Halter F, Garner A, Tytgat GNJ, eds.: *Mechanisms of Peptic Ulcer Healing*. Falk Symposium No. 59. 1991   ISBN: 0-7923-8955-7
60. Goebell H, Ewe K, Malchow H, Koelbel Ch, eds.: *Inflammatory Bowel Diseases – Progress in Basic Research and Clinical Implications*. Falk Symposium No. 60. 1991   ISBN: 0-7923-8956-5
61. Falk Symposium No. 61 not published
62. Dowling RH, Folsch UR, Löser Ch, eds.: *Polyamines in the Gastrointestinal Tract*. Falk Symposium No. 62. 1992   ISBN: 0-7923-8976-X
63. Lentze MJ, Reichen J, eds.: *Paediatric Cholestasis: Novel Approaches to Treatment*. Falk Symposium No. 63. 1992   ISBN: 0-7923-8977-8
64. Demling L, Frühmorgen P, eds.: *Non-Neoplastic Diseases of the Anorectum*. Falk Symposium No. 64. 1992   ISBN: 0-7923-8979-4
64B. Gressner AM, Ramadori G, eds.: *Molecular and Cell Biology of Liver Fibrogenesis*. International Falk Symposium. 1992   ISBN: 0-7923-8980-8

*These titles were published under the MTP Press imprint.

Falk Symposium Series

65. Hadziselimovic F, Herzog B, eds.: *Inflammatory Bowel Diseases and Morbus Hirschprung.* Falk Symposium No. 65. 1992   ISBN: 0-7923-8995-6
66. Martin F, McLeod RS, Sutherland LR, Williams CN, eds.: *Trends in Inflammatory Bowel Disease Therapy.* Falk Symposium No. 66. 1993   ISBN: 0-7923-8827-5
67. Schölmerich J, Kruis W, Goebell H, Hohenberger W, Gross V, eds.: *Inflammatory Bowel Diseases – Pathophysiology as Basis of Treatment.* Falk Symposium No. 67. 1993   ISBN: 0-7923-8996-4
68. Paumgartner G, Stiehl A, Gerok W, eds.: *Bile Acids and The Hepatobiliary System: From Basic Science to Clinical Practice.* Falk Symposium No. 68. 1993   ISBN: 0-7923-8829-1
69. Schmid R, Bianchi L, Gerok W, Maier K-P, eds.: *Extrahepatic Manifestations in Liver Diseases.* Falk Symposium No. 69. 1993   ISBN: 0-7923-8821-6
70. Meyer zum Büschenfelde K-H, Hoofnagle J, Manns M, eds.: *Immunology and Liver.* Falk Symposium No. 70. 1993   ISBN: 0-7923-8830-5
71. Surrenti C, Casini A, Milani S, Pinzani M , eds.: *Fat-Storing Cells and Liver Fibrosis.* Falk Symposium No. 71. 1994   ISBN: 0-7923-8842-9
72. Rachmilewitz D, ed.: *Inflammatory Bowel Diseases – 1994.* Falk Symposium No. 72. 1994   ISBN: 0-7923-8845-3
73. Binder HJ, Cummings J, Soergel KH, eds.: *Short Chain Fatty Acids.* Falk Symposium No. 73. 1994   ISBN: 0-7923-8849-6
73B. Möllmann HW, May B, eds.: *Glucocorticoid Therapy in Chronic Inflammatory Bowel Disease: from basic principles to rational therapy.* International Falk Workshop. 1996   ISBN 0-7923-8708-2
74. Keppler D, Jungermann K, eds.: *Transport in the Liver.* Falk Symposium No. 74. 1994   ISBN: 0-7923-8858-5
74B. Stange EF, ed.: *Chronic Inflammatory Bowel Disease.* Falk Symposium. 1995   ISBN: 0-7923-8876-3
75. van Berge Henegouwen GP, van Hoek B, De Groote J, Matern S, Stockbrügger RW, eds.: *Cholestatic Liver Diseases: New Strategies for Prevention and Treatment of Hepatobiliary and Cholestatic Liver Diseases.* Falk Symposium 75. 1994.   ISBN: 0-7923-8867-4
76. Monteiro E, Tavarela Veloso F, eds.: *Inflammatory Bowel Diseases: New Insights into Mechanisms of Inflammation and Challenges in Diagnosis and Treatment.* Falk Symposium 76. 1995.   ISBN 0-7923-8884-4
77. Singer MV, Ziegler R, Rohr G, eds.: *Gastrointestinal Tract and Endocrine System.* Falk Symposium 77. 1995.   ISBN 0-7923-8877-1
78. Decker K, Gerok W, Andus T, Gross V, eds.: *Cytokines and the Liver.* Falk Symposium 78. 1995.   ISBN 0-7923-8878-X
79. Holstege A, Schölmerich J, Hahn EG, eds.: *Portal Hypertension.* Falk Symposium 79. 1995.   ISBN 0-7923-8879-8
80. Hofmann AF, Paumgartner G, Stiehl A, eds.: *Bile Acids in Gastroenterology: Basic and Clinical Aspects.* Falk Symposium 80. 1995   ISBN 0-7923-8880-1
81. Riecken EO, Stallmach A, Zeitz M, Heise W, eds.: *Malignancy and Chronic Inflammation in the Gastrointestinal Tract – New Concepts.* Falk Symposium 81. 1995   ISBN 0-7923-8889-5
82. Fleig WE, ed.: *Inflammatory Bowel Diseases: New Developments and Standards.* Falk Symposium 82. 1995   ISBN 0-7923-8890-6

Falk Symposium Series

82B. Paumgartner G, Beuers U, eds.: *Bile Acids in Liver Diseases*. International Falk Workshop. 1995 ISBN 0-7923-8891-7

83. Dobrilla G, Felder M, de Pretis G, eds.: *Advances in Hepatobiliary and Pancreatic Diseases: Special Clinical Topics*. Falk Symposium 83. 1995. ISBN 0-7923-8892-5

84. Fromm H, Leuschner U, eds.: *Bile Acids – Cholestasis – Gallstones: Advances in Basic and Clinical Bile Acid Research*. Falk Symposium 84. 1995 ISBN 0-7923-8893-3

85. Tytgat GNJ, Bartelsman JFWM, van Deventer SJH, eds.: *Inflammatory Bowel Diseases*. Falk Symposium 85. 1995 ISBN 0-7923-8894-1

86. Berg PA, Leuschner U, eds.: *Bile Acids and Immunology*. Falk Symposium 86. 1996 ISBN 0-7923-8700-7

87. Schmid R, Bianchi L, Blum HE, Gerok W, Maier KP, Stalder GA, eds.: *Acute and Chronic Liver Diseases: Molecular Biology and Clinics*. Falk Symposium 87. 1996 ISBN 0-7923-8701-5

88. Blum HE, Wu GY, Wu CH, eds.: *Molecular Diagnosis and Gene Therapy*. Falk Symposium 88. 1996 ISBN 0-7923-8702-3

88B. Poupon RE, Reichen J, eds.: *Surrogate Markers to Assess Efficacy of TReatment in Chronic Liver Diseases*. International Falk Workshop. 1996 ISBN 0-7923-8705-8

89. Reyes HB, Leuschner U, Arias IM, eds.: *Pregnancy, Sex Hormones and the Liver*. Falk Symposium 89. 1996 ISBN 0-7923-8704-X

89B. Broelsch CE, Burdelski M, Rogiers X, eds.: *Cholestatic Liver Diseases in Children and Adults*. International Falk Workshop. 1996 ISBN 0-7923-8710-4

90. Lam S-K, Paumgartner P, Wang B, eds.: *Update on Hepatobiliary Diseases 1996*. Falk Symposium 90. 1996 ISBN 0-7923-8715-5

91. Hadziselimovic F, Herzog B, eds.: *Inflammatory Bowel Diseases and Chronic Recurrent Abdominal Pain*. Falk Symposium 91. 1996 ISBN 0-7923-8722-8

91B. Alvaro D, Benedetti A, Strazzabosco M, eds.: *Vanishing Bile Duct Syndrome – Pathophysiology and Treatment*. International Falk Workshop. 1996 ISBN 0-7923-8721-X

92. Gerok W, Loginov AS, Pokrowskij VI, eds.: *New Trends in Hepatology 1996*. Falk Symposium 92. 1997 ISBN 0-7923-8723-6

93. Paumgartner G, Stiehl A, Gerok W, eds.: *Bile Acids in Hepatobiliary Diseases – Basic Research and Clinical Application*. Falk Symposium 93. 1997 ISBN 0-7923-8725-2

94. Halter F, Winton D, Wright NA, eds.: *The Gut as a Model in Cell and Molecular Biology*. Falk Symposium 94. 1997 ISBN 0-7923-8726-0

94B. Kruse-Jarres JD, Schölmerich J, eds.: *Zinc and Diseases of the Digestive Tract*. International Falk Workshop. 1997 ISBN 0-7923-8724-4

95. Ewe K, Eckardt VF, Enck P, eds.: *Constipation and Anorectal Insufficiency*. Falk Symposium 95. 1997 ISBN 0-7923-8727-9

96. Andus T, Goebell H, Layer P, Schölmerich J, eds.: *Inflammatory Bowel Disease – from Bench to Bedside*. Falk Symposium 96. 1997 ISBN 0-7923-8728-7

97. Campieri M, Bianchi-Porro G, Fiocchi C, Schölmerich J, eds. *Clinical Challenges in Inflammatory Bowel Diseases: Diagnosis, Prognosis and Treatment*. Falk Symposium 97. 1998 ISBN 0-7923-8733-3

98. Lembcke B, Kruis W, Sartor RB, eds. *Systemic Manifestations of IBD: The Pending Challenge for Subtle Diagnosis and Treatment*. Falk Symposium 98. 1998 ISBN 0-7923-8734-1

Falk Symposium Series

99. Goebell H, Holtmann G, Talley NJ, eds. *Functional Dyspepsia and Irritable Bowel Syndrome: Concepts and Controversies.* Falk Symposium 99. 1998
ISBN 0-7923-8735-X

100. Blum HE, Bode Ch, Bode JCh, Sartor RB, eds. *Gut and the Liver.* Falk Symposium 100. 1998
ISBN 0-7923-8736-8

101. Rachmilewitz D, ed. *V International Symposium on Inflammatory Bowel Diseases.* Falk Symposium 101. 1998
ISBN 0-7923-8743-0

102. Manns MP, Boyer JL, Jansen PLM, Reichen J, eds. *Cholestatic Liver Diseases.* Falk Symposium 102. 1998
ISBN 0-7923-8746-5

102B. Manns MP, Chapman RW, Stiehl A, Wiesner R, eds. *Primary Sclerosing Cholangitis.* International Falk Workshop. 1998.
ISBN 0-7923-8745-7

103. Häussinger D, Jungermann K, eds. *Liver and Nervous System.* Falk Symposium 102. 1998
ISBN 0-7924-8742-2

103B. Häussinger D, Heinrich PC, eds. *Signalling in the Liver.* International Falk Workshop. 1998
ISBN 0-7923-8744-9

103C. Fleig W, ed. *Normal and Malignant Liver Cell Growth.* International Falk Workshop. 1998
ISBN 0-7923-8748-1

104. Stallmach A, Zeitz M, Strober W, MacDonald TT, Lochs H, eds. *Induction and Modulation of Gastrointestinal Inflammation.* Falk Symposium 104. 1998
ISBN 0-7923-8747-3

105. Emmrich J, Liebe S, Stange EF, eds. *Innovative Concepts in Inflammatory Bowel Diseases.* Falk Symposium 105. 1999
ISBN 0-7923-8749-X

106. Rutgeerts P, Colombel J-F, Hanauer SB, Schölmerich J, Tytgat GNJ, van Gossum A, eds. *Advances in Inflammatory Bowel Diseases.* Falk Symposium 106. 1999
ISBN 0-7923-8750-3

107. Špičák J, Boyer J, Gilat T, Kotrlik K, Mareček Z, Paumgartner G, eds. *Diseases of the Liver and the Bile Ducts – New Aspects and Clinical Implications.* Falk Symposium 107. 1999
ISBN 0-7923-8751-1

108. Paumgartner G, Stiehl A, Gerok W, Keppler D, Leuschner U, eds. *Bile Acids and Cholestasis.* Falk Symposium 108. 1999
ISBN 0-7923-8752-X

109. Schmiegel W, Schölmerich J, eds. *Colorectal Cancer – Molecular Mechanisms, Premalignant State and its Prevention.* Falk Symposium 109. 1999
ISBN 0-7923-8753-8

110. Domschke W, Stoll R, Brasitus TA, Kagnoff MF, eds. *Intestinal Mucosa and its Diseases – Pathophysiology and Clinics.* Falk Symposium 110. 1999
ISBN 0-7923-8754-6

110B. Northfield TC, Ahmed HA, Jazwari RP, Zentler-Munro PL, eds. *Bile Acids in Hepatobiliary Disease.* Falk Workshop. 2000
ISBN 0-7923-8755-4

111. Rogler G, Kullmann F, Rutgeerts P, Sartor RB, Schölmerich J, eds. *IBD at the End of its First Century.* Falk Symposium 111. 2000
ISBN 0-7923-8756-2

112. Krammer HJ, Singer MV, eds. *Neurogastroenterology: From the Basics to the Clinics.* Falk Symposium 112. 2000
ISBN 0-7923-8757-0

113. Andus T, Rogler G, Schlottmann K, Frick E, Adler G, Schmiegel W, Zeitz M, Schölmerich J, eds. *Cytokines and Cell Homeostasis in the Gastrointestinal Tract.* Falk Symposium 113. 2000
ISBN 0-7923-8758-9

114. Manns MP, Paumgartner G, Leuschner U, eds. *Immunology and Liver.* Falk Symposium 114. 2000
ISBN 0-7923-8759-7

Falk Symposium Series

115. Boyer JL, Blum HE, Maier K-P, Sauerbruch T, Stalder GA, eds. *Liver Cirrhosis and its Development.* Falk Symposium 115. 2000   ISBN 0-7923-8760-0
116. Riemann JF, Neuhaus H, eds. *Interventional Endoscopy in Hepatology.* Falk Symposium 116. 2000   ISBN 0-7923-8761-9
116A. Dienes HP, Schirmacher P, Brechot C, Okuda K, eds. *Chronic Hepatitis: New Concepts of Pathogenesis, Diagnosis and Treatment.* Falk Workshop. 2000   ISBN 0-7923-8763-5
117. Gerbes AL, Beuers U, Jüngst D, Pape GR, Sackmann M, Sauerbruch T, eds. *Hepatology 2000 – Symposium in Honour of Gustav Paumgartner.* Falk Symposium 117. 2000   ISBN 0-7923-8765-1
117A. Acalovschi M, Paumgartner G, eds. *Hepatobiliary Diseases: Cholestasis and Gallstones.* Falk Workshop. 2000   ISBN 0-7923-8770-8
118. Frühmorgen P, Bruch H-P, eds. *Non-Neoplastic Diseases of the Anorectum.* Falk Symposium 118. 2001   ISBN 0-7923-8766-X
119. Fellermann K, Jewell DP, Sandborn WJ, Schölmerich J, Stange EF, eds. *Immunosuppression in Inflammatory Bowel Diseases – Standards, New Developments, Future Trends.* Falk Symposium 119. 2001   ISBN 0-7923-8767-8
120. van Berge Henegouwen GP, Keppler D, Leuschner U, Paumgartner G, Stiehl A, eds. *Biology of Bile Acids in Health and Disease.* Falk Symposium 120. 2001   ISBN 0-7923-8768-6
121. Leuschner U, James OFW, Dancygier H, eds. *Steatohepatitis (NASH and ASH).* Falk Symposium 121. 2001   ISBN 0-7923-8769-4
121A. Matern S, Boyer JL, Keppler D, Meier-Abt PJ, eds. *Hepatobiliary Transport: From Bench to Bedside.* Falk Workshop. 2001   ISBN 0-7923-8771-6
122. Campieri M, Fiocchi C, Hanauer SB, Jewell DP, Rachmilewitz R, Schölmerich J, eds. *Inflammatory Bowel Disease – A Clinical Case Approach to Pathophysiology, Diagnosis, and Treatment.* Falk Symposium 122. 2002   ISBN 0-7923-8772-4
123. Rachmilewitz D, Modigliani R, Podolsky DK, Sachar DB, Tozun N, eds. *VI International Symposium on Inflammatory Bowel Diseases.* Falk Symposium 123. 2002   ISBN 0-7923-8773-2
124. Hagenmüller F, Manns MP, Musmann H-G, Riemann JF, eds. *Medical Imaging in Gastroenterology and Hepatology.* Falk Symposium 124. 2002   ISBN 0-7923-8774-0
125. Gressner AM, Heinrich PC, Matern S, eds. *Cytokines in Liver Injury and Repair.* Falk Symposium 125. 2002   ISBN 0-7923-8775-9
126. Gupta S, Jansen PLM, Klempnauer J, Manns MP, eds. *Hepatocyte Transplantation.* Falk Symposium 126. 2002   ISBN 0-7923-8776-7
127. Hadziselimovic F, ed. *Autoimmune Diseases in Paediatric Gastroenterology.* Falk Symposium 127. 2002   ISBN 0-7923-8778-3
127A. Berr F, Bruix J, Hauss J, Wands J, Wittekind Ch, eds. *Malignant Liver Tumours: Basic Concepts and Clinical Management.* Falk Workshop. 2002   ISBN 0-7923-8779-1
128. Scheppach W, Scheurlen M, eds. *Exogenous Factors in Colonic Carcinogenesis.* Falk Symposium 128. 2002   ISBN 0-7923-8780-5
129. Paumgartner G, Keppler D, Leuschner U, Stiehl A, eds. *Bile Acids: From Genomics to Disease and Therapy.* Falk Symposium 129. 2002   ISBN 0-7923-8781-3
129A. Leuschner U, Berg PA, Holtmeier J, eds. *Bile Acids and Pregnancy.* Falk Workshop. 2002   ISBN 0-7923-8782-1